Perspectives on Complementary and Alternative Medicines

Perspectives on Complementary and Alternative Medicines

Editors

Ian Olver

Cancer Council Australia and University of Sydney, Australia

Monica Robotin

Cancer Council NSW and University of Sydney, Australia

ICP

Imperial College Press

Published by

Imperial College Press
57 Shelton Street
Covent Garden
London WC2H 9HE

Distributed by

World Scientific Publishing Co. Pte. Ltd.
5 Toh Tuck Link, Singapore 596224
USA office: 27 Warren Street, Suite 401-402, Hackensack, NJ 07601
UK office: 57 Shelton Street, Covent Garden, London WC2H 9HE

British Library Cataloguing-in-Publication Data
A catalogue record for this book is available from the British Library.

PERSPECTIVES ON COMPLEMENTARY AND ALTERNATIVE MEDICINES

ISBN-13 978-1-84816-556-4
ISBN-10 1-84816-556-0

Typeset by Stallion Press
Email: enquiries@stallionpress.com

Printed by FuIsland Offset Printing (S) Pte Ltd Singapore

Contents

Contributors

Deborah Black, BSc, Dip Ed, MStat, PhD
Faculty of Health Sciences
The University of Sydney
C42 – Cumberland Campus
Lidcombe, NSW 2141, Australia

Lesley Braun, PhD, BPharm, DipAppSciNaturopathy
Pharmacy Department, Alfred Hospital
Department of Surgery, Monash University
Level 6, The Alfred Centre
99 Commercial Road
Melbourne, VIC 3004, Australia

Stephen J. Clarke, MBBS, PhD, FRACP, FAChPM
Professor of Medicine, The University of Sydney
Senior Staff Specialist in Medical Oncology
Royal North Shore Hospital
Reserve Road
St. Leonards, NSW 2065, Australia

Haryana M. Dhillon, PhD
Post-doctoral Research Fellow
Survivorship Research Group, Centre for Medical Psychology and Evidence-Based Decision-Making, Central Clinical School
School of Psychology
The University of Sydney

Brennan MacCallum Building (A18)
Sydney, NSW 2006, Australia

Jaklin A. Eliott, PhD
Social Scientist, Cancer Council Australia
Affiliate Lecturer, Discipline of Public Health
The University of Adelaide
Level 11, 178 North Tce
Adelaide, SA 5005, Australia

James Flowers, MA
Department of Medical History
College of Oriental Medicine
Wonkwang University
344-2 Shinyongdong
Iksan, Chonbuk, Korea

Deborah Gray
Author and Broadcaster
DeborahGrayMagic
P.O. Box 229
Woollahra, NSW 2025, Australia

Ken Harvey, MBBS, FRCPA
Adjunct Senior Lecturer
School of Public Health
La Trobe University
Medreach Pty. Ltd.
35a Mary St.
Hawthorn, VIC 3122, Australia

Craig Hassed, MBBS, FRACGP
Senior Lecturer
Deputy Head, Department of General Practice
School of Primary Health Care
Faculty of Medicine, Nursing and Health Sciences
Monash University
Bldg 1, 270 Ferntree Gully Rd
Notting Hill, VIC 3168, Australia

David Joske, MBBS, FRACP, FRCPA
Founder and Chairman, SolarisCare Foundation Cancer Support Centres
Clinical Professor of Medicine, University of Western Australia
Head, Department of Haematology
Sir Charles Gairdner Hospital
Hospital Avenue
Nedlands, WA 6009, Australia

Ray Lowenthal, AO, MBBS, MD, FRCP, FRACP, FAChPM
Consultant Haematologist/Oncologist, Royal Hobart Hospital
Honorary Member, Menzies Research Institute
Clinical Professor, Faculty of Health Science
School of Medicine, University of Tasmania
Hobart CBD Campuses
Medical Science 1, Private Bag 68
Hobart, TAS 7001, Australia

Ramesh Manocha, MBBS, BSc(Med), PhD
Senior Lecturer, Discipline of Psychiatry
Sydney Medical School
The University of Sydney
Edward Ford Building A27
Sydney, NSW 2006, Australia

Loretta Marron, BSc, Assoc Dip Bus(Accnt), AAII, MACS
Cancer Survivor and Author
Email: health.info@bigpond.com

Andrew J. McLachlan, Bpharm, PhD, FPS, FACP, MCPA, MSHPA
Professor of Pharmacy (Aged Care)
Faculty of Pharmacy and Centre for Education and Research on Ageing
The University of Sydney and Concord Hospital
A15 Science Rd
Sydney, NSW 2006, Australia

Vivienne O'Callaghan, BA, BHlthSc(ComplMed)
Publications Editor
Cancer Council New South Wales
153 Dowling Street
Woolloomooloo, NSW 2011, Australia

Byeongsang Oh, PhD
Clinical Senior Lecturer, Sydney Medical School
The University of Sydney
Edward Ford Building A27
Sydney, NSW 2006, Australia

Ian N. Olver, AM, MD, PhD
Clinical Professor, Sydney Medical School
The University of Sydney
CEO, Cancer Council Australia
120 Chalmers Street, Surry Hills
New South Wales 2010, GPO Box 4708
Sydney, NSW 2001, Australia

Liz Paslawsky, PhD, MHA, BSc(Hons1)
International Health Business Consultant
G11/1 Clement Place
Rushcutters Bay, 2011 NSW, Australia

Kerryn Phelps, AM, MBBS (Syd), FRACGP, FAMA
President, Australasian Integrative Medicine Association
Conjoint Professor, University of New South Wales
Adjunct Professor, Sydney Medical School
c/o Cooper Street Clinic
1a Cooper St
Double Bay, NSW 2028, Australia

Carlo Pirri, BSc, BPsych, MPsych(Clinical)
Research and Statistical Consultant / PhD Candidate
Faculty of Health Sciences (Psychology)
Murdoch University
90 South Street
Murdoch, WA 6150, Australia

Veronica M. Raszeja, BA(Hons), GradDipPsych
M.Phil.(Medicine) Candidate at the Centre for Values, Ethics and the Law in Medicine
The University of Sydney
Level 1, Medical Foundation Building
92-94 Parramatta Road
Camperdown, NSW, Australia

Tom Reeve, AC, CBE
Emeritus Consultant in Surgery, Royal North Shore Hospital
Emeritus Professor of Surgery, Sydney Medical School
The University of Sydney
Edward Ford Building A27
Sydney, NSW 2006, Australia

Monica C. Robotin, MBBS, FRACS, MBA, A Appl Epid, M Int Health
Medical Director, Cancer Council New South Wales
Senior Lecturer, School of Public Health
The University of Sydney School of Medicine
Kings Cross, NSW 1340
Sydney 2011, Australia

Leigh Wilson, MPH, Grad Cert Clin Res Mgmt, DPH
Faculty of Health Sciences
The University of Sydney
C42 – Cumberland Campus
Lidcombe, NSW 2141, Australia

Preface

The subject of complementary and alternative medicines attracts controversy. There is often great passion expressed by proponents of both conventional and complementary and alternative therapies.

The current paradigm in "Western" medicine is that it must be evidence-based. There are established scientific methodologies, epitomised by the randomised controlled trial, which govern the investigation of new treatments. The results of this research are used by practitioners to balance the known risks and benefits when advising patients about treatment options.

In contrast, the principles of Chinese medicine, for example, are part of a culture that has evolved over centuries and belief in that system is part of the healing experience. Other complementary and alternative medicines are promoted through collections of single case reports.

Central to the discussion of any treatment is the patients. Patients differ widely in their understanding of evidence-based medicine, and for them there is a singular personal experience of illness. They receive information from multiple sources, including friends and relatives, and weigh many factors, beyond the medical facts, into treatment decisions. They use complementary and alternative therapies to a similar degree as conventional medicines. They often seek to maintain control over their therapy. If they feel that their doctor disapproves of a complementary or alternative medicine choice they simply do not discuss it and therefore never receive the doctor's perspective. They can be left with a confusing array of opinions.

My co-editor, Monica Robotin from Cancer Council New South Wales, joined with me at Cancer Council Australia to collect together a broad spectrum of perspectives on complementary and alternative medicines. We chose authors who practised complementary and alternative medicine, those who practised conventional medicine, researchers, educators and consumers. We asked each to present their perspective on complementary and alternative medicines, and gave them the freedom to express themselves in their own styles. The result is a lively mixture of poignant stories, strong opinions and scientific reviews. By reading 20 different perspectives on complementary and alternative medicines we trust that readers will then be able to form their own opinions, their perspectives.

We are most grateful that all the authors agreed to give their time and expertise voluntarily, and indeed the proceeds will go towards cancer control and support activities at the Cancer Councils. It also reflects a passion that we all share for improving the lives of those with cancer.

Ian Olver, AM
Cancer Council Australia

1

Complementary and Alternative Medicines — The Introductory Perspective

Ian N. Olver

'Two roads diverged in a wood and I took the road less travelled by, And that has made all the difference'

Robert Frost: *The Road Not Taken*

ABSTRACT

This book aims to provide views of complementary and alternative medicines (CAMs) from multiple perspectives to enable the reader to come to their own informed conclusions. Practitioners of conventional medicine range from those who highlight the dangers of treatments that lack conventional evidence to those who wish to integrate CAMs into conventional practice. The authorship also includes educators and researchers into CAMs, those involved in public policy, regulators and consumers. The term CAMs encompasses a wide range of treatments from the biological and the physical to the mental and energy therapies. Mechanisms of action may not be known and should not be subject to pseudoscientific explanations. There are methodological challenges in researching CAMs. Also, CAMs are regulated differently to conventional medicines and yet the public must understand that CAMs can have side-effects and should know upon what evidence claims of efficacy are based and how often it is known to be effective. Medical practitioners should be familiar with CAMs so they can respond to their patients' questions and know if there are any problematic interactions between CAMs and conventional therapies. How to integrate CAMs and conventional medicine is a challenge being explored by some medical centres.

Keywords: Complementary; Alternative; Conventional; Integrative Medicine.

INTRODUCTION

This book about complementary and alternative medicines (CAMs) could have easily followed the well-trodden path of reviewing the available evidence and provided yet another set of tedious arguments over the definition of CAMs, and the use of the term itself. We could have followed with a discussion of countless papers estimating the usage of CAMs to treat a variety of illnesses, the relative merits (or otherwise) of complementary treatments and the reasons they are chosen by patients the world over. Instead we chose to 'take the road less travelled by' and let different writers give their own perspective on what makes CAM different, special or challenging.

This is not because the above topics do not warrant special consideration, as many of these issues are found somewhere within the pages of this collection, but all as part of a variety of perspectives on CAMs. Given that there is a confusing and often polarising array of opinions on CAMs, this book is designed to encapsulate a wide array of views, so that the readers can form their own perspectives, by comparing the views expressed, or drawing wisdom from the contributions made by authors from different walks of life.

The contributors range from practitioners of CAMs to several specialists practising conventional 'Western' medicine. Even the latter span those signalling the potential danger of CAMs, because they lack conventional evidence of their efficacy, to those wishing to integrate CAMs into conventional practice. The authorship includes educators and researchers, those involved in public policy and regulators. Consumers who have had illnesses such as cancer have also given their perspectives, as they have been faced with choices of whether to use CAMs, and they have contributed their insights, although they have not always chosen to display that label.

Complementary and alternative medicines are controversial and there is a confusing array of sincerely held opinions, and of practitioners; some are motivated by a desire to do the best for their patients, some wanting to integrate CAMs and conventional medicine, and others exploiting the uncertainty in these therapies for personal gain.

Consumers can also hold strong opinions for and against CAMs. My research group interviewed patients being treated for cancer about end-of-life decision-making and then analysed their speech to ascertain their views on a variety of issues. CAMs were mentioned by many spontaneously and yet there was a clear distinction between users and non-users.[1]

Against a discourse that holds individuals responsible for their health, users of CAMs valued them as being of both physical and psychological benefit, as part of a desired holistic approach to their care to complement conventional treatment, and were upset at themselves if they failed to continue CAMs, even in the face of practical or financial difficulties. Non-users devalued CAMs for their inability to cure their cancer, although they did not similarly devalue conventional medicine, even if the final outcome was strikingly similar. Moreover, they regarded CAMs users as desperate, or as challenging conventional medical wisdom.

WHAT DO WE MEAN BY CAM?

I will have to admit to not liking the term CAMs, but its use has become widespread and in general people know what is meant. It would be better to use the broader term 'therapies' as this encompasses both medicines and other therapeutic endeavours, such as mind/body or energy treatments. There is also no real distinction between complementary and alternative therapies, as the same non-conventional therapy could be added to, or complement, traditional evidence-based medicine or promoted as an alternative to it. It may be acceptable to conventional medicine practitioners to use such a therapy as complementary, but not as an alternative to evidence-based effective therapy. So, lumping complementary and alternative together may not be helpful.

Moreover, in Veronica Raszeja's chapter on classification she makes the point that CAMs can be only two positive randomised trials away from being accepted as conventional, which in essence is true. So the same treatment could over time be regarded as alternative, complementary and conventional!

THE CLASSIFICATION OF CAM

Some of the authors in this book have outlined classification schemes by the type of therapy, i.e. whether it is a biological medicine or diet, involves touch (as is the case with forms of massage), tries to influence the body with the mind (as with meditation) or involves tapping into some external energy (as with Qi Gong). Of course, even having classified a therapy as a CAM classifies it as outside the accepted medical paradigm of the culture in which it is found. In China, for example, it was Western medicine that had to be integrated with traditional Chinese medicines, not the other way around.

I could speculate about other possible classification schemes. What if we classified therapies by mechanism of action? That would provide two major problems. Firstly, it would reflect the culture from which the therapy came. Western scientific method and understanding, for example, may seek to identify molecular targets by which a treatment retards the growth of a tumour or to measure a hormonal change that impacts on hormone-sensitive tumours to satisfy itself of a mechanism, but the meridians used in acupuncture or forms of universal energy do not fit that paradigm. Secondly, where would that leave Western medical practices that have developed empirically without knowing precisely how they work (the case for many cytotoxic drugs, where the mechanism was found well after efficacy was established by observation in clinical trials)?

Another claim is that there is a distinction between 'natural' therapies and others. Again this does not stand up to scrutiny. A vitamin may well be natural, but at many times its normal dose it takes on the characteristics of a drug, often with side-effects to balance against benefit. The body may well find it 'natural' to absorb such nutrients from food, but how natural is it to take a vitamin or antioxidant in the form of a tablet or injection? Furthermore, several cytotoxics are derived from plants, including the taxanes from yew trees and the vinca alkaloids from the periwinkle plant.[2,3] These drugs have a full range of side-effects, which should hardly be considered natural.

I contend that classification may be helpful in communicating what type of therapy is being discussed. It is not helpful if it carries a value judgement about that treatment. For example, having been trained in the Western scientific model I am more comfortable with treatments that fit within that model and I will want to know the level of evidence of efficacy based upon the results of randomised clinical trials that the treatment carries within that model. I will make my judgements about the value of a treatment from that viewpoint. If I came from another culture, however, I may judge as satisfactory a remedy that has been handed down through generations of my ancestors, based upon observations of its efficacy, according to the understanding of illness that is much older than Western medicine. Now, one treatment may actually have better outcomes than the other, but just comparing the background evidence for each may not allow that decision to be made without referring to one's value system. Can research differentiate between what should be regarded as conventional and what should be called a CAM?

RESEARCHING CAM

A possible method of reducing the gulf between conventional Western medicine and CAMs would be to test CAMs using the standards of evidence and methodology required for treatments to be accepted under the Western system. Certainly some CAMs have been accepted as having efficacy as a result of doing just that. Monica Robotin, in her chapter, shows how conventional drugs can evolve from knowledge of herbal remedies. Taking examples from a field of interest of mine (chemotherapy-induced nausea), acupuncture and acupressure, hypnosis and ginger have all shown efficacy in randomised controlled trials.[4–6]

Life, however, isn't always that simple. Take traditional Chinese medicine, for example, where as part of the treatments, various combinations of naturally occurring substances are offered. As we have discussed, conventional chemotherapy has several drugs also derived from plants. In Western medicine the active ingredient of the plant is sought, purified, often synthesised and then submitted to clinical trial. You could adopt the same techniques for traditional Chinese medicines, but that would be assuming that the activity was due to a single active agent and not the interplay between several components of the plant, an assumption that should not be made. Moreover, reproducible dosing, if this is desired, is more straightforward for a purified single agent than for a mixture of raw plants. Again using nausea as an example in Western practice, the investigation of the anecdotal reports that smoking marijuana helped alleviate post-chemotherapy nausea was fraught with such problems as standardising the dose, let alone being able to do a blinded study with such distinctive side-effects.[7]

When faced with CAMs where the explanation of the activity has no counterpart in Western scientific understanding, as is the case with some of the 'energy' therapies, design of a study becomes highly problematic. Even if a randomised trial is positive, that does not demonstrate that the ascribed mechanism of action is correct. I have addressed these issues in the chapter that describes a study of intercessory prayer. In that situation some may call for prospectively randomised clinical trials that satisfy Consolidated Standards of Reporting Trials (CONSORT) guidelines to test its efficacy, whereas others reject the possibility that metaphysical phenomena should or could be investigated using these traditional methodologies.[8,9] Emerging fields such as psychoneuroimmunology also provide difficult design issues, as immunological endpoints that can be influenced by so many things may be impacted upon by psychological symptoms such as stress and the research must cross disciplines to explore the interactions.

Do all complementary therapies have to be subjected to randomised trials before they are integrated into clinical practice? Take aromatherapy, for example. I have seen this used by nursing staff to improve the comfort of patients based upon their anecdotal experience that patients find it helpful, which is further reinforced by positive feedback from individual patients. Given that the chance of harm is minimal, interactions with conventional therapy are unlikely and this is a supplement to evidence-based treatments, an argument could be made for its use without a randomised trial, given that the resources required to provide randomised controlled trial evidence may be better allocated elsewhere.

Having said that, it has often been claimed that no money is available to conduct research into CAMs. However, the NHMRC (National Health and Medical Research Council) has, of recent years, earmarked money specifically for CAMs research. That aside, what is required in general is very basic. Keeping a record of the outcome and the side-effects of a CAM and particularly knowing the denominator; how many were treated to obtain any allegedly positive effect seen is a good way to make a start in the evaluation of the outcome.

REGULATION OF CAM

Ken Harvey has given us his perspective on the regulation of CAMs in Australia and Loretta Marron has expressed a critical perspective, especially when the regulation of CAMs is compared with the regulation of pharmaceuticals and medical devices. In my opinion, Australia has a very good drug regulation system, where detailed data are scrutinised to assess proof of a drug's efficacy and acceptable toxicity before a drug can be registered. Further scrutiny occurs about its cost-effectiveness when a drug is assessed for listing on the Pharmaceutical Benefits scheme. This process has served the public well, protecting them from untested drugs, poorly manufactured drugs and extravagant claims of efficacy and ensuring, as far as possible, that a drug or device is safe. This extensive process of review is costly and the aim is to largely recover the cost from the drug companies that will reap the financial rewards of a successful product.

Such a scheme is not in place for complementary and alternative medicines and devices, despite the fact that the use of such products is just as extensive as that of conventional drugs. There are many reasons for this. Firstly, as we have discussed, the scientific evidence of efficacy may not exist, beyond anecdotes and testimonials for CAMs. Some CAMs may not be classified as drugs, but as foods or food supplements. There may be different commercial imperatives for CAMs, depending on what can be patented and this may impact on the willingness of a commercial sponsor to pay for a process of evaluation as extensive as that required for pharmaceutical products. The government, however, does have a concern for the welfare of the population, and its initial priority is to assess, as far as possible, the safety of a product and whether it meets satisfactory manufacturing standards. This does not address the question of efficacy; however, there are restrictions on what a manufacturer of a CAM can claim about efficacy if data are not available. Short of assessing efficacy, the collection of data about a CAM's pedigree may be useful, as an indication of the likelihood of efficacy. If I was trying to make a decision about using a CAM, I would certainly be more impressed with the claims associated with a drug that had been handed down through generations of a cultural group, as compared with something concocted in someone's back yard last Friday.

WHAT TO TELL THE PUBLIC ABOUT CAM

The information about CAMs seems to me to travel faster through a population than that about conventional evidence-based therapies. There may be many reasons for this. On the positive side, often CAMs can be administered by the patient, which is empowering. Sometimes this leads to unfounded conspiracy theories purporting that information about CAMs has been purposely suppressed, to keep doctors and the pharmaceutical industry in business! There is also often the perception that because a product is deemed 'natural' it will not have any side-effects. Many in the general public do not understand the nature of the evidence required for conventional medicines, and may therefore believe claims about CAMs, without realising that they lack similar evidence to support them.

There can be a harmful side to patients accepting concepts such as being able to use mental powers to rid themselves of cancer, because failure to control the tumour can lead to patients feeling guilty over not trying hard enough. It is rather cruel to add that suggestion to the distress that accompanies a diagnosis of cancer.

So what I suggest here is that rather than discussing with the public the details of each CAM (something they can obtain readily anyway), we focus the discussion on the nature and extent of the available evidence, so that they can make an informed choice about any treatment, conventional or CAMs, that is being offered. I used to encourage my patients to ask the same questions of any treatment.

The first of these is what is the denominator? A treatment that works for one in every two people who try it is quite different from a treatment that works for one in ten, or one in a thousand. Often if an alternative treatment has only been promoted by anecdote and testimonial, the information about the denominator will not be available, and that should sound a note of caution, unless individuals are willing to abandon the Western scientific paradigm. The second issue is to examine the rationale behind a treatment. It is simply not the case that if something is good for you, twice as much is twice as good and yet that is often behind therapies such as high-dose vitamins, for example. Conversely, if too much of something is damaging to your health, it does not mean that it should be cut out altogether, which is the rationale for some extreme diets.

A third piece of advice is to be careful of pseudo-scientific explanations. The immune system is often referred to as though it is a simple system that can overall be stimulated or suppressed by a specific treatment. We know, through the advent of targeted treatments, that to be effective, very specific parts of the immune system need to be targeted to obtain the shrinkage of a cancer.

Another common target claimed for various CAMs is their ability to detoxify the body. My medical training taught me about the important role of the liver and kidneys in removing toxic waste products from the body. So, I am totally at a loss to explain how manoeuvres such as coffee enemas could detoxify anything. And what are these toxins anyway? Incidentally, the coffee enema fails my next test. If it doesn't even sound sensible, don't do it. Ray Lowenthal shares with us, in this book, his experience of a lifetime of collecting unorthodox therapies and bizarre claims for their mode of action. I can only conclude that if you don't know why something works, and there are many examples in orthodox medicine where that is the case, perhaps it is better just to admit that you don't know, rather than construct a mechanism of action. In summary, I encourage patients to ask many questions about any treatment they are offered, and even question the answers they receive until they understand enough to make an informed choice.

WHAT MEDICAL PRACTITIONERS AND STUDENTS SHOULD KNOW ABOUT CAM

Craig Hassed, in his chapter, has stressed the importance of medical students having a good working knowledge of CAMs in order to be able to communicate with their patients, the majority of whom will be taking some form of CAM in addition to their conventional therapy. What I would like to stress, however, is that even medical practitioners who are not particularly interested in exploring treatments outside orthodox medical practice must be aware of which CAMs interact with conventional treatments, such is the widespread use of CAMs. Unfortunately there is a propensity for patients not to report use of CAMs to their medical practitioners if they perceive that the practitioner will disapprove of their choice.

Indeed, the enhanced communication with patients that may result from having some knowledge of CAMs may be very useful, both in the therapeutic relationship and in guiding a patient through the mass of information about both CAMs and conventional treatment options. Also, keeping up with CAMs will mean being more aware when, as a result of trials, a CAM treatment has crossed to the mainstream. Clinicians with a research bent may also gain cues for fruitful investigations in patients who report the outcomes of their CAMs use.

INTEGRATE CAM ON WHAT BASIS?

Consumers who use CAMs would like to experience some integration of conventional medicine and CAMs. Some conventional medical practitioners are trying to integrate the two, for example David Joske relates his perspective on how to do this in his chapter. How do we choose what to integrate? It is tempting to say that we should integrate those CAMs for which the evidence of efficacy has been demonstrated in randomised trials, but that is not really integration, that is just a CAM crossing over to being accepted by conventional criteria. We could integrate certain types of CAMs as complementary therapies, like massage or aromatherapy where the toxicity is very low, even if their efficacy has not been demonstrated by more than individual case reports of patients gaining comfort from them. However, we should be encouraged to gather data about potentially useful CAMs. It is also important to realise that harm not only refers to side-effects, but may also be measured in terms of the opportunity cost for an individual to use time and money in pursuits other than on an ineffective CAM.

What integration should be able to achieve is better communication with patients, thereby allowing them to make choices outside conventional medicine of using complementary therapies, although mainstream medicine would not accept the use of a CAM as an alternative to a conventional therapy that was known to be effective.

These choices are difficult and individuals often hold passionate views on this topic. There is rarely, however, a complete separation between CAMs and conventional medicine, but evidence-based medicine is currently the prevailing paradigm in the West. I understand that individuals are the products of their social background and education, which leads to different views on what represents mainstream. I am very much influenced by my orthodox medical training and accept this as a basis for recommending treatments. Yet, I can share the experience of investigating a CAM, with surprising results within that paradigm. My only personal use of CAM was as a result of my mother swearing by tincture of myrrh for aphthous ulcers, and without knowing the evidence I tried it and found it effective. I suspect that personal experiences dictating opinions on specific CAMs are not uncommon. I also suspect that personal experience motivates many to adopt various CAMs, and integrating is not about suddenly overturning the principles of orthodox practice, but recognising individual experience as legitimate. These are not necessarily sufficient grounds on which to recommend a CAM more widely, but a willingness to accommodate an individual's viewpoint and strengthen the therapeutic relationship as a result.

The purpose of this book was to present a wide range of perspectives on CAMs, so that the readers can hear the opinions and come to their own position. I will not have accommodated every viewpoint, but 22 chapters-worth is a good place to begin to understand the complexity of this topic. I invite you to join me in this exploration, where the path chosen is the 'road less travelled by'.

REFERENCES

1. Eliott JA, Kealey CP, Olver IN. (Using) complementary and alternative medicine: the perceptions of palliative patients with cancer. *J Palliat Med* **11**(1):58–67 (2008).
2. Houghton PJ. The role of plants in traditional medicine and current therapy. *J Altern Complement Med* **1**:131–143 (1995).
3. Noble RL, Beer CT, Cutts JH. Role of chance observations in chemotherapy: Vinca rosea. *Ann N Y Acad Sci* **76**:882–894 (1958).
4. Melcahrt D, Ihbe Heffinger A, Leps B, *et al.* Acupuncture and acupressure for the prevention of chemotherapy-induced nausea — a randomised cross-over pilot study. *Support Care Cancer* **14**:878–882 (2006).
5. Ryan JL, Heckler C, Dakhil SR, *et al.* Ginger for chemotherapy-related nausea in cancer patients: a URCC CCOP randomized, double-blind, placebo-controlled clinical trial of 644 cancer patients. *J Clin Oncol* **27**:15s (2009) (suppl; abstr 9511).
6. Richardson J, Smith JE, McCall G, *et al.* Hypnosis for nausea and vomiting in cancer chemotherapy: a systematic review of the research evidence. *Eur J Cancer Care* **16**:402–412 (2007).
7. Gralla RJ, Tyson LB, Bordin LA, *et al.* Antiemetic therapy: a review of recent studies and a report of a random assignment trial comparing metoclopramide with delta-9-tetrahydrocannabinol. *Cancer Treat Rep* **68**:163–172 (1984).
8. Moher D, Hopewell S, Schulz KF, *et al.* CONSORT 2010 explanation and elaboration: updated guidelines for reporting parallel group randomised trials. *BMJ* **340**:c869 (2010).
9. Halperin EC. Should academic medical centres conduct clinical trials of the efficacy of intercessory prayer? *Acad Med* **76**:791–797 (2001).

2

Beyond the Classification of Complementary and Alternative Medicine (CAM): Towards a Systematic Approach to Understanding CAM

Veronica M. Raszeja

ABSTRACT

Large numbers of people with cancer use complementary and alternative medicines (CAMs), either alongside or instead of conventional medical treatments. To be able to make informed decisions about the use of CAMs, it is important that consumers of CAMs, health-care professionals, policy-makers and government bodies understand something about what CAMs are, how they work and what their risks and benefits may be in different settings. Although a number of systems for classifying CAMs are available, they are generally unable to account for the complex, multifunctional and dynamic nature of CAMs. A more systematic approach to classifying CAMs, which incorporates the use of modern computer technology, could provide an additional, flexible and comprehensive information resource for the benefit of patients, carers, health professionals and policy-makers alike.

Keywords: Complementary and Alternative Medicine (CAM); CAM Classification; CAM Definition; CAM Taxonomy; CAM Use in Cancer; CAM Information Resource; CAM Computer Technology.

INTRODUCTION

Classification is a fundamental part of human experience. All phenomena perceived by humankind are subject to classification — whether objects, events or behaviour — and systems of classification are constructed to make sense of, and bring order to, what otherwise may be experienced as a chaotic world.[1] The myriad forms of healing are no exception to this.

The classification of all forms of healing serves to define the medicines and therapies acceptable to the dominant healing system in that particular time and place. Thus, *conventional* healing practices are those of the dominant healing system, whereas *complementary* practices are those that aid, or at least do not interfere with, the conventional medical therapies of the dominant healing system, and *alternative* practices are those that are offered and used instead of the therapies approved by the dominant healing system.

In the modern industrialised world, classifying the different modalities of healing in this way enables the systematic collection, comparison and provision of information to health professionals, consumers, policy-makers and all others who require this information. However, the nature of these classifications is fluid and changeable, reflecting changes in time and circumstances. Yesterday's complementary or alternative medicine may, through an accumulating body of affirmative evidence, become tomorrow's mainstream medicine. A specific application of a complementary or alternative medicine may be an accepted part of conventional medical practice, and one culture's complementary or alternative medicine may be another's conventional medicine.

TOWARDS THE CLASSIFICATION OF CAM — A GLOBAL AND HISTORICAL VIEW

The World Health Organisation (WHO) describes and categorises this large and diverse group of medicines and therapies as traditional and complementary medicine (TCAM), and further divides this into the categories traditional medicine (TM) and complementary and alternative medicine (CAM). TM is defined as being 'the sum total of the knowledge, skills, and practices based on the theories, beliefs, and experiences indigenous to different cultures, whether explicable or not, used in the maintenance of health as well as in the prevention, diagnosis, improvement or treatment of physical and mental illness'.[2] CAM, however, is regarded as an 'industrialised world' adaptation of TM — 'a broad set of health care practices that are not part of that country's own tradition and are not integrated into the dominant health care system'.[3]

But the WHO's definition of CAM is perhaps not quite the case. Many CAMs used in the Western industrialised world, while indeed not being 'integrated into the dominant health care system', are modern-day applications or interpretations of that industrialised world's folkloric and historical medical traditions. For instance, herbalism or homeopathy — both currently considered to be CAMs in Western societies — were both widely used systems of healing practised alongside the healing system that has become modern, conventional scientific medicine, or 'bio-medicine'.

Before the legislated ascendancy — in the Western industrialised world — of bio-medicine over many other competing medical systems in the second half of the 19th century, [a]the practice of medicine was open to all healers — be they herbalists, midwives, mesmerists, bone-setters, apothecaries, or barber-surgeons, amongst others. However, as the new scientific medicine became increasingly dominant, practices that were once considered part of the normal healing battery were moved outside the boundaries of 'modern medicine'. Practices such as treatments with herbs or minerals, dietary and exercise regimens, homeopathic remedies and naturopathic therapies all became tainted with the terms 'unorthodox' or even 'quackery'.[4,5,b]

---

[a] In 1858 the Medical Registration Act was passed in Britain. In Australia, the colonies and states introduced various legislation and regulations throughout the 19th century regarding the practice of medicine.

[b] Although 'quackery' certainly wasn't a newly minted derogatory term — as clearly demonstrated by one Thomas Jones of England in his 1676 vitriolic treatise: *The Character of a Quack Doctor, or the Abusive Practices of Impudent Illiterate Pretenders to Physick Exposed*, Thomas Jones, London (1676).

Although now deemed 'non-scientific', many of these modes of healing did not disappear, and even more therapies that were 'non-scientific' continued to be developed and practised. During the early part of the 20th century, treatments such as enzyme therapy, light therapy and specific cancer therapies such as the Gerson therapy emerged, and entire systems of healing, such as anthroposophical medicine, which considered itself to be an extension of modern 'scientific' medicine,[6] were introduced.

While the old 'non-scientific' therapies continued to be used and new 'non-scientific' therapies emerged, during the latter part of the 19th century and the first 60 years of the 20th century, modern bio-medicine reigned supreme. This was the so-called 'golden age of doctoring'.[7] In the 1960s, however, modern medicine increasingly began to be seen as conservative, dogmatic and reductionist, and there was a resurgence of interest in what were perceived as the more 'holistic' healing therapies. Healing systems such as naturopathy and traditional Chinese medicine (TCM), plus individual practices such as acupuncture, aromatherapy, yoga and meditation experienced a boom, and a multitude of new therapies appeared, many of them specifically targeting cancer. Although not necessarily holistic, therapies such as the Burzynski protocol, kinesiology and microwave therapy were developed, and the use of substances such as 714-X, DMSO and hydrozine sulphate to treat cancer were employed. All of these were classed together as being 'unorthodox' or 'unscientific' by modern bio-medicine, and there was much official opprobrium for them all.

Despite this disapproval from mainstream medicine, 'unscientific' therapies continued to rise in popularity. In response, the American National Institutes of Health (NIH) Office of Alternative Medicine (OAM) was established in 1992 to more rigorously investigate the scientific basis of these healing modalities.[4,8] After the establishment of the OAM, the more neutral term for these treatments, 'alternative medicine', began to be more widely used.[4,8] The renaming of the OAM as the National Center for Complementary and Alternative Medicine (NCCAM) in 1998 saw a corresponding increase in the use of the term 'complementary therapies' and the introduction of the acronym 'CAM' to encompass all complementary and alternative medicines and therapies.[4] Today, NCCAM's definition of CAM: 'CAM is a group of diverse medical and health care systems, practices, and products that are not presently considered to be part of conventional medicine',[9] and NCCAM's classification system of CAMs are widely referenced.

Throughout the period of the dominance of bio-medicine (from the late 18th century to the present), some of the healing modalities deemed 'unorthodox', 'unscientific' or 'alternative' have been taken back into the bio-medical fold, as scientific advances — or practical or political necessities — demonstrated that these practices were useful. An example of this is acupuncture.

Developed over 2,000 years ago in China as an integral part of TCM, acupuncture today is an established part of the therapeutic armamentarium of medical treatment in China. Described to Europeans in the 17th century, the first records of acupuncture being practised in Europe didn't appear until the late 18th century.[10] By the early 19th century, acupuncture was being written about approvingly in the medical journals of the time; in 1836 the *Lancet* described acupuncture as an exotic and valuable new medical technique.[10] But with the rise of scientific medicine during the second half of the 19th century, and perhaps also affected by the deterioration of Sino–British relations, acupuncture became progressively more marginalised, although some 'Europeanised' versions were still practised by a few individual practitioners. By the early 20th century acupuncture had virtually disappeared from Western medical practice.[10]

It wasn't until the second half of the 20th century that there was a resurgence of Western interest in acupuncture. This has been variously attributed to the rising interest in all alternate modes of healing, and to the resumption of Chinese–American relations in the 1970s. Since that time, various levels of scientific evidence of acupuncture's efficacy have been published in scholarly journals. In Australia this has led to various health fund rebates for the procedure, and, in 1984, Medicare rebates when acupuncture is performed by registered conventional medical practitioners.[11] Acupuncture (when practised by conventional medical practitioners) has again become a part of conventional practice. [12,c]

As the example of acupuncture ably demonstrates, history, geographical location and politics are all central to the definition and

[c] According to the American Medical Association (AMA) in their 2002 Position Statement, at least 15% of Australian GPs were practising acupuncture.

classification of CAM. Today's complementary or alternative therapy may be only a few random controlled trials away from tomorrow's orthodox medicine therapy, and what is considered a dangerous alternative 'quackery' in one country or culture, can be considered an orthodox medical practice in another. Time and place specific, the definition of CAM is, by necessity, a fluid and changeable one.

SOME EXAMPLES OF DIFFERENT SYSTEMS OF CAM CLASSIFICATION

Given the degree to which our understanding of healing modalities is historically and culturally determined, it is unsurprising that there exist a number of different classification systems for CAM. One of the most widely referenced definition and classification systems of CAM is that of the US NCCAM. NCCAM defines CAM as 'a group of diverse medical and health care systems, practices, and products that are not presently considered to be part of conventional medicine'.[9] For NCCAM, 'conventional medicine' is 'medicine as practiced by holders of M.D. (medical doctor) or D.O. (doctor of osteopathy) degrees and by their allied health professionals, such as physical therapists, psychologists, and registered nurses'.[9]

Acknowledging that there can be some overlap, NCCAM categorises CAMs by four broad 'domains' — and includes a 'whole medical systems' category. This category can encompass individual CAMs from each of the four 'domains'.[13]

- 'Whole medical systems' include systems from non-Western cultures such as TCM and Ayurveda, and systems that have developed in Western cultures such as homeopathy and naturopathy.
- The domain of 'mind–body medicine' includes practices such as meditation, prayer, art and music therapies.
- The 'biologically based practices' domain includes herbs, vitamins, minerals, dietary supplements and dietary changes.
- 'Manipulative and body-based practices' include massage, chiropractic and osteopathic manipulation.
- 'Energy therapies' include acupuncture, reiki, Qi Gong and therapeutic touch.

Demonstrating the fluid and changeable nature of CAM classification systems, NCCAM has recently removed two therapies, cognitive behavioural therapy and support groups, from its CAM listings, as both are now considered part of conventional mainstream medicine.[d]

Other large organisations, such as the American Cancer Society (ACS), also have their own classification systems. Designed as an information resource, the ACS system also uses five categories, currently with descriptions of over 200 CAMs allocated to one of each of these groups[14]:

- Mind, body and spirit
- Manual healing and physical touch
- Herbs, vitamins and minerals
- Diet and nutrition
- Pharmacological and biological treatment

Unlike NCCAM, the ACS doesn't specifically acknowledge that there can be overlap between these groups, nor that a specific CAM (and especially a whole healing system) can have practices that fit into more than one discrete category. Although the method of classification of CAMs employed by the ACS prevents duplication of information, it fails to capture the complexity and fluidity of CAMs.

In contrast to most classification systems, such as those of NCCAM and the ACS, researches and authors Cant and Sharma — making the point that most of the non-biomedical modes of healing are not new — categorise CAMs by historical origin.[15] In their schema, CAMs are categorised into:

- Those developed before, or at the same time as, modern biomedicine. Included here are homeopathy, herbalism and a variety of folk medicines.
- Those developed in the 'period of medical individualism' in the late 19th and early 20th centuries. Included in this category are chiropractic and osteopathy.
- Those derived from practices of the 19th century central European health spas, such as naturopathy, exercise and diet.

---

[d]These CAMs were removed between the author's accessions of the NCCAM website on 30th January 2008 and 20th January 2010.

- Those imported by Westerners from Asia, such as TCM and acupuncture.
- Those that entered Western society via immigration from other cultures, such as Ayurveda and Unani Tibb.

Cant and Sharma's system of classifying CAM brings an added dimension to the typology of CAM. It provides a more complete context for the understanding of particular CAMs, as well as providing a history of the changes in healing in the modern Western world.[15]

With each definition of CAM and each classification system, researchers and government bodies are creating forms of order out of a culturally diverse and constantly changing field. But each definition or taxonomy by itself does not give the whole picture because a CAM may operate on many levels — mind/body, pharmacological, spiritual, manipulative — either at the same time or at different times. A particular healing practice may also be considered both a CAM and a conventional medical treatment (e.g. acupuncture), depending upon the aim of the treatment and by whom it is practised. And a healing modality considered to be a CAM may have many elements of conventional medicine within it (such as osteopathy or anthroposophical medicine). It may come from a tradition older than that of modern bio-medicine, or be a healing system that developed alongside modern bio-medicine. It may have been derived from — or be a different use of — procedures or substances employed by modern bio-medicine, such as certain light therapies when used to treat cancer, or substances like insulin when used in the alternative cancer, therapy 'Insulin potentiation therapy'.

There are, therefore, no hard and fast categories to which a CAM can be assigned. Adopting a more 'holistic' way of viewing CAMs could perhaps better capture the many aspects of many CAMs and provide those who need to access information about CAMs with a number of different ways of viewing them.

TOWARDS A SYSTEMATIC APPROACH TO UNDERSTANDING CAM

Despite the fact that it is difficult to be clear about what CAMs are, it is, nonetheless, crucial that we have some way of classifying healing modalities into categories such as conventional, complementary and alternative. Health professionals, policy-makers and government bodies need data about CAM usage to be able to make informed decisions about the legislation and regulation of CAM, the allocation of health resources and the place of CAM in healthcare. And consumers and health professionals alike need information about CAMs in order to be able to make informed decisions about treatments.

The wide variety of views about how CAMs can be defined or categorised has meant that there is a lack of meaningfully comparable statistics on CAM use. A meta-analysis of 26 surveys of CAM use in cancer from 13 countries in the Western industrialised world recorded CAM usage rates between 7 and 64%.[16] Likewise, the 2005 Australian Senate Inquiry into services and treatment options for people with cancer commented that CAM use by cancer patients in Australia is reported to vary between 7 and 83.3%.[17] As Cassileth and Vickers point out, the prevalence of CAM usage 'depend[s]on the definition of CAM used.'[18] For instance, some may include all non-conventional medical activities used by cancer patients as examples of CAM — activities such as psychological counselling, exercise, prayer and other spiritual practices, whereas others may set narrower limits, with lower CAM usage figures as a result.

For example, a US survey, published in 2005, of 752 oncology patients found that 91% of respondents used at least one form of CAM, with the most widely used CAM being prayer (77%).[19] A larger study conducted in 2002 by the US NIH, surveyed 31,000 people and found that 62% used at least one CAM, including prayer for health reasons, in the previous 12 months. Excluding prayer, 36% had used CAM.[20] In the subsequent NIH survey in 2007, 38.3% used at least one form of CAM, but this time prayer (and various folk-healing practices) were excluded from the survey.[21]

It is clear, therefore, that a universal system of categorising CAM usage needs to be agreed upon. Substantial work in this area has been done by Kristoffersen and colleagues.[22] These researchers have developed a model incorporating various levels of CAM usage from Level 1, where users have demonstrated their commitment to CAM, with multiple visits to a CAM practitioner, to

Level 6, where a user need only have tried CAM once, and that CAM could be any medicine or therapy (including activities such as prayer or exercise) not considered to be conventional medical therapy for that particular complaint.

Systems for the classification of CAM are important not only because they help provide a picture of overall CAM usage, but because they also form the basis of information resources. Regardless of the way that one defines CAM, there can be no doubt that large numbers of people with cancer use CAM.[17] And in cancer care, where all therapies — whether conventional or non-conventional — may have significant risks or benefits, it is especially important that reliable and up-to-date information about CAM is readily available. Recognising this need for information, the AMA considers that it 'is essential that consumers have improved access to well researched information about Complementary Medicine so that they are empowered to question and to raise relevant issues with any complementary therapist they consult and to make well informed choices'.[12] And that it 'is important that medical practitioners are informed about the potential benefits and any potentially adverse effects of complementary medicines and therapies'.[12]

A number of studies have shown that people gather information about CAM from a variety of sources, including conventional medical professionals, CAM practitioners, friends, relations, magazines, books and, increasingly, the Internet.[23–26] (In 2002 it was estimated that in the US the Internet had over 600 million users, with up to 55% of these using the internet to access health information and 48% of these health information seekers seeking information about CAM.[23] But current, reliable, easily accessible and comprehensive information about CAMs is not easy to find, and the current applications of existing systems of classification do not readily lend themselves to the tasks of providing this.

A systematic approach to presenting or interpreting CAM would go a long way to answering some of the complex questions about them. Questions such as: what is the current scientific research on this therapy; what are the possible contraindications in a particular health condition or if used with conventional medicines; how long has this therapy been in use and where does it come from? Although it may not be possible to print and publish detailed information about CAMs that is constantly up-to-date, computer technology, however, is well placed to fulfil such requirements. A computer application can simultaneously handle the multiple tasks of display, organisation, categorisation, information retrieval, search and research, and provide all this required information on, or from, one display page. Figure 1 is an example of such a computer application.

In this application a scrollable list of all known CAMs is provided, to which CAMs can be added or amended as appropriate at any time. There is no need to actually remove a CAM from a system such as this, as therapies that are no longer considered to be CAMs can remain on the list with an amended status. In this way, all information about the therapy is still accessible.

As CAMs can have multiple therapeutic actions,[13] information about this can be provided in a single, in-line display. For instance, acupuncture is at once an example of body work, an energy therapy and an invasive technique. Likewise, apitherapy, a CAM technique using various products of the common honey bee, can be simultaneously viewed as a dietary or supplementation CAM (through ingesting honey or pollen for its nutritional value), a pharmacological CAM (when using bee venom), and can also be considered to be an invasive type of CAM (when using live bee stings).[14]

As any one therapy may have several uses, in the display shown in Fig. 1 each therapy is classified as complementary, alternative or orthodox, or some combination of all three. For example, the herb aloe can be used topically as a complementary therapy for minor skin burns or irritations, or ingested to relieve constipation. However, when it is promoted as a cancer therapy (sometimes with injections directly into tumours), available scientific evidence has not, to date, shown this practice to be of any benefit; indeed, it has shown it to be harmful in several cases.[14] The use of aloe is therefore classified here as both a complementary and an alternative medicine. By comparison, acupuncture is classified as both an orthodox and complementary therapy, and the substance 714-X (only used in healing therapies as a non-conventional treatment for serious diseases, including cancer) is classified only as an alternative medicine.

There are many reasons why people with cancer use CAMs. They may be used as a cure for the cancer, to prolong life, to relieve

CONTEMPORARY CAMS																				
		TYPES OF THERAPEUTIC ACTION									Orthodox/ complementary/ alternative			Whole system						
CAM NAME	Click for more info	Body work; body-> mind work	Mind work; mind-> bodywork	Religious/ spiritual	Manipu lative	Dietary/ sup plement	Pharma cological	Energy therapy	Invasive	Biological therapy	OM	CM	AM		Use in cancer	Click for PubMed	Click for herb info	Click for possible benefits and risks	Recorded first use and/or resurgence	Click for history
714-X	More									•			AM		3	More		More	1960s	More
Aconite	More						•					CM	AM		3,4	More	More	More	Ancient	More
Aloe	More						•					CM	AM		3,4	More	More	More	Ancient/1930s/ 1960s	More
Arnica	More						•					CM	AM		3	More	More	More	Medieval	More
Astralagus	More						•					CM	AM		3	More	More	More	Medieval	More
Australian Aboriginal healing	More		•	•			•					CM	AM	Yes	1,2,3	More		More	<2000 BCE	More
Acupressure	More	•						•				CM			1,2	More		More	<2000 BCE	More
Acupressure – Shiatsu	More	•			•			•				CM			1,2,	More		More	1900s	More
Acupressure – Jin-Shin Jyutsu	More	•						•				CM			1,2	More		More	1900s	More
Acupressure – Tui-Na	More	•						•				CM			1,2	More		More	<2000 BCE	More
Acupressure – Ohashiatsu	More	•						•				CM			1,2	More		More	1974	More
Acupressure – Watsu	More	•						•				CM			1,2	More		More	Mid-1970s	More
Acupuncture	More	•						•	•		OM	CM			1,2	More		More	<2000 BCE	More
Alexander technique	More	•			•							CM				More		More	1890s	More
Anthroposophical medicine (see also iscador, mistletoe)	More		•			•	•				OM	CM	AM	Yes	1,2,3	More		More	1920s	More
Antineoplaston treatment (see also Burzynski protocol)	More								•	•			AM		3	More		More	1970s	More
Apitherapy	More					•	•		•			CM	AM		3,4	More		More	Ancient	More
Applied kinesiology	More				•								AM		3	More		More	1964	More
Aromatherapy	More	•					•					CM			1	More		More	1928,1960s	More
Art therapy	More	•										CM			1	More		More	1920s	More
Aveloz	More						•						AM		4	More	More	More	Ancient/1970s	More
Ayurveda	More	•	•	•		•	•		•			CM	AM	Yes	1,2,3	More		More	Ancient	More
Bach flowers	More	•					•					CM	AM		1	More		More	1900s	More
Behaviour therapy	More		•				•					CM			1	More		More	1950s	More
Biofeedback	More		•								OM	CM			1	More		More	1970s	More
Black cohosh	More						•					CM	AM		2,3	More	More	More	Ancient	More
Bromelain	More						•					CM	AM		2,3	More	More	More	c. 1500s	More
Burzynski protocol	More								•	•			AM		3	More		More	1970s	More

Fig. 1. Example of a CAM classification screen. *Note*: This example is for illustrative purposes only. It should not be considered complete, and the information contained therein should not be relied upon. It has not been reviewed and approved by the relevant health practitioner bodies.

symptoms of the cancer itself or to alleviate the side-effects of conventional therapies. They may also be used to enhance conventional treatments, to improve quality of life or for cultural reasons.[27–29] The 'Use in cancer' column in Fig. 1 shows, using numbers, the way in which conventional medicine regards these CAMs when used in cancer treatment.

- One: Use is complementary to conventional medical treatment, and is either approved of, or considered harmless, by conventional medicine.
- Two: Use is complementary to conventional medical treatment, but use is not approved of by conventional medicine.
- Three: Use is alternative to conventional medical treatment, and the CAM may be promoted as a cure for cancer. Use is not approved of by conventional medicine.
- Four: Use is alternative to conventional medical treatment, and where the CAM may be promoted as a cure for cancer there is documented scientific evidence of severe harm. Use is not approved of by conventional medicine.

Some CAMs are assigned more than one number. This indicates that there may be several different uses of the same CAM when used in cancer treatment, each with a differing level of medico-scientific regard. For instance, the whole healing system, Ayurvedic medicine, comprises many different therapies. The Ayurvedic dietary regimes, yoga, meditation and some of the Ayurvedic herbal medicines may have some degree of medico-scientific support, but procedures such as bowel purging and induced vomiting in cancer patients may lead to serious medical complications, and may therefore not be approved, or may be actively discouraged, by conventional medicine. More information about the uses, risks and benefits, and levels of approval of these CAMs in cancer treatment can be provided in pop-up windows, or via the link in the 'Possible benefits and risks' column.

The use of a computer application, such as that displayed in Fig. 1, not only provides a view of CAMs according to their types of therapeutic action, but it also enables the user to reorganise the display of CAMs by either therapeutic action or various other categories. For instance, a list of all CAMs with a component of

'Energy Therapy' can be created by selecting the 'Energy Therapy' column. This list can then be further organised by choosing to exclude, for example, any therapy that is classified as 'Manipulative', and 'Alternative'. It can then be further selected to only include those therapies whose use in cancer is rated as a '1'. In this case, the user who was searching for all non-manipulative complementary energy therapies would now only see the list displayed in Fig. 2. This sort of functionality would therefore enable each user of such a system to construct groups, or taxonomies, of CAMs according to their needs.

There are many benefits to be gained from using a computer-driven taxonomy of CAMs, not the least being that it can provide immediate access to the latest scientific information. A portal-type solution, such as that displayed in Fig. 1, enables access to a variety of many of the existing, reliable sources of information about CAMs. Direct links can be made to sites such as the ACS (which has comprehensive CAM information), the search already being primed with the appropriate ACS website page and name of the CAM being queried. A list of the latest published scientific research from the US NIH search engine 'PubMed' could be displayed, and links to herbal medicines databases (such as HerbMed or Medline Plus) could also be included.[e] If required, a wide variety of further information, such as the history of the therapy in question, could also be accessed via hyperlink.

Providing information about CAM in such a way allows the individual user — whether patient or clinician — to access the level of complexity of information that they need. Definitions of and information about CAMs could also be added, deleted or revised as necessary by the hosting organisation, and their classification and gradings updated regularly. The provision of links to reputable sites such as the ACS and PubMed can provide access to the latest scientific research and opinion for those who desire it. A computer-driven CAM taxonomy can provide a more flexible and informative mechanism for meeting the different information needs of consumers, patients, carers and health professionals.

---

[e] NOTE: Issues of access and licensing for some websites will need to be negotiated by the CAM information website hosting organization.

CONTEMPORARY CAMS																				
		TYPES OF THERAPEUTIC ACTION									Orthodox/ complementary/ alternative			Whole system						
CAM NAME	Click for more info	Body work; body-> mind work	Mind work; mind-> bodywork	Religious/ spiritual	Manipu lative	Dietary/ sup plement	Pharma cological	Energy therapy	Invasive	Biological therapy	OM	CM	AM		Use in cancer	Click for PubMed	Click for herb info	Click for possible benefits and risks	Recorded first use and/or resurgence	Click for history
Acupressure	More							*				CM			1,2	More		More	<2000 BCE	More
Acupressure – Jin-Shin Jyutsu	More							*				CM			1,2	More		More	1900s	More
Acupressure – Tui-Na	More							*				CM			1,2	More		More	<2000 BCE	More
Acupressure – Ohashiatsu	More							*				CM			1,2	More		More	1974	More
Acupressure – Watsu	More							*				CM			1,2	More		More	Mid-1970s	More
Acupuncture	More							*	*		OM	CM			1,2	More		More	<2000 BCE	More
Reflexology	More							*				CM			1,2	More		More	Ancient/1900s	More

Fig. 2. Selection list of energy therapies. *Note*: This example is for illustrative purposes only. It should not be considered complete, and the information contained therein should not be relied upon. It has not been reviewed and approved by the relevant health practitioner bodies.

CONCLUSION

Large numbers of patients with cancer use CAMs, and as such there is a clear need for easily accessible, comprehensive and reliable information about these therapies and practices. In order to make informed decisions about CAMs — whether these are policy or treatment decisions — it is essential firstly to understand something about what they are, how they work and what their risks and benefits may be in a variety of different settings. Although this requires some means for classifying CAMs, existing systems for classifying CAMs are unable to account for their complex multi-functional and dynamic nature. Adopting a different approach to the classification of CAMs, which takes advantage of modern computer technology, could provide a more flexible and comprehensive information resource for all those who need it.

ACKNOWLEDGEMENTS

I would like to acknowledge the support of my research supervisors Associate Professor Ian Kerridge and Dr Chris Jordens of the Centre for Values, Ethics and the Law in Medicine at the University of Sydney. I would also like to express my appreciation to the Centre for Clinical Research Excellence — Infection and Bioethics in Haematological Malignancies (CCRE–IBHM) for the scholarship that provided support for my early research in the area of CAMs.

REFERENCES

1. Tyler SA. Introduction to cognitive anthropology. In McGee RJ, Warms RL (eds.) *Anthropological Theory: An Introductory History*, McGraw Hill, Boston, pp. 368–383 (2008).
2. World Health Organisation *General Guidelines for Methodologies on Research and Evaluation of Traditional Medicine*, Geneva (2000). http://whqlibdoc.who.int/hq/2000/WHO_EDM_TRM_2000.1.pdf [Accessed July 2008].
3. World Health Organisation. *Traditional Medicine — Fact Sheet No. 134* (2003). http://www.who.int/mediacentre/factsheets/fs134/en/index.html. [Accessed July 2008].

4. Cohen MH. *Beyond Complementary Medicine: Legal and Ethical Perspectives on Health Care and Human Evolution*, University of Michigan Press, Michigan (2003).
5. Winnick TA. From quackery to "complementary" medicine: the American medical profession confronts alternative therapies. *Social Problems* **52**(1):38–61 (2005).
6. Keinle GS, Kiene H, Albonico H-U. *Anthroposophical Medicine: Effectiveness, Utility, Costs, Safety*, Schattauer GmbH, Stuttgart (2006).
7. McKinlay JB, Marceau LD. The end of the golden age of doctoring. *Int J Health Services* **32**(2):379–416 (2002).
8. Baer HA. The growing interest of biomedicine in complementary and alternative medicine: a critical perspective. *Med Anthropol Quart* **16**(4):403–405 (2002).
9. US National Institutes of Health. *National Center for Complementary and Alternative Medicine website*. http://nccam.nih.gov/ [Accessed 30 January 2008].
10. Bivins R. *Alternative Medicine? A History*, Oxford University Press, Oxford (2007).
11. Easthope G, Gill VF, Beilby JJ, *et al*. Acupuncture in Australian general practice: patient characteristics. *Med J Aust* **170**:259–262 (1999).
12. Australian Medical Association (AMA). *Complementary Medicine Position Statement* (2002). http://www.ama.com.au/web.nsf/doc/WEEN-6L74GC [Accessed 13 April 2007].
13. US National Institutes of Health. *National Center for Complementary and Alternative Medicine website*. http://nccam.nih.gov/ [Accessed 20 January 2010].
14. American Cancer Society. *American Cancer Society website*, http://www.cancer.org/ [Accessed 20 January 2010].
15. Cant S, Sharma U. *A New Medical Pluralism? Alternative Medicine, Doctors, Patients and the State*, UCL Press, London (1999).
16. Ernst E, Cassileth BR. The prevalence of complementary/alternative medicine in cancer: a systematic review. *Cancer* **83**(4): 777–782 (1998).
17. Senate Community Affairs Committee, Parliament of Australia. *The Cancer Journey: Informing Choice* (23 June 2005).
18. Cassileth BR, Vickers AJ. High prevalence of complementary and alternative medicine use among cancer patients: implications for research and clinical care (editorial). *J Clin Oncol* **23**(12): 2590–2592 (2005).

19. Yates JS, Mustian KM, Morrow GR, *et al.* Prevalence of complementary and alternative medicine use in cancer patients during treatment. *Support Care Cancer* **13**(10): 806–811 (2005).
20. Barnes PM, Powell-Griner E, McFann K, *et al.* National Institutes of Health. *Complementary and Alternative Medicine Use Among Adults: United States, 2002* (27 May 2004).
21. Barnes PM, Bloom B, Nahin RL. National Institutes of Health. *Complementary and Alternative Medicine Use Among Adults and Children: United States, 2007*, 12 December 2008.
22. Kristoffersen AE, Fonnebo V, Norheim AJ. Use of complementary and alternative medicine among patients: classification criteria determine level of use. *J Altern Complement Med* **14**(8): 911–919 (2008).
23. Fox S, Rainie L. Pew Research Center. *Vital Decisions: How Internet Users Decide What Information to Trust When They or Their Loved Ones are Sick*, 22 May 2002.
24. Metz J, Devine P, DeNittis A, *et al.* A multi-institutional study of Internet utilization by radiation oncology patients. *Int J Radiat Oncol* **56**(4):1201–1205 (2003).
25. Newnham GM, Burns WI, Snyder RD, *et al.* Information from the Internet: attitudes of Australian oncology patients. *Int Med J* **36**(11): 718–723 (2006).
26. Schmidt K, Ernst E. Assessing websites on complementary and alternative medicine for cancer. *Ann of Oncol* **15**(5):733–742 (2004).
27. Begbie SD, Kerestes ZL, Bell DR. Patterns of alternative medicine use by cancer patients. *Med J Aust* **165**(10):545–548 (1996).
28. Correa-Velez I, Clavarino A, Eastwood H. Surviving, relieving, repairing, and boosting up: reasons for using complementary/alternative medicine among patients with advanced cancer: a thematic analysis. *J Palliat Med* **8**(5):953–961 (2005).
29. Miller M, Boyer MJ, Butow PN, *et al.* The use of unproven methods of treatment by cancer patients. Frequency, expectations and cost. *Support Care Cancer* **6**(4):337–347 (1998).

3

Complementary and Alternative Medicine Used by Patients with Cancer: Evidence for Efficacy and Safety

Carlo Pirri

ABSTRACT

In Australia the overall prevalence for complementary medicine use is 14–65% among adults diagnosed with cancer (with estimates as high as 80–91% in the US and Europe), and 8–14% for alternative medicine use among adult cancer patients. Given the increasing desire of cancer patients to use complementary and alternative medicine (CAM), it is important that clinicians have a good understanding of the levels of evidence available for the efficacy and safety of specific complementary and alternative therapies. This systematic review aims to evaluate the efficacy and safety of a range of CAMs in each of five categories used by cancer patients (upon diagnosis, during conventional treatment, in response to disease progression or recurrence, or during remission/survivorship) in Australia and elsewhere. Where possible, evidence from meta-analytic and systematic reviews is utilised. Currently, there is evidence from high-quality clinical trials that some complementary therapies, used as adjuncts to conventional medical treatments, are beneficial in reducing disease or treatment symptoms and improving quality of life and psychological functioning. There is also evidence of potential harm. It is therefore imperative that those involved in the medical care of cancer patients are equipped with the skills and knowledge to help patients appropriately evaluate complementary and alternative therapies. Additionally, clinicians are strongly encouraged to routinely ask patients about complementary and alternative therapy use. Offering evidence-based complementary therapies alongside conventional treatments in cancer services can influence patients' decisions to continue with mainstream care and help avoid any potential harm that may occur with autonomous CAM use.

Keywords: Complementary and Alternative Medicines; Efficacy; Safety; Systematic Review.

POPULAR CAM APPROACHES AND EVIDENCE FOR USE

Whole Medical Systems

Whole medical systems are complete systems of diagnosis and practice, developed in both Western cultures (e.g. homeopathy), and other cultures [e.g. traditional Chinese medicine (TCM) and ayurveda].

Homeopathy

Homeopathy is based on the proposed law of similars that "like cures like", whereby low concentrations of substances that cause symptoms in healthy individuals can be used to treat patients with similar symptoms. Homeopathic medicines are generally safe in terms of adverse effects and interactions with conventional treatments. A systematic review of 53 studies found that homeopathic medicines prescribed by trained practitioners in low concentrations are probably safe and unlikely to cause serious adverse events, with the main risks being indirect, stemming from practitioner inexperience (e.g. misdiagnosis).[1]

Systematic reviews of controlled trials have found that homeopathic medicines appeared to improve symptom management during chemotherapy and radiotherapy (specifically chemotherapy-induced stomatitis and acute radiotherapy-induced dermatitis).[2]

Although producing encouraging preliminary evidence, the authors of both reviews expressed concern about the general lack of evidence and the clinical heterogeneity of identified homeopathy studies and cautioned that further research was required before any definitive recommendations on use by cancer patients could be made.

Naturopathy

Naturopathy is an alternative medical system based on the core beliefs that nature has the ability to heal and that the human body has the vital ability to maintain and heal itself. Naturopaths favour natural remedies and minimally-invasive approaches in preference to surgery and drugs. Practitioners use a wide variety of treatment modalities, including dietary and lifestyle changes (e.g. eating more whole and unprocessed foods, abstaining from alcohol and sugar, stress reduction); using vitamins, minerals and nutritional supplements; herbal medicine; homeopathy; mind–body techniques (e.g. meditation, yoga, counselling); and manipulative and body-based therapies (e.g. hydrotherapy, physical exercise). Given the overlap of naturopathic remedies with other categories of complementary and alternative medicine (CAM), they will be reviewed in their respective sections below.

Traditional Chinese medicine

Traditional Chinese medicine (TCM) is based upon the concept that the human body is a dynamic universe of interconnected energy systems and aims to maintain balance, harmony and order of these systems to ensure healthy body functioning. TCM treatments include acupuncture and related techniques (e.g. acupressure, moxibustion), Chinese herbal medicine (CHM), massage (e.g. tui na, cupping), exercise and breathing techniques (e.g. Qigong), and dietary and lifestyle advice.

TCM is predominantly used by cancer patients to improve immune function, for symptom management (i.e. of general constitutional symptoms such as fatigue, pain and depression, and for specific symptoms such as gastrointestinal distress, or appetite loss) and overall well-being, as well as to enhance the effects of conventional treatments in chemotherapy and radiotherapy. In a review of randomised controlled trials (RCTs) and observational studies of TCM in supportive cancer care,[3] the authors concluded that overall there was sufficient preliminary evidence to suggest that further clinical trials were warranted to evaluate the effects on quality of life (QoL) and survival of integrating TCM into conventional oncology care (see below for discussion of specific TCM treatments).

Mind–Body Techniques

Mind–body techniques involve individuals learning coping strategies to deal with emotional distress that may be manifest in physical symptoms. Techniques include practitioner-administered therapies such as hypnotherapy and mindfulness-based stress reduction (MBSR), and self-help strategies such as relaxation, meditation and creative therapies (including art, music and dance therapy). Some techniques that were considered as CAM in the past have become mainstream (e.g. patient support groups), but they are discussed below nonetheless, because they complement conventional anticancer treatment.

Relaxation

Relaxation techniques originated in the early 1900s in the US and Europe. They are designed to elicit a state of mental and physical relaxation, most commonly by focusing attention on the sensations associated with systematically tensing and relaxing muscle groups, as in progressive muscle relaxation (PMR), or to achieve a hypometabolic state of reduced sympathetic arousal (e.g. via autogenic training, PMR augmented with diaphragmatic breathing and/or guided imagery). Relaxation techniques often involve diaphragmatic or deep breathing (slow, deep rhythmic breathing) to aid in the release of muscle tension, and may incorporate guided imagery/visualisation (evoking images, usually sensory or affective) to calm the mind. Relaxation is generally safe and adverse events are rare.

Turning to efficacy, a meta-analysis of 15 RCTs involving patients undertaking acute non-surgical cancer treatment (chemotherapy, radiotherapy, bone marrow transplantation, hyperthermia) revealed that relaxation exerted significant positive effects on nausea, pain, physiological arousal (blood pressure, heart rate), anxiety, depression and hostility.[4] A more recent meta-analysis of 25 controlled trials and observational studies also found reasonably strong evidence for the efficacy of relaxation-based interventions in reducing cancer pain,[5] and recent systematic reviews showed some support for relaxation reducing pain,[6] nausea and vomiting,[7] and anticipatory nausea and vomiting,[8] respectively.

Meditation

Meditation is an ancient Eastern practice that has been popularly adopted worldwide. It involves training the mind to focus on breathing or a specific object/image in an effort to free it of all thought (concentrative meditation), or to focus on sensations experienced in the present moment in a non-judgemental and accepting manner, to establish a stable, non-reactive awareness to the physical or psychological symptoms associated with them (mindfulness meditation).[9] Most meditation practices were developed within a religious or spiritual context and the ultimate goal is to achieve some form of spiritual/personal growth or transcendental experience and to find a system of values and philosophy of life, whereas many approaches in behavioural medicine (e.g. relaxation, biofeedback) are designed as treatments for particular disorders.[10] There are many forms of meditation (e.g. Sahaja yoga meditation, Vipassana meditation), but the two most researched practices are mindfulness and transcendental meditation [the latter involves a silent word or phrase (a mantra) being repeated in order to calm (and ultimately transcend) the ordinary flow of internal mental dialogue].[11]

Meditation is generally safe and serious adverse events are rare, but it is not without some side-effects. Common adverse effects include relaxation-induced anxiety and panic, restlessness, frustration, paradoxical increases in tension, depersonalisation or derealisation (which can recur after meditation), antisocial behaviour and flattened affect.[12,13] Other adverse effects during and after meditation may include reduced motivation, boredom, difficulty in returning to normal life after meditation retreats, pain, impaired reality testing, disorientation, feeling "spaced out", depression, other psychological sequelae and feeling addicted to meditation.[12]

In any case, most studies reporting safety concerns about meditation have involved transcendental or Vipassana meditation and most side-effects have been observed in longer-term retreats (e.g. 10 days) and/or intensive meditation (e.g. 3 hour sessions) which are not formally recommended for "novice" patients of some meditation practices such as mindfulness.[14,15] Moreover, only 7.4% of long-term meditators in one study reported severe adverse effects.[12] Nevertheless, meditation practices (transcendental or Vipassana meditation, in particular) should be used with caution or are best avoided in cancer patients with (a history of) psychosis, personality/bipolar/dissociative/hypochondrial/somatisation disorders, or with physical exhaustion.[14–16]

A meta-analysis of three RCTs and seven observational studies suggested that MBSR may improve breast cancer patients' psychological adjustment to illness (i.e. ameliorating anxiety, stress, fatigue, general mood and sleep disturbance), but it found less convincing evidence to support improvement in physical health.[17] Additional larger RCTs involving other cancer populations were recommended. Similar conclusions were also drawn in recent systematic reviews involving cancer patients using MBSR or mindfulness meditation alone.[6,18,19]

Hypnotherapy

Hypnotherapy is a psychological approach that induces a state of aroused consciousness in which suggestions are made to an individual to facilitate behaviour change or symptom relief. An induction procedure, often involving relaxation/imagery techniques, is used prior to suggestion. The efficacy of hypnotherapy is associated with an individual's level of suggestibility, particularly in achieving long-term symptom relief.[20] Hypnotherapy is generally safe when administered by qualified practitioners, but some individuals might experience transient side-effects during or after hypnosis.[21,22] These adverse effects include headaches, drowsiness, confusion, dizziness, or nausea and, less frequently, anxiety or panic;[22] they occur in 5–31% of individuals who undertake hypnotherapy.[21] Serious adverse events are rare and typically involve exacerbation of psychological symptoms, which is usually caused by the misapplication of hypnotherapeutic techniques or poor clinical practice (e.g. not preparing patients sufficiently).[21] Nevertheless, the World Health Organization and others caution against the use of hypnotherapy in individuals with (a history of) psychosis, personality disorders or organic psychiatric conditions.[23]

A meta-analysis of six RCTs (one in adults, five in children) has suggested that hypnotherapy is effective in reducing anticipatory and chemotherapy-induced nausea and vomiting in paediatric patients alone.[24] Furthermore, a more recent systematic review found that hypnotherapy improved cancer pain without exception in a small number of controlled and observational studies;[6] and systematic reviews of RCTs and observational studies have demonstrated that hypnotherapy is a potentially valuable treatment for acute procedural pain and distress in adult and paediatric cancer patients,[25,26] although large RCTs are needed.

Yoga

Yoga is a series of practices that incorporate eight disciplines, including physical poses and postures, breath control and meditation, with the goal of uniting the mind, body and spirit for improved physical/mental health and self-awareness. There are many types of yoga, with Hatha yoga (a gentle form most commonly practised in Western countries) and Tibetan yoga being the most studied in recent years. Yoga has been well-tolerated in studies with no serious adverse effects. Nevertheless, yoga should be avoided or used in a gentler, modified form by individuals with balance problems; uncontrolled hypertension, symptomatic anaemia or postural hypotension; infection or significant thrombocytopenia; certain eye conditions (e.g. glaucoma); severe osteoporosis and bone injury, vertebral damage or cervical spondylosis; artificial joints or prosthetic devices (e.g. infusaport, colostomy bag), pregnancy; and psychosis.[27]

Two systematic reviews of RCTs and observational studies provide preliminary support for the efficacy of yoga interventions in cancer patients and survivors.[28,29] Positive effects were reported for a range of outcomes including sleep quality, mood, stress and overall QoL, but more RCTs are needed.

Tai Chi

Sometimes referred to as "moving meditation", tai chi is derived from TCM and incorporates slow movements and postures (similar to aerobic exercise), controlled breathing and meditation. Tai chi appears to be generally safe and no serious adverse effects have been reported in cancer and other chronic disease populations.[30,31]

Tai chi has been used by cancer patients to improve QoL, mood, flexibility, and balance.[31] Two systematic reviews of controlled studies in supportive breast cancer care, however, have found insufficient evidence for the positive impact of tai chi on physical or psychological outcomes and QoL in patients.[30,31] Large RCTs involving breast and other cancer populations are required.

Music Therapy

Music therapy is designed to facilitate communication and achieve therapeutic goals through the creative use of music alone or in combination with relaxation/imagery techniques. A recent meta-analysis of 183 studies across 11 medical specialties (with a heavy emphasis on cancer patients) revealed that music therapy resulted in significant improvements in pain, well-being, mood, and nausea and vomiting.[32] Nevertheless, more large RCTs are required, although music therapy could be supported for use in cancer patients in the interim given its association with few (if any) adverse events.

Support Groups

Support groups enable patients at any stage of their cancer experience to gain emotional support from others with similar experiences (and to reciprocate in kind) by sharing. Cancer support groups include a variety of different approaches (e.g. psychotherapy, psychoeducation, cognitive–behavioural therapy), types (e.g. face-to-face, telephone or internet support) and settings (e.g. community centres or hospitals, the patient's home) encompassing health professional-led support groups and self-help groups.

A meta-analysis of 20 RCTs has suggested that participation in professional-led support groups results in significant improvements in cancer patients' emotional well-being (depression, anxiety), adjustment to illness, QoL and marital satisfaction, but not survival.[33] Similarly, a more recent systematic review of 32 RCTs and 12 descriptive studies revealed that professional-led support groups produced positive effects in psychosocial functioning (less social isolation, felt more understood and hopeful) and morale and other QoL dimensions, but not improved survival.[34] Further RCTs of professional-led support groups involving different cancer populations, preferably in community settings, are required.

Benefit from peer/volunteer support programmes, however, is less apparent for cancer patients. A systematic review of 16 controlled trials and 26 descriptive studies indicated a high level of satisfaction with individual/group peer support programmes, but mixed evidence for psychosocial benefit.[35] A systematic review of ten controlled trials and ten descriptive studies also found a high level of satisfaction among participants in individual volunteer support programmes, but very limited evidence for psychosocial benefit given the lack of RCTs performed.[36] Again, more large RCTs involving different cancer populations are needed.

Spirituality, Religion and Prayer

Spirituality and religion are overlapping concepts that involve a search for the sacred, in which individuals seek to discover, hold on to, and, when necessary, transform whatever they hold sacred in their lives.[37] Spirituality differs from religion in that religion is a search for significance in ways related to the sacred[38] and, in instances of popular usage, places spirituality within the context of beliefs, values and practices of an organised institution.[39]

A systematic review of seven longitudinal and ten cross-sectional studies found some evidence for improved adjustment to illness or reduced distress from religious/spiritual coping with cancer, but could not draw any firm conclusions,[40] A more recent review of four longitudinal and 36 cross-sectional studies drew similar conclusions regarding spirituality and emotional well-being in cancer patients.[41] Further large longitudinal studies are required.

Researchers have argued that prayer can be separated from religion in the same way as related activities such as meditation.[42] A systematic review of seven prospective cohort studies, 14 cross-sectional studies and three qualitative studies involving hospitalised populations (including cancer patients) found a positive association between private prayer and emotional well-being (anxiety, depression), optimism and functioning, respectively, in patients with religious faith who engage in regular devoted prayer, and some evidence that prayer out of desperation (e.g. in response to pain, poor prognosis or post-operative trauma) in the absence of faith is associated with poorer emotional well-being and functioning.[43] However, more rigorous studies involving cancer patients across different religions are needed.

Studies examining the effects of intercessory prayer on well-being are rarer and reported in another chapter of this book. Additionally, a systematic review of 17 epidemiological studies (including a subgroup analysis of 11 studies adjusted for demographic and lifestyle factors) revealed no significant reduction in cancer risk among members of Christian communities compared with the general population, and concluded that a healthy lifestyle was the most important mediating factor in explaining any correlation observed between religious membership and cancer risk.[44] Finally, two meta-analyses of randomised trials involving medical populations (including leukaemia patients) have found insufficient evidence that distant intercessory prayer has any beneficial effects on clinical outcomes (health, mortality, hospital readmission).[45,46]

Biologically-Based Practices

Biologically-based practices involve supplementing a person's normal diet with additional extracts, nutrients, herbs and/or certain foods. Examples include nutritional supplements, herbal and other plant-based preparations (botanicals), animal-derived extracts, vitamins, minerals, fatty acids, amino acids, proteins, pre-biotics and pro-biotics (live bacteria often found in whole grains, yoghurt and functional foods), whole diet therapies, functional foods, and other so-called natural therapies (e.g. shark cartilage for cancer treatment).[47]

Nutritional Supplements (Dietary Supplements, Food Supplements)

Nutrients in dietary supplements may include vitamins, minerals, herbs or other plant-based substances (botanicals), amino acids, fatty acids and substances such as enzymes. Nutritional supplements may be extracts or concentrates sold as tablets/capsules, liquids or powders.

Antioxidants

Free radicals are unstable molecules produced when the body breaks down food, or is exposed to environmental influences (e.g. tobacco smoke, radiation). Although free radicals are essential for various biological functions including the removal of damaged cells, they are also highly reactive and can damage healthy cells via oxidation. Excessive free radicals may play a role in the development and progression of certain diseases, such as cancer, cardiovascular disease and liver disease.[48] Antioxidants neutralise free radicals and may protect cells in the body from damage caused by oxidative stress.[49] Broadly, antioxidants take the form of nutrients [e.g. vitamins C (ascorbic acid) and E (alpha-tocopherol); minerals such as selenium and zinc] and non-nutrients (e.g. phytochemicals such as lycopene, beta-carotene and indole-3-carbinol; zoochemicals in red meat and fish products). Although present in food and beverages, they are commonly taken as nutritional supplements (capsules/tablets, powders) alone or in combination with vitamins and minerals.

Proponents argue that antioxidants are beneficial to cancer patients because they enhance the efficacy of chemotherapy, as well as alleviate treatment toxicity and thus allow patients to tolerate full courses of chemotherapy and/or radiotherapy with fewer dose reductions.[50] Others are concerned that antioxidants may not only reduce the efficacy of some chemotherapy agents and radiotherapy, but may protect cancer cells as well as healthy cells from oxidative damage.[51]

A recent systematic review of 33 RCTs found that concurrent use of antioxidants with chemotherapy resulted in reduced toxicity in the majority of studies (which involved mostly advanced or recurrent cancer patients), and that patients in five studies completed more full doses of chemotherapy or had fewer dose reductions when receiving antioxidants than control patients.[52] Similarly, another review suggested that antioxidants may mitigate the adverse effects of radiotherapy,[53] whereas a meta-analysis of 14 RCTs showed that amifostine (a synthetic antioxidant) significantly reduced the side-effects of radiotherapy.[54] In contrast, however, a systematic review of 22 controlled trials and observational studies involving breast cancer patients found insufficient evidence that individual antioxidant supplements reduced toxicity during conventional breast cancer treatment.[55] Other systematic reviews have also revealed insufficient evidence that selenium supplementation alleviates chemotherapy- or radiotherapy-induced toxicity or post-operative side-effects in cancer patients,[56] or that selenium or lycopene supplementation relieves symptoms in prostate cancer patients.[57,58] Similarly, a systematic review of six controlled trials found inconclusive evidence that coenzyme Q10 (synthetic antioxidant) reduced chemotherapy-induced toxicity.[59] Further large, well-designed RCTs are advised. The formation of free radicals is the primary mechanism by which radiotherapy and many chemotherapy drugs act in destroying cancer cells. One systematic review of 21 randomised trials and 31 observational studies of antioxidants and chemotherapy observed such great diversity across studies (study design, cancer diagnoses, chemotherapy regimens, type/dose/schedule of antioxidant supplementation) that definitive conclusions could not be made about the efficacy and safety of antioxidant supplementation.[60] Similarly, a systematic review of 22 controlled trials and observational studies could not draw any conclusions regarding the effects of antioxidants during breast cancer treatment (chemotherapy, radiotherapy and/or hormonal therapy) on tumour response, survival or recurrence,[55] and nor could the authors in a systematic review of lycopene supplementation in prostate cancer patients.[58] Another review of 44 randomised trials, however, went further and concluded that concurrent use of antioxidants with chemotherapy and/or radiotherapy should be discouraged, due to the possibility of tumour protection and reduced survival, despite limited evidence of these negative outcomes during radiotherapy and limited evidence that some antioxidant supplements may actually enhance the efficacy of chemotherapy.[61] In contrast, a systematic review found that the great majority of 19 RCTs demonstrated either statistically significant or non-significantly greater survival and/or treatment response for concurrent use of antioxidants with free radical-generating chemotherapy, in patients with predominantly advanced or recurrent cancer.[62] Additionally, no evidence was found that antioxidant supplementation reduced the efficacy of chemotherapy. Again, further large, well-designed studies are recommended.

More unequivocal, though, were the results of three meta-analyses. One meta-analysis of seven RCTs (with no evidence of heterogeneity) found that amifostine (a synthetic antioxidant) had no effect on tumour response in locally advanced non-small cell lung cancer in patients treated with radiotherapy with or without chemotherapy.[63] Another meta-analysis and systematic review of 38 studies found no support for vitamin E or C supplementation helping to treat or prevent cancer.[64] The third meta-analysis of ten unblinded RCTs (with no evidence of heterogeneity), however, demonstrated consistent positive effects on 1-year survival across melatonin dose and diagnosis for advanced solid tumour patients receiving melatonin alone or combined with cancer treatment.[65]

With regard to chemoprevention, a meta-analysis of 22 RCTs indicated no evidence for the primary or secondary prevention of cancer through use of antioxidant supplements.[66] Another meta-analytic and systematic review of 12 RCTs (predominantly high quality) revealed that antioxidant supplementation did not significantly reduce total cancer incidence or mortality or any site-specific cancer incidence in primary prevention.[67] Similarly, meta-analytic and systematic reviews do not support the supplementation of antioxidants (vitamins A, C, E; selenium; beta-carotene) alone or in combination to prevent colorectal cancer[68] or gastrointestinal cancers;[69] of vitamin C or E individually to prevent cancer overall;[64,67,70,71] or of vitamin C or E, folate or beta-carotene individually to prevent lung cancer.[72,73] Vitamin E and selenium may have preventative effects for prostate cancer and gastrointestinal cancers or cancer in men, respectively, although confirmation is required in further RCTs.[67,69,70]

Despite the lack of clinical trial data, antioxidants in foods are generally considered safe and few studies of antioxidant supplements have reported adverse effects. Common minor adverse effects include mild diarrhoea and gastrointestinal upset for vitamin C,[74] and carotenodermia (yellowish discolouration of the skin) following heavy, chronic intake of beta-carotene.[69] However, high-dose beta-carotene appears to increase lung cancer incidence and cancer mortality among smokers;[67,75] antioxidant supplementation may increase the risk of bladder cancer;[66] and high vitamin E supplementation may increase bleeding in individuals with drug-induced vitamin K deficiency.[74] Given the lack of long-term safety data, antioxidant supplementation during cancer treatment is not recommended without guidance from the treating oncology team.

Omega-3 fatty acids (n-3 polyunsaturated fatty acids)

Omega-3 fatty acids [eicosapentaenoic acid (EPA), docosahexaenoic acid (DHA), alpha-linolenic acid (ALA)] influence many physiological functions, including fertility, cell division, angiogenesis, apoptosis and immune cell function, thus suggesting that they may protect against cancer or alter the response to cancer treatment.[76,77] Omega-3 fatty acids are found naturally in fish, fish oil, vegetable oils (mainly canola and soybean), walnuts, wheat germ, and other foods or as supplements. They are also available as nutritional supplements in fish oil preparations in both capsule and liquid form. EPA and, to a lesser extent, DHA have demonstrated anticancer and anticachectic effects in human studies.[78,79]

A meta-analytic and systematic review of 38 studies, involving 20 different prospective cohorts across seven countries with different demographics, revealed that data across 11 different types of cancer suggested that nutritional supplementation with omega-3 fatty acids is unlikely to prevent cancer.[80] Additionally, a recent meta-analysis of five prospective studies found a weak protective association between high dietary ALA intake (1.5 g/day) and prostate cancer risk.[81] In contrast, two other recent meta-analyses of prospective and case-control studies revealed that high intake or blood level of ALA (but not EPA or DHA intake) is weakly associated with an increased risk of prostate cancer.[82,83] Clearly, further *in-vitro* and epidemiological studies are needed.

Many advanced cancer patients develop cachexia and treatment of associated weight loss and other symptoms has proven difficult. More recently, novel approaches have included the use of fish oils containing EPA and DHA. A Cochrane systematic review of five RCTs found insufficient data to establish whether oral EPA was better than placebo in improving symptoms associated with cachexia in advanced cancer patients.[78] Similarly, a meta-analytic and systematic review of 19 studies demonstrated no effect of omega-3 fatty acids on weight loss, nutritional status, post-operative complications, mortality or length of hospital stay after surgery for upper gastrointestinal cancers.[80] A more recent systematic review of 17 clinical trials and prospective studies, however, suggested that dietary or supplemental intake of omega-3 fatty acids (EPA and/or DHA; 1.5 g/day) for prolonged periods (8 weeks) by advanced cancer patients is associated with improved clinical (nutritional status, tolerance, survival, hospital stays), biological and QoL outcomes.[79] Further large RCTs are recommended. Finally, omega-3 fatty acids are generally well-tolerated and cause few adverse effects in low to moderate doses. Gastrointestinal symptoms (e.g. diarrhoea, heartburn, bloating, nausea) are the most common side-effects.

Shark cartilage and AE-941 (neovastat)

Shark cartilage use by cancer patients became popular in the 1980s after several poor quality studies claiming "miracle" cancer cures were reported by the US media,[84] many of which were generated by a single manufacturer (Lane Labs-USA, producer of BeneFin). Use of shark cartilage in cancer patients originally stemmed from and has been perpetuated by the popular belief that sharks do not develop cancer because of the high proportion of cartilage in their body (about 6% by body weight).[85] Scientifically, this has been shown to be untrue (several tumours in sharks have subsequently been detailed in a review article).[86]

Shark cartilage preparations are not standardised and there is no generally accepted recommended dosage or duration for administration. The only standardised source of shark cartilage is Neovastat (AE-941, manufactured by AEterna Zentaris), a matrix metalloproteinase inhibitor specifically developed as a highly purified liquid shark cartilage extract for evaluation in clinical drug trials. Generally, shark cartilage is well-tolerated. The most common adverse effects reported are gastrointestinal symptoms (nausea, vomiting, stomach upset, constipation, diarrhoea, flatulence) and taste alteration.[87]

Although some pre-clinical studies of shark cartilage and preliminary clinical studies of Neovastat have demonstrated antiangiogenic and anticancer properties,[88] and it has been observed that cartilage lacks blood vessels and that human cancer rarely invades cartilage,[89,90] no controlled study has demonstrated that crude cartilage extracts are beneficial in the treatment of cancer in humans (or animals).[91,92] In a double-blind RCT of 83 incurable breast and colorectal carcinoma patients (with good performance status and organ function), no differences in overall survival or QoL were observed between patients receiving standard conventional care (including chemotherapy for some patients) with powdered liquid shark cartilage extract (BeneFin nutritional supplement, three to four times daily until unacceptable toxicity developed) versus standard conventional care with placebo.[91] These results mirrored those of a previous uncontrolled phase I/II trial involving 60 advanced cancer patients.[87]

Larger RCTs involving the use of Neovastat in cancer patients have been similarly disappointing. In a double-blind RCT of 305 metastatic renal cell carcinoma patients refractory to immunotherapy, no survival advantage was observed in patients treated with Neovastat versus placebo.[93] More recently, a comprehensive double-blind RCT of 379 locally advanced non-small cell lung cancer patients (newly-diagnosed, unresectable and previously untreated) found no differences in overall survival, tumour response rates, time to disease progression and progression-free survival between patients receiving chemoradiation with Neovastat (120 ml orally, twice daily until disease progression or unacceptable toxicity developed) versus chemoradiation with placebo.[92] It was concluded that the results do not support the use of shark cartilage-derived products for lung cancer patients, and this has prompted the pharmaceutical manufacturer of Neovastat to cease clinical development.

Laetrile and amygdalin (vitamin B17)

Laetrile has been popularly used by cancer patients worldwide since the 1970s in the hope that it might cure or slow the growth of cancer. The term "laetrile" is an amalgam of laevorotatory and mandelonitrile, which is used to describe a purified form of amygdalin (cyanogenic glycoside plant compound).[94] Amygdalin is found in the stones of many fruits and nuts (e.g. almonds, cashews).[95] Laetrile may be taken as an oral supplement (dubbed vitamin B17, although it is not a real vitamin), or injected intravenously, intraperitoneally or intramuscularly. Despite frequent interchangeable use, the intravenous form of laetrile (D-mandelonitrile-beta-glucuronide) is a US-patented semi-synthetic derivative of amygdalin, whereas laetrile produced in Mexico (D-mandelonitrile-beta-gentiobioside) is usually amygdalin naturally produced from crushed apricot stones.

Laetrile/amygdalin is typically used as an adjunct to conventional anticancer treatments or in combination with other alternative therapies, such as metabolic therapy.[96] *In-vitro* studies suggest that amygdalin has anticancer properties,[94,97] but no RCTs have been performed on amygdalin or laetrile in humans.[95] A limited uncontrolled phase II trial, performed by the US National Cancer Institute in 1982, found that 95 of 178 (53%) of mixed, non-metastatic cancer patients experienced disease progression and only one patient exhibited a partial tumour response (lasting 10 weeks) following 21 days of intravenous laetrile plus oral maintenance therapy combined with metabolic therapy (pancreatic enzymes, high vitamin doses, dietary changes employed by metabolic practitioners).[96] Furthermore, all remaining patients experienced disease progression within 7 months post-treatment, and no significant difference in survival was observed compared with historical controls who had inactive or no treatment.

Better evidence, however, is offered by a systematic review of 36 studies (25 case reports, six best case series of case reports, three non-consecutive case series, two consecutive case series) involving 352 cancer patients treated with laetrile/amygdalin.[95] Despite the likelihood of positive bias in case reports, only 3.1% of patients reportedly had a complete response and 9.4% had a partial response (although some of these patients may have received conventional treatments and no detailed follow-up information was reported for complete response patients), whereas 36.4% exhibited disease progression; symptomatic benefits were also reported in 22.9% of cases. The authors concluded that the claim that laetrile has beneficial effects for cancer patients is not supported by sound clinical evidence.

Possible adverse effects of laetrile/amygdalin are of particular concern, given the belief that the cyanide produced when it is broken down kills cancer cells. In the aforementioned systematic review, 14.4% of patients experienced adverse reactions consisting mainly of nausea, vomiting, headache, fever and abdominal pain.[95] The most important concern with toxicity, however, involves several reports of cyanide poisoning (including deaths) from the use of laetrile/amygdalin by cancer patients in North America in the 1970s and 80s, which prompted the US to ban its use.[95]

Chinese Herbal Medicine

Chinese herbal medicine (CHM) is a key part of TCM and is used to normalise imbalanced energy that runs through invisible meridians in the body. CHM includes any mixture of herbs (mainly plant-based, but also including minerals or animal extracts) and decoction (liquid extraction of boiled herbs), which may take the form of tablets/capsules, powders, tonics, lotions and pastes. There are a number of issues associated with the safety and quality of CHMs, including herb–drug interactions [via induction or inhibition of enzyme systems (e.g. cytochrome P450) or by affecting efflux proteins (e.g. P-glycoprotein)], resulting in a reduced efficacy or increased toxicity of chemotherapy and prescription medications; direct (pharmacological) or indirect (e.g. free radical-mediated) toxicities; allergic responses; contamination with heavy metals, pesticides, micro-organisms or other impurities; deliberate substitution or adulteration with prescription or non-prescription drugs (e.g. corticosteroids, hormones, salicylates, antihistamines, caffeine); and reactivation of viruses or disease (e.g. hepatitis B or C, herpes simplex, varicella zoster, tuberculosis).[98] The safety and quality of CHMs are regulated by the Therapeutic Goods Administration (TGA) in Australia, but limitations of *The Therapeutic Goods Act 1989* do not subject individual practitioners to the standards that companies selling CHMs are required to meet.[99]

Consequently, practitioners can import raw herbs that may not meet the TGA standards and legally dispense them over the counter, without registering with the TGA.

Astragalus (Astragalus membranaceus, Astragalus mongolicus, Astragalus propinquus, Radix astragali)

Astragalus is usually combined with other Chinese herbs, particularly as part of an immune-enhancing herbal regimen known in TCM as Fu Zheng therapy. It is typically administered as a dried root, a powder or in a decoction, although it may also be given by intraperitoneal injection. Human and *in-vitro* studies have demonstrated the immunostimulatory properties of astragalus polysaccharides and triterpinoid saponins in both healthy individuals and cancer patients (e.g. by stimulating macrophage and natural killer cell activity, and inhibiting T-helper cell type 2 cytokines), as well as anticancer activity.[100–103]

In China, astragalus-based Chinese herbs (e.g. Jin Fu Kang) combined with platinum-based chemotherapy is a standard treatment for non-small cell lung cancer. A meta-analysis of 34 Chinese RCTs found evidence that astragalus-based herbal medicine (oral Jin Fu Kang, Aidi injection, other preparations) may enhance the treatment outcomes (improved survival, tumour response and performance status) and reduce the toxicity (leukopenia, haemoglobin toxicity) of standard platinum-based chemotherapy for advanced non-small cell lung cancer patients.[104] Similarly, a more recent meta-analysis and systematic review of 45 RCTs revealed that oral astragalus-based herbal medicine enhanced complete/partial tumour response, survival rates and symptom control (abdominal pain, fatigue, appetite loss), and reduced the risk of disease progression (also for astragalus alone) in unresectable liver cancer patients receiving transcatheter arterial chemoembolisation.[105] Another systematic review of 14 Chinese RCTs suggested that Aidi injection improved the tumour response and QoL of non-small cell lung cancer patients receiving chemotherapy involving vinorelbine and cisplatin injections or cobalt-60 (but not etoposide or paclitaxel combined with cisplatin injections).[106] Finally, a Cochrane meta-analytic review of four RCTs involving colorectal patients suggested that astragalus (huang qi) compound decoctions as an adjunct to chemotherapy may decrease chemotherapy toxicity (nausea and vomiting, leukopenia) and stimulate immunocompetent cells.[101] The authors in each review, however, concluded that larger, more rigorous RCTs were needed to confirm these benefits given the poor quality of the studies examined.[101,104–106]

Attributing specific adverse events or drug interactions to astragalus is difficult, however, given that it is predominantly used in combined herbal preparations. Nevertheless, side-effects of oral astragalus-based preparations reported in two phase II studies involving incurable cancer patients receiving standard care (including chemotherapy and radiotherapy) and incurable non-small lung cancer patients undergoing adjuvant chemotherapy with paclitaxel included grade 3 lymphopenia, grade 3/4 hyperglycaemia and grade 1/2 gastrointestinal symptoms (e.g. diarrhoea, dyspepsia).[106,107] Finally, direct ingestion of certain toxic astragalus plants (locoweed) containing swainsonine and selenium may cause neurological symptoms, some of which are irreversible.[108]

Ginseng (Panax ginseng, Panax quinquefolium, Eleutherococcus senticosus, Angelica sinensis)

Although the immunostimulatory properties of ginseng (and its ginsenosides) in recent reviews[109,110] have suggested a possible role as an adjuvant or immunotherapeutic agent, to enhance immunological function and improve QoL in cancer patients during chemotherapy and radiotherapy, RCTs are yet to be performed to confirm these benefits. Ginseng is associated with a relatively low incidence of adverse events, with reports being attributed to adulterated or contaminated preparations.[111,112] Common side-effects of ginseng include insomnia if taken in the evening, and agitation/overstimulation if excessively used.[111] Possible contraindications of Asian ginseng (*Panax ginseng*) and American ginseng (*Panax quinquefolium*) include hypertension, diabetes, coagulation disorders and surgery,[111,113] and use of anticoagulants (e.g. warfarin) or antiplatelet medications (aspirin), phenelzine (monoamine oxidase inhibitor antidepressant), hypoglycaemics, oestrogens, corticosteroids or alcohol.[112–114] Possible contraindications of Siberian ginseng/eleuthero (*Eleutherococcus senticosus*) include cardiovascular disease,[115] and concomitant use of digoxin (heart drug) and antihypertensive medications.[98] Finally, ginseng, particularly dong quai/female ginseng (*Angelica sinensis*), has oestrogenic effects, which may interfere with the treatment of hormone-sensitive conditions, such as breast cancer (e.g. hormonal therapy) and pregnancy.[116]

Ginger (Zingiber officinale)

Ginger may be used by cancer patients to alleviate postoperative and chemotherapy-induced nausea and vomiting, as well as gastrointestinal symptoms including diarrhoea. A meta-analysis of five RCTs demonstrated that a fixed dose of ≥ 1 g of ginger is more effective than placebo in reducing acute post-operative nausea and vomiting.[117] Studies examining the efficacy of ginger for chemotherapy-induced nausea and vomiting, however, have produced mixed results and are still in their infancy.[118] More RCTs comparing ginger with current antiemetics are required.

Ginger causes few adverse effects when taken in small doses. Gastrointestinal symptoms (e.g. heartburn, bloating, flatulence) are the most common side-effects. Additionally, ginger inhibits thromboxane synthase (platelet enzyme) and platelet aggregation, thus the risk of bleeding is increased in individuals taking anticoagulant/antiplatelet medications (e.g. warfarin, aspirin), those with coagulation disorders and surgical patients.[113]

Lingzhi/Reishi mushroom (Ganoderma lucidum, Ganoderma tsugae)

Lingzhi is a traditional medicinal mushroom that has been used extensively in cancer treatment in Asia. Lingzhi polysaccharides have demonstrated anticancer and immunostimulatory properties.[119] Reviews of preliminary clinical data suggest that Lingzhi extracts or powders may have some potential in cancer treatment, but more rigorous RCTs are required.[119,120] Adverse effects from medicinal mushrooms are rare. Dry throat and nose and gastrointestinal symptoms are the most common side-effects of Lingzhi. Caution is warranted, however, as Lingzhi causes platelet inhibition, thus the risk of bleeding is increased in individuals taking anticoagulant/antiplatelet drugs (e.g. warfarin, aspirin), those with coagulation disorders and surgical patients.[121] Additionally, Lingzhi can increase antioxidant capacity and may interact with chemotherapy agents that rely on free radicals.[122]

Green tea (Camellia sinensis, Thea sinensis)

Green tea and its extracts have a long history of use as a traditional cancer treatment in Asian cultures. Polyphenols in green tea known as catechins, particularly epigallocatechin gallate (EGCG), have demonstrated anticancer, antioxidant and chemopreventive properties.[123] The US Food and Drug Administration (FDA) in a review of studies concluded that there is no supportive evidence for green tea decreasing the risk of gastric, lung, colorectal, oesophageal, pancreatic, ovarian and combined cancers, but weak evidence for decreased risk in breast and prostate cancer.[124] Similarly, more recent systematic reviews have suggested that green tea may reduce cancer risk and slow or prevent progression in cancer patients, but found the overall evidence to be inconclusive[125,126] and counselled that use of green tea alone to treat cancer may be ill-advised given its limited cytotoxic effects.[126] Further large prospective cohort studies and RCTs are recommended.

Green tea is generally safe when consumed in moderate amounts (three to nine cups per day). Excessive consumption (five to six litres per day) may cause gastrointestinal and central nervous system disturbances (e.g. nausea, insomnia, irritability, frequent urination, cardiac arrhythmia), however, predominantly as a result of the caffeine content, rather than the tannin content of green tea.[127,128] Finally, EGCG and other polyphenols in green tea are potent blockers of boronic acid-based proteasome inhibitors and can reduce the efficacy of bortezomib during chemotherapy for multiple myeloma and mantle cell lymphoma.[129]

Ginkgo (Ginkgo biloba, EGb 761)

Ginkgo is one of the most popular herbal medicines worldwide; it is used for a wide range of conditions including cardiovascular disease, stress, neurodegenerative diseases such as Alzheimer's, cognitive impairment including memory loss and psychiatric disorders such as schizophrenia, as well as cancer. Ginkgo is contained in the leaves and seeds of the ginkgo tree and is available as a standardised extract (EGb 761), taken orally or, rarely intravenously. Amongst others, the flavonoids and the terpenoids (gingkolides, bilobalide) of ginkgo have been reported to have anticancer, antioxidant, cardioprotective, antiplatelet, stress-alleviating, cognitive-improving and sexually-enhancing effects.[130] Nonetheless, RCTs are yet to confirm these benefits in cancer patients.

Side-effects of excessive ginkgo consumption include headache, gastrointestinal disturbances (e.g. nausea, diarrhoea), dizziness, palpitations, convulsions (due to 4-methoxypyridoxine in ginkgo seeds), allergic skin reactions (by handling ginkgo seeds), and anaphylaxis-like reactions (intravenous administration only).[130] Additionally, ginkgo enhances anticoagulant/antiplatelet activity and increases the risk of bleeding.[113,130]

Western Herbal Medicine

Western herbal medicine (WHM) includes any mixture of herbs that are primarily native to Europe, which may take the form of tablets/capsules, infusions (teas), concentrated liquid extracts (requiring dilution) and lotions. WHMs share the same safety and quality issues associated with TCMs.

St. John's wort (Hypericum perforatum)

St. John's wort (SJW) is well-known for its antidepressant activity. Although a Cochrane meta-analytic review of 29 RCTs suggests that SJW has similar efficacy to standard prescription antidepressants and fewer side-effects,[131] numerous herb–drug interactions preclude its safe use in cancer patients and other populations. In fact, SJW is the most implicated herbal product in herb–drug interactions reported in the literature to date.[132] Human studies suggest that SJW can interact with medicines by affecting drug metabolism (via induction of cytochrome P450 enzymes, particularly cytochrome P450 3A4, and P-glycoprotein) or levels of neurotransmitters (primarily serotonin).[114,123] Consequently, SJW is contraindicated with the use of opioids, anaesthetics (e.g. fentanyl and propofol), benzodiazepines (e.g. midazolam) and anticoagulants (e.g. warfarin) in surgical patients, and opioid use for cancer pain in (palliative) patients (e.g. morphine, fentanyl).[123] Additionally, SJW taken in combination with other antidepressants by cancer patients may result in reduced efficacy of the antidepressants or serotonin syndrome [cognitive, autonomic and somatic effects ranging from mild symptoms (e.g. hypervigilance, agitation, muscle twitching) to severe symptoms (e.g. tachycardia and hypertension that may lead to shock and death)].[123] Finally, SJW can reduce the efficacy of imatinib during chemotherapy for chronic myeloid leukaemia, gastrointestinal stromal tumours and other malignancies, while having the same effect accompanied by greater myelosuppression in advanced colorectal and lung cancer patients receiving irinotecan.[123]

Garlic (Allium sativum)

Garlic has had a long history of use worldwide for general health, as well as in a variety of conditions including infections and cancer. Garlic can be eaten raw or cooked, may be dried or powdered and used in tablets/capsules, or taken in the form of oils and liquid extracts. Amongst others, garlic has been reported to have antimicrobial, antithrombotic, immune-enhancing, and anticancer/chemopreventive effects.[133,134] A meta-analysis of 18 observational studies suggested that high consumption of raw and/or cooked garlic (but not garlic supplements) may be associated with reduced risk of colorectal and gastric cancers, although a review of intervention studies was recommended given that many of the studies identified did not control for dietary differences.[135] A more recent meta-analysis of two small RCTs and eight observational studies also found an inverse relationship between high garlic intake and colorectal cancer risk, despite great heterogeneity of measures of intake and lack of control for dietary differences in the studies examined.[136] In contrast, a recent large RCT found that long-term garlic supplementation has no beneficial effects on the incidence of gastric cancer or the prevalence of pre-cancerous gastric lesions.[137] Further large prospective cohort studies and RCTs are needed.

Garlic appears to be generally safe, but may cause mild to severe gastrointestinal symptoms (stomach upset, heartburn, bloating) and allergic reactions (e.g. contact dermatitis, garlic burns and anaphylaxis resulting in possible death with topical or oral use).[138] Human clinical trials using well-established probe drugs have demonstrated that oral garlic inhibits cytochrome P450 2E1 enzymes (but not 1A2, 3A4 or 2D6 enzymes),[139,140] which may reduce the efficacy of chemotherapy involving dacarbazine (metastatic melanoma, Hodgkin's lymphoma and other malignancies) and other drugs (e.g. anaesthetics).[114,141] Finally, due to its anticoagulant properties, garlic should be avoided by patients undergoing surgery and should be used with caution by those taking anticoagulant/antiplatelet medications (e.g. warfarin, fluindione, aspirin).[142]

Kava (Piper methysticum)

Kava, a psychoactive substance, is derived from the pepper plant and has been traditionally consumed as a beverage in cultural practices of Pacific countries. It has gained popularity in Western countries in recent years as a medicinal herb because of its anxiolytic, stress-relieving and sedative properties.[143] The roots and rhizomes of kava are used to prepare beverages, extracts, tablets/capsules, and topical solutions. Complementary medicine practitioners commonly prescribe kava for anxiety, sleep disorders and menopausal symptoms. A recent Cochrane meta-analytic review of seven RCTs suggests that kava extract is a safe, effective treatment for anxiety in the short term (1–24 weeks) compared with placebo, but recommended that more rigorous studies be performed to clarify uncertainties about long-term efficacy and safety.[144]

Possible adverse effects of kava are of concern. Chronic and/or heavy use (300–400 g per week) may cause appetite loss, leading to malnutrition and weight loss, shortness of breath, skin conditions (e.g. dry, scaly skin; yellow or white ulcer-like lesions known as kani or kava dermopathy), blood and metabolic abnormalities, loss of muscle control (ataxia/dystonia), and pulmonary hypertension.[145] The most important concern with toxicity, however, involves several reports of hepatotoxicity (including those resulting in death and liver transplants) from use of concentrated kava extracts (but not beverages) in Europe and North America, which prompted several European countries to ban its use in 2002 and other countries (including Australia and the US) to issue health warnings to health-care professionals and consumers advising of the potential (albeit rare) outcome of severe liver injury.[146]

Valerian (Valeriana officinalis)

Valerian, although native to Europe and Asia, grows in most parts of the world and has a long history of use as a sedative for sleep disturbance. The roots and rhizomes of valerian can be prepared to make supplements including capsules/tablets and liquid extracts, as well as infusions (teas). Short-term use (≤ 4–6 weeks) of valerian in recommended doses is generally well tolerated. Common side-effects include central nervous system (e.g. headache, nervousness, dizziness) and gastrointestinal (notably diarrhoea, but also nausea, heartburn and epigastric pain) symptoms.[147] As with conventional sleep medications, chronic use of valerian (≥ 2–4 months) may result in insomnia, as well as withdrawal effects (e.g. delirium, tachycardia) if also used heavily.[148]

Valerian is often used for the treatment of insomnia, fatigue and anxiety/stress, which are common symptoms experienced by cancer patients. A Cochrane review found only one small RCT evaluating the treatment of anxiety disorders using valerian and recommended that more, larger RCTs be performed before drawing any conclusions about its efficacy for anxiety.[149] One systematic review of 29 controlled trials found no significant differences between valerian pills and placebo, overall, in healthy individuals or in individuals with general sleep disturbances or insomnia.[150] A more recent meta-analysis of 18 RCTs, however, found that valerian resulted in significant improvement on subjective measures of sleep quality, but that the effect was not mirrored in objective sleep measures.[147] Further RCTs are required. Overall, short-term use of valerian could be considered for some cancer patients (e.g. non-surgical patients who prefer not to take conventional sleep medications), particularly given that there is no evidence of potential interactions with chemotherapy agents.

Evening primrose oil (Oenothera biennis)

Evening primrose, although native to North America, grows in Europe and parts of the southern hemisphere. Flowers and seeds are pressed to make evening primrose oil (EPO), which contains gamma-linolenic acid, an omega-6 essential fatty acid believed to be the active ingredient. EPO is commercially available in capsule or liquid form and is widely used to treat menopausal symptoms, pre-menstrual syndrome and chronic mastalgia (breast pain associated with menstruation).[151]

Breast cancer patients may experience symptoms of (premature) menopause (e.g. hot flashes, night sweats, vaginal dryness) as a result of chemotherapy, which may be exacerbated by therapy with tamoxifen in patients with hormone-receptor positive tumours.[152] Non-hormonal therapies in the form of herbal medicines such as EPO have become a popular alternative for women (including breast cancer survivors) for the treatment of menopausal symptoms, particularly since health risks were cast over prolonged use (> 5 years) of hormone replacement therapy by the Women's Health Intervention study published in 2002.[153] The menopausal benefits of EPO, however, have yet to be confirmed in RCTs involving post-menopausal women or breast cancer patients.[154,155] Few studies examining the safety of EPO have been conducted. Common adverse effects include headache and gastrointestinal symptoms (e.g. stomach upset, nausea, mild diarrhoea).[156] Limited evidence suggests that EPO may lower the seizure threshold and increase the risk of seizures in individuals taking phenothiazines (e.g. fluphenazine).[151] Finally, despite the absence of reported herb–drug interactions of EPO, it may be prudent to monitor use by patients receiving chemotherapy.[141]

Black cohosh (Actaea racemosa, Cimicifuga racemosa)

Black cohosh, a member of the buttercup family, was traditionally used by the North American Indians and in 19th-century America for a variety of conditions ranging from gynaecological disorders to rheumatism, but has more recently been adopted for use in Europe and Western countries for the treatment of menopausal symptoms and dysmenorrhoea. The roots and rhizomes of black cohosh are commonly used fresh or dried to make infusions (strong teas), capsules, solid extracts used in pills, or liquid extracts.

Like EPO, black cohosh is used by breast cancer survivors for the treatment of menopausal symptoms. Alternatively, prostate cancer patients may use black cohosh to control hot flushes after surgical or medical castration (e.g. hormonal ablation).[152] Systematic reviews of RCTs, however, have found inconclusive evidence to support the use of black cohosh for menopausal symptom relief in peri-/post-menopausal women[157,158] and breast cancer patients.[159] More rigorous RCTs of longer duration (> 6 months) are needed.

Black cohosh appears to be relatively safe despite reports that it may be associated with hepatotoxicity.[158] The most important safety concern with black cohosh, however, is the fear that it has oestrogenic effects and may promote breast or uterine cancer in women. Early studies suggested an oestrogenic mechanism of action for black cohosh, but this may have been due to phytoestrogen contamination.[160] More recent *in-vitro* and human studies of unadulterated black cohosh extracts, however, have demonstrated no oestrogenic activity.[159] Nevertheless, women with oestrogen-dependent cancers may want to avoid black cohosh until its long-term effects on breast or uterine tissue are more clearly established in epidemiological studies. Finally, no herb–drug interactions have been reported for black cohosh.[161]

Echinacea (Echinacea purpurea, Echinacea angustifolia, Echinacea pallida)

Echinacea is an immunostimulant commonly used by cancer patients to boost their immune system and to prevent or treat upper respiratory tract infections. However, RCTs are yet to confirm these benefits in cancer patients.[111] Short-term use of echinacea is relatively safe, although there is some concern about allergic reactions including rashes, increased asthma and, in rare cases, anaphylaxis.[111,162] Echinacea use is contraindicated in individuals with asthma or atopy (a genetic tendency towards allergic reactions), given the greater risk of an allergic reaction.[111] Currently, there are no verifiable reports of herb–drug interactions for any echinacea products.[163,164]

Milk thistle (Silybum marianum, Carduus marianum)

The principal constituent of milk thistle is silymarin, which is a mixture of flavonolignans (silychristin, silydianin, silybin and others) isolated mainly from the seeds (fruit) of the plant. The seeds are used to prepare capsules, extracts, and infusions (strong teas). Evidence suggests that milk thistle has hepatoprotective, anticancer, tissue-regenerative, hypoglycaemic and cardioprotective properties.[165,166] Milk thistle is being increasingly used by cancer patients for liver protection during chemotherapy[167] and for detoxification between chemotherapy cycles or after chemotherapy, as well as an adjuvant treatment and chemopreventive agent.

A Cochrane meta-analytic review of 13 RCTs involving alcoholic and/or hepatitis B or C liver disease patients found significant benefits of milk thistle on mortality or hepatic complications across low-quality trials alone, but not across all trials or high-quality trials alone.[168] High-quality RCTs involving liver disease patients (including those with chemotherapy-induced hepatotoxicity) are needed. Reviews of pre-clinical studies and preliminary clinical trials also suggest that milk thistle extract may potentiate the antitumour action of certain chemotherapy drugs (e.g. doxorubicin, cisplatin) and radiotherapy[169] and have chemopreventive potential (e.g. skin cancer, colorectal cancer),[169,170] but rigorous RCTs are required to establish its efficacy and safety as an adjuvant or chemopreventive treatment.

Finally, reviews have established that the chronic use (≤ 41 months) of milk thistle is generally safe and well-tolerated in recommended doses.[168,171] Gastrointestinal problems are the most common complaint, but are infrequent.[172] Allergic reactions, ranging from itchiness to eczema and anaphylaxis, are rare. Large doses (> 1.5 g/day) may cause diarrhoea, and very high doses (10–20 g/day) can result in asymptomatic hepatotoxicity (hyperbilirubinaemia) in cancer patients.[173] Drug interactions do not appear to be problematic either,[165] although further study of mistletoe at higher doses is required.

European mistletoe (Viscum album L.)

Mistletoe has a long tradition of folk remedy use in Europe, but has been used extensively in recent years in adjuvant cancer treatment or as a standalone alternative therapy, by and large in German-speaking countries (Switzerland, Austria, Germany). Its use in cancer treatment stems from anthroposophic medicine developed in the early 1900s, which approaches disease as an imbalance in the biological organism and utilises treatment strategies designed to restore this balance. Anthroposophic doctors believe that regular injections of mistletoe will inhibit or stop tumour growth and improve QoL in cancer patients.[174] The stem and leaves of the semi-parasitic mistletoe plant are used to make commercial preparations (e.g. extracts, pressed sap) that are often administered by subcutaneous injection (near or directly into the tumour), but may be taken orally, intravenously or intrapleurally.

In-vitro studies indicate that mistletoe or its main constituents (lectins, viscotoxins, polysaccharides, alkaloids) have antiangiogenic, anticancer and immunostimulatory properties.[175] In 2003, a systematic review of 10 RCTs found some benefits of mistletoe extract as an adjuvant or standalone treatment for cancer patients, particularly in relation to QoL, across low-quality trials alone; however, no benefits in terms of QoL, survival and other outcomes were demonstrated in higher quality trials.[176] In contrast, another systematic review in 2003 involving 16 RCTs and seven quasi-/non-RCTs of mistletoe preparations revealed that 12 studies exhibited significantly positive results on at least one clinically-relevant outcome measure, seven studies indicated a positive trend on at least one measure, three showed no significant results and one demonstrated a negative trend.[177] In 2007, a systematic review of 16 RCTs and nine non-RCTs involving mistletoe use as an adjuvant or standalone treatment found arguable benefits for cancer survival, but better evidence for the efficacy of anthroposophic mistletoe preparations in improving QoL and reducing toxicity of conventional treatments.[178] Despite similar observations, a 2008 Cochrane systematic review of 21 RCTs found weak evidence to support that mistletoe extract improves survival and QoL or reduces the adverse effects of chemotherapy and radiotherapy, although the conclusions for QoL were qualified by stating that a small number of higher quality trials suggested possible benefits for breast cancer patients during chemotherapy.[179]

Seeking to minimise the problems of previous reviews (e.g. heterogeneity), a more recent systematic review limited to 18 RCTs and observational studies[180] found inconsistent evidence for the efficacy of mistletoe preparations as an adjuvant or standalone treatment in increasing cancer survival and tolerance to chemotherapy and radiotherapy, but concluded that there was clear evidence for enhanced QoL and that these benefits were not limited to specific mistletoe preparations or cancer populations. The latest systematic review (26 RCTs, ten non-RCTs) has further also confirmed the QoL benefits.[181] Nevertheless, more high-quality prospective trials are needed to consolidate the positive QoL effects of mistletoe preparations in cancer patients.

Mistletoe preparations are usually well-tolerated and serious adverse effects are rare (cf. mistletoe plants and berries, which are poisonous) when used as directed under the supervision of health professionals.[179,180] Depending on the dose, local reactions (e.g. pruritus, erythema or induration at the injection site) have been observed in 0.9–43% of cancer patients[182] and systemic reactions (e.g. headaches, fever, influenza-like symptoms) in up to 10% of patients.[179] Allergic reactions (e.g. breathing difficulties, anaphylaxis) have been reported, but are rare (< 1%).[182] Also, long-term use of mistletoe extracts may reduce T-cell function in cancer patients without local reactions, thus use should be suspended periodically to allow T-cell reactivity to recover.[183] Finally, herb–drug interaction studies involving mistletoe use in cancer patients are required, given their virtual non-existence.

Manipulative and Body-Based Practices

Manipulative and body-based practices focus primarily on body structures and systems including bones and joints, soft tissue, and the circulatory and lymphatic systems.[184] They involve manipulation or movement of one or more parts of the body in order to heal the body and achieve good health. Examples include massage, acupuncture/acupressure, chiropractic and osteopathic manipulation, tui na, reflexology, and Bowen therapy. There is considerable variation in the level of formal training and approaches taken by practitioners both across and within modalities (e.g. chiropractic and osteopathic manipulation primarily involve rapid movements, whereas massage therapy involves slower application of force). Despite this heterogeneity, manipulative and body-based practices share some common principles (e.g. the human body is self-regulating, parts of the body are interdependent) and features (e.g. therapies tend to be tailored to the specific needs of patients).

Massage Therapy

Massage therapy involves the systematic manipulation of soft tissues of the body; examples include Swedish massage, aromatherapy, shiatsu, reflexology and acupressure. The common goal of most massage techniques is to promote relaxation and general well-being. Overall, therapeutic massage administered by trained practitioners is very safe. Two reviews, one focusing on cancer patients, found few reported adverse events.[185,186] Although there is no evidence that massage therapy can spread cancer, applying direct pressure over known tumours is best avoided. Reduced pressure and/or avoidance of direct or deep tissue massage is also advisable for cancer patients with coagulation disorders (and those using anticoagulant/antiplatelet medications, such as warfarin and aspirin), bone metastases or severe osteoporosis, open wounds or radiation dermatitis, and prosthetic devices (e.g. infusaport, colostomy bag, stents).[186] Additionally, caution is advised with use of aromatherapy essential oils in cancer patients with renal or liver disorders, and direct application should be avoided in those with wounds, skin conditions or allergies to essential oils.[187]

A Cochrane meta-analytic review of eight RCTs found limited evidence for short-term benefits of massage/aromatherapy on anxiety in cancer patients, but inconclusive results for other symptoms.[188] More recent systematic reviews of RCTs and observational studies have also suggested that massage may alleviate anxiety, as well as other symptoms such as pain, nausea, depression and stress.[186,189] Larger RCTs are required, but massage therapy should be supported for use by patients in the interim given the encouraging evidence for symptom control and safety.

Acupuncture

Acupuncture, a key aspect of TCM, is a family of procedures that involves the application of needles, pressure, heat and other treatments to the skin at particular sites called acupuncture points for therapeutic purposes. Acupuncture performed by competent and experienced practitioners is safe.[190,191]

Systematic reviews revealed that there is no convincing evidence that acupuncture alleviates cancer pain[192,193] or hot flushes in breast and prostate cancer patients,[194,195] although further RCTs were recommended. In contrast, a Cochrane meta-analytic review of 11 RCTs concluded that acupuncture-point stimulation (manual acupuncture, electroacupunture, self-/practitioner-administered acupressure) in combination with antiemetics demonstrated benefits for acute chemotherapy-induced nausea and/or vomiting and complemented the positive evidence for postoperative nausea and vomiting.[196] Additionally, an exploratory meta-analysis of 11 Chinese non-randomised clinical trials of poor quality found that acupuncture was associated with an increase in leukocytes during chemotherapy and chemoradiation, suggesting that acupuncture may be effective in reducing leukopenia in patients undertaking such treatments.[197] Finally, several pilot studies suggest that acupuncture may improve radiation-induced xerostomia in head and neck cancer patients (e.g. Cho *et al.*,[198] and Garcia *et al.*),[199] although RCTs are needed to further confirm these promising results.

Exercise Interventions

There are two broad categories of exercise. Aerobic or cardiorespiratory exercise involves large muscle groups performing continuous or intermittent physical activity over an extended period of time, whereas anabolic or resistance exercise involves performing sets of repetitive movements against a resistance during which neuromuscular fatigue occurs within 6–12 repetitions.[200] Exercise may be home-based or take the form of highly structured, supervised interventions. Cancer survivors and patients undergoing treatment are generally prescribed aerobic and/or resistance exercise of low to moderate intensity and regular frequency (three to five times per week) for at least 20 minutes per session.[201]

Aerobic and resistance exercise appear to be relatively safe in cancer patients during treatment or survivorship, even in home-based programmes and older or advanced cancer patients.[202,203] Recent meta-analytic and systematic reviews have found that serious adverse events (e.g. back injury; falls; development or exacerbation of lymphoedema, anaemia or cachexia) are rare, and that the most common minor adverse effects (e.g. hip/calf pain, pulled hamstring, shoulder tendonitis) of exercise interventions were no more frequent compared with control interventions in RCTs.[203–205]

A meta-analysis and systematic review of exercise-based and psychological interventions revealed in a subgroup analysis of 17 RCTs that there were no significant decreases in cancer-related fatigue (CRF) during treatment or survivorship for predominantly non-metastatic cancer patients who completed various exercise-based interventions.[206] In contrast, a Cochrane meta-analytic review of 28 RCTs found a small beneficial effect of exercise in reducing symptoms of CRF during treatment or survivorship in patients (predominantly diagnosed with breast cancer) who completed various exercise-based interventions compared with control interventions.[207] A more recent meta-analysis of 18 RCTs examined the effects of different exercise parameters on CRF symptoms experienced during cancer treatment.[208] Overall, exercise produced small significant reductions in CRF for breast cancer patients and moderate significant reductions in prostate cancer patients. Supervised aerobic exercise interventions proved more effective in reducing CRF during breast cancer treatment than home-based programmes, which did not significantly decrease CRF. Clearly, further large RCTs comparing different forms of exercise interventions across settings and patient populations with CRF are needed.

Looking beyond CRF, a meta-analysis of 16 randomised and 14 non-randomised trials found that exercise interventions resulted in small positive effects on clinical and QoL outcomes (physical functioning, symptoms other than fatigue, body composition, fatigue, mood, overall QoL) during cancer treatment, although larger effects were generally contributed by poorer quality studies.[209] Similarly, a systematic review of three RCTs and five non-randomised trials found positive effects on QoL and physical outcomes in metastatic cancer patients, although heterogeneity was problematic and limited the generalisability of results.[210] Also, a Cochrane meta-analytic review of nine RCTs revealed a moderate positive effect of exercise interventions on physical functioning during adjuvant breast cancer treatment (and insufficient evidence for other outcomes, such as fatigue, mood disturbance, immune function and weight gain), although heterogeneity again was problematic.[211] A more recent meta-analysis of exercise and behavioural interventions revealed in a subgroup analysis of 17 RCTs that physical exercise produced small positive effects on fatigue, depression, body image and QoL in breast cancer survivors or patients receiving treatment.[212]

Finally, in the most comprehensive evaluation to date, a meta-analysis and systematic review of 74 RCTs and eight non-randomised trials (including 66 judged to be of high quality) showed a large beneficial effect of exercise interventions for cancer survivors on lower and upper body strength and moderate effects on fatigue and breast cancer-specific concerns.[205] Small to moderate positive effects in cancer patients undergoing treatment were observed for physical activity level, aerobic fitness, muscular strength, functional QoL, anxiety and self-esteem. More large RCTs, as prescribed for CRF, are recommended in evaluating exercise interventions targeting other clinical and QoL outcomes.

Energy Therapies

Energy therapies involve the use of two types of energy fields. Veritable energy fields, which can be measured, employ mechanical vibrations (e.g. sound) and electromagnetic forces including visible light, magnetism, monochromatic radiation (e.g. laser beams), and rays from other parts of the electromagnetic spectrum. Specific, measurable wavelengths and frequencies are used to treat individuals.[213] In contrast, putative energy fields or biofields are theorised to surround the body and have yet to be scientifically measured. Biofield therapies are based on the concept that humans are infused with a subtle form of energy or life force (termed differently in different cultures; e.g. qi in TCM, ki in the Japanese Kampo system, doshas in ayurvedic medicine, and elsewhere as prana, etheric energy and other names) that can be manipulated to effect changes in the physical body and influence health.[214,215]

Biofield Therapies

Biofield therapies refer to techniques that use energy fields that purportedly surround the human body to stimulate one's own healing (internal practices; e.g. internal Qigong) or healing in others (external practices; e.g. external Qigong, therapeutic touch, healing touch, Reiki, Johrei, polarity therapy). Energy fields are sometimes manoeuvred by manipulating the body using light touch or placing the hands above the body. The broad goal of biofield therapies is to heal mental or physical disorders by rebalancing the energy fields in the body or by drawing upon spiritual energies for such healing. Cancer patients may use them to improve general well-being and QoL (e.g. pain relief), particularly in palliative and supportive care settings. Biofield therapies are generally safe when administered by trained practitioners. Although few (if any) adverse events have been reported for touch therapies (healing touch, therapeutic touch, Reiki),[216] use of Reiki is not advised for individuals with (a history of) psychosis, personality disorders or bipolar disorder.

Qigong

Qigong is the most studied biofield therapy among cancer patients and refers to a whole host of different meditative exercises (sometimes combined with breathing techniques, imagery and/or vocalisation of sounds) from TCM used to prevent or slow disease and maintain health. Medical Qigong, however, has been specifically developed for the treatment and cure of disease (e.g. hypertension, arthritis, cancer, HIV), and may be used as an adjunct to conventional medical treatments. Given its utilisation of meditation, imagery and breathing techniques and dependence on regular practice, Qigong has many parallels to Western behavioural medicine.

Qigong is generally safe for most individuals when instructed by qualified practitioners and practised correctly according to standard moderate principles.[217–219] Abnormal psychosomatic responses and culture-bound psychiatric disorders (specific to individuals of Chinese or other Asian ethnicities, even when living in Western countries) may be induced, however, when Qigong is practised inappropriately, excessively and/or unguided, particularly on psychologically vulnerable individuals.[218–220] Serious adverse events are rare, but Qigong-induced psychiatric disorders are becoming more prevalent in China.[221] Adverse effects may include sensory or somatic disturbances (e.g. headache, dizziness, chest tightness, tachycardia, breathlessness); motor disturbances (e.g. muscle twitching, tremors, odd limb movements, uncontrolled motor activity); cognitive impairment (e.g. memory, attention); psychological symptoms (e.g. anxiety, irritability, hypochondriasis, obsessive thoughts or images, delusions, visual/auditory hallucinations, disorganised speech, dissociation, altered consciousness, disorientation, mania, depression, suicidal or bizarre behaviour); and allergic skin reactions.[217,220,222,223]

An exploratory review of 21 Chinese studies (mostly controlled) revealed that cancer patients predominantly treated with internal Qigong and conventional medical treatment exhibited a consistent tendency for greater improvement on biological indicators and/or longer survival time than those who received conventional treatment alone, but concluded that there was much need for replication and improved methodological quality in future studies.[224] A more recent systematic review of nine controlled studies involving palliative/supportive care cancer patients, however, was less positive and concluded that the efficacy of internal Qigong (alone or combined with conventional medical treatment) in cancer care is not yet supported due to the poor methodological quality of existing studies, and recommended that large-scale RCTs be performed along with studies investigating possible scientific mechanisms.[225] Finally, a systematic review of 66 RCTs and observational studies examining a variety of practitioner-administered biofield therapies (external Qigong, therapeutic touch, Reiki, spiritual healing, healing touch and others) in different medical populations found moderate (level 2) evidence for their efficacy in reducing acute pain in cancer patients and post-operative and hospitalised patients, but mixed (level 4) evidence for chronic pain, fatigue, physiological arousal (heart/respiratory rate, blood pressure) and QoL in cancer patients.[226] Again, larger high-quality studies were advised.

Bioelectromagnetic-Based Therapies

Bioelectromagnetic-based therapies involve the unconventional use of electromagnetic fields, such as magnetic, pulsed or alternating-/direct-current fields.[214] Examples include magnetic, millimetre wave, sound energy (vibrational or frequency), and light therapy.

Microwave (ultra-high-frequency radiowave)/tronado therapy

Microwave or ultra-high-frequency (UHF) therapy is designed to treat cancer via exposure of tumorous tissue to electromagnetic radiation delivered using frequencies ranging from 300 MHz to 3 GHz (although super-high and extra-high frequencies ranging up to 300 GHz have reportedly also been utilised).[227] UHF frequencies commonly used include 200–300, 434, 915 and 2450 MHz.[228] Microwave therapy is generally thought to exert therapeutic effects via direct or indirect heating of cancer cells, thus thermometry is typically undertaken at the time of treatment to measure intratumour temperature. Microwave therapy is usually combined with conventional radiotherapy or uncommonly with infusions of glucose-blocking agents (e.g. cyclophosphamide, cystine disulphide or penicillamine disulphide), and is often administered 5 days per week over a period of weeks.[228]

A systematic review of 58 controlled and uncontrolled studies (mostly poor quality due to the absence of single- or double-blind RCTs and inadequate patient follow-up, and exhibiting significant clinical heterogeneity), largely comparing microwave therapy and radiotherapy combined with microwave therapy alone in relation to tumour response and overall survival, found minimal evidence to support the routine use of microwave therapy for cancer treatment.[228] Additionally, in the same review, a limited clinical audit of the medical records of 179 cancer patients treated in Western Australia suggested that microwave therapy with radiotherapy resulted in greater toxicity than radiotherapy alone or microwave therapy with glucose-blocking agents for patients with bladder or other invasive cancers. Some of the more common adverse effects associated with microwave therapy appear to be pain, erythema, fibrosis, necrosis, ulcerations, blisters and thermal burns. Third-degree burns, arterial rupture and development of fistulae have been reported on occasions, as have deaths (often related to inadvertent heating of blood vessels or infections following invasive thermometry).[228,229]

SUMMARY CONCLUSIONS

The complementary and alternative therapies used by cancer patients are diverse in their origin, premise (including proposed or actual mechanisms of action), practice, efficacy and safety. Cancer patients and other members of the public are mostly unaware of distinctions between conventional drugs *registered* by the TGA and may believe that a CAM *listed* by the TGA has been assessed as both effective and safe and approved for such use by the Federal Government. Additionally, many complementary and alternative therapies have long histories as components of ancient traditional medical practices, but have only been subjected to rigorous scientific investigation in the last 10–20 years. More research is required to evaluate or confirm the efficacy and safety of many of these therapies.

Currently, however, there is evidence from high-quality clinical trials that some complementary therapies, used as adjuncts to conventional medical treatments, are beneficial in reducing disease or treatment symptoms and improving QoL and psychological functioning (e.g. relaxation). There is also evidence of potential harm. Nutritional supplements, herbal preparations, and other natural therapies among the biologically-based practices may pose direct safety risks because of their potential adverse effects or interactions with conventional anticancer treatments (chemotherapy, radiotherapy, surgery, hormonal therapies) and other medications. Some should not be used under any circumstances in cancer patients, irrespective of potential benefit (e.g. SJW), whereas others may be beneficial when patients are not undergoing these treatments and have no other contraindications (e.g. valerian for short-term amelioration of sleep problems in non-surgical cancer patients). Alternative therapies promoted as "cures" in place of conventional treatments (e.g. shark cartilage) have the potential to cause patients (and their loved ones) the most harm, however, when they forego evidence-based cancer treatments that are likely to be more effective.

In conclusion, whether termed complementary medicine or integrative oncology, cancer physicians in Australia should strongly consider offering evidence-based complementary therapies (or at least safe forms of them) alongside conventional treatments through their own cancer services.[230] Conceivably, this may influence patients to continue with mainstream care and help them avoid any potential harm that may occur with autonomous CAM use. In this way, optimal holistic care will be ensured for cancer patients by clinicians providing conventional oncology treatment and care.

ACKNOWLEDGEMENTS

I would like to thank Professor Ian Olver (editor), Professor Peter Drummond and Mr Paul Katris for their comments on early drafts of this chapter. Finally, I would like to thank my loved ones for the patience they showed during the writing of this chapter.

REFERENCES

1. Dantas F, Rampes H. Do homeopathic medicines provoke adverse effects? A systematic review. *Br Homeopath J* **89**(suppl 1):S35–S38 (2000).
2. Kassab S, Cummings M, Berkovitz S, *et al.* Homeopathic medicines for adverse effects of cancer treatments. *Cochrane Database Syst Rev* **2**:CD004845 (2009).
3. Wong R, Sagar CM, Sagar SM. Integration of Chinese medicine into supportive cancer care: a modern role for an ancient tradition. *Cancer Treat Rev* **27**(4):235–246 (2001).
4. Luebbert K, Dahme B, Hasenbring M. The effectiveness of relaxation training in reducing treatment-related symptoms and improving emotional adjustment in acute non-surgical cancer treatment: a meta-analytical review. *Psychooncology* **10**(6):490–502 (2001).
5. Devine EC. Meta-analysis of the effect of psychoeducational interventions on pain in adults with cancer. *Oncol Nurs Forum* **30**(1):75–89 (2003).
6. Kwekkeboom KL, Cherwin CH, Lee JW, *et al.* Mind-body treatments for the pain-fatigue-sleep disturbance symptom cluster in persons with cancer. *J Pain Symptom Manage* **39**(1):126–138 (2010).
7. Lotfi-Jam K, Carey M, Jefford M, *et al.* Nonpharmacologic strategies for managing common chemotherapy adverse effects: a systematic review. *J Clin Oncol* **26**(34):5618–5629 (2008).
8. Figueroa-Moseley C, Jean-Pierre P, Roscoe JA, *et al.* Behavioral interventions in treating anticipatory nausea and vomiting. *J Natl Compr Canc Netw* **5**(1):44–50 (2007).
9. Shapiro DH Jr. Overview: clinical and physiological comparison of meditation with other self-control strategies. *Am J Psychiatry* **139**(3):267–274 (1982).

10. Astin JA, Shapiro SL, Eisenberg DM, *et al*. Mind-body medicine: state of the science, implications for practice. *Mind-Body Med* **16**(2):131–147 (2003).
11. Alexander CN, Robinson P, Orme-Johnson DW, *et al*. The effects of transcendental meditation compared to other methods of relaxation and meditation in reducing risk factors, morbidity, and mortality. CIANS-ISBM Satellite Conference Symposium: lifestyle changes in the prevention and treatment of disease (1992, Hannover, Germany). *Homeostasis Health Dis* **35**:243–263 (1994).
12. Shapiro DH Jr. Adverse effects of meditation: a preliminary investigation of long-term meditators. *Int J Psychosom* **39**:62–67 (1992).
13. Castillo RJ. Depersonalization and meditation. *Psychiatry* **53**:158–168 (1990).
14. Melbourne Academic Mindfulness Interest Group. Mindfulness-based psychotherapies: a review of conceptual foundations, empirical evidence and practical considerations. *ANZ J Psychiatry* **40**:285–294 (2006).
15. Kuijpers HJH, van der Heijden FMMA, Tuinier S, *et al*. Meditation-induced psychosis. *Psychopathology* **40**:461–464 (2007).
16. Shapiro DH Jr. Examining the content and context of meditation: a challenge for psychology in the areas of stress management. *Psychother Religious Values* **34**(4):101–135 (1994).
17. Ledesma D, Kumano H. Mindfulness-based stress reduction and cancer: a meta-analysis. *Psychooncology* **18**(6):571–579 (2009).
18. Smith JE, Richardson J, Hoffman C, *et al*. Mindfulness-based stress reduction as supportive therapy in cancer care: systematic review. *J Adv Nurs* **52**(3):315–327 (2005).
19. Ott MJ, Norris RL, Bauer-Wu SM. Mindfulness meditation for oncology patients: a discussion and critical review. *Integr Cancer Ther* **5**(2):98–108 (2006).
20. Patterson DR, Jensen MP. Hypnosis and clinical pain. *Psychol Bull* **129**(4):495–521 (2003).
21. Lynn SJ, Martin DJ, Frauman DC. Does hypnosis pose special risks for negative effects? A master class commentary. *Int J Clin Exp Hypn* **44**:7–19 (1996).
22. MacHovec F. Hypnosis complications, risk factors, and prevention. *Am J Clin Hypn* **31**:40–49 (1988).
23. Vickers A, Zollman C. ABC of complementary medicine. Hypnosis and relaxation therapies. *BMJ* **319**(7221):1346–1349 (1999).

24. Richardson J, Smith JE, McCall G, *et al*. Hypnosis for nausea and vomiting in cancer chemotherapy: a systematic review of the research evidence. *Eur J Cancer Care (Engl)* **16**(5):402–412 (2007).
25. Flory N, Lang E. Practical hypnotic interventions during invasive cancer diagnosis and treatment. *Hematol Oncol Clin North Am* **22**(4):709–725 (2008).
26. Richardson J, Smith JE, McCall G, *et al*. Hypnosis for procedure-related pain and distress in pediatric cancer patients: a systematic review of effectiveness and methodology related to hypnosis interventions. *J Pain Symptom Manage* **31**(1):70–84 (2006).
27. Oestreicher P. Help patients integrate yoga into cancer care. *ONS Connect* **23**(4):20–21 (2008).
28. Bower JE, Woolery A, Sternlieb B, *et al*. Yoga for cancer patients and survivors. *Cancer Control* **12**(3):165–171 (2005).
29. Smith KB, Pukall CF. An evidence-based review of yoga as a complementary intervention for patients with cancer. *Psychooncology* **18**(5):465–475 (2009).
30. Lee MS, Pittler MH, Ernst E. Is tai chi an effective adjunct in cancer care? A systematic review of controlled clinical trials. *Support Care Cancer* **15**(6):597–601 (2007).
31. Lee MS, Choi TY, Ernst E. Tai chi for breast cancer patients: a systematic review. *Breast Cancer Res Treat* **120**(2):309–316 (2010).
32. Dileo C. Effects of music and music therapy on medical patients: a meta-analysis of the research and implications for the future. *J Soc Integr Oncol* **4**(2):67–70 (2006).
33. Zabalegui A, Sanchez S, Sanchez PD, *et al*. Nursing and cancer support groups. *J Adv Nurs* **51**(4):369–381 (2005).
34. Gottlieb BH, Wachala ED. Cancer support groups: a critical review of empirical studies. *Psychooncology* **16**(5):379–400 (2007).
35. Hoey LM, Ieropoli SC, White VM, *et al*. Systematic review of peer-support programs for people with cancer. *Patient Educ Couns* **70**(3):315–337 (2008).
36. Macvean ML, White VM, Sanson-Fisher R. One-to-one volunteer support programs for people with cancer: a review of the literature. *Patient Educ Couns* **70**(1):10–24 (2008).
37. Pargament KI. The psychology of religion and spirituality? Yes and no. *Int J Psych Religion* **9**:3–16 (1999).
38. Pargament KI. *The Psychology of Religion and Coping: Theory, Research, Practice*, Guilford Press, New York (1997).

39. Belzen JA. Spirituality, culture and mental health: prospects and risks for contemporary psychology of religion. *J Religion Health* **43**:291–316 (2004).
40. Thuné-Boyle IC, Stygall JA, Keshtgar MR, *et al*. Do religious/spiritual coping strategies affect illness adjustment in patients with cancer? A systematic review of the literature. *Soc Sci Med* **63**(1):151–164 (2006).
41. Visser A, Garssen B, Vingerhoets A. Spirituality and well-being in cancer patients: a review. *Psychooncology* **19**(6):565–572 (2010).
42. Rossiter-Thornton JF. Prayer in your practice. *Complement Ther Nurs Midwifery* **8**(1):21–28 (2002).
43. Hollywell C, Walker J. Private prayer as a suitable intervention for hospitalised patients: a critical review of the literature. *J Clin Nurs* **18**(5):637–651 (2009).
44. Hoff A, Johannessen-Henry CT, Ross L, *et al*. Religion and reduced cancer risk: what is the explanation? A review. *Eur J Cancer* **44**(17):2573–2579 (2008).
45. Masters KS, Spielmans GI. Prayer and health: review, meta-analysis and research agenda. *J Behav Med* **30**(4):329–338 (2007).
46. Roberts L, Ahmed I, Hall S, *et al*. Intercessory prayer for the alleviation of ill health. *Cochrane Database Syst Rev* **15**(2):CD000368 (2009).
47. National Center for Complementary and Alternative Medicine (NCCAM). Biologically based practices: an overview (NCCAM Publication No. D237). http://www.umbwellness.org/PDF_files/biobasedprac.pdf [Accessed 15 June 2010].
48. Ames BN, Gold LS, Willett WC. The causes and prevention of cancer. *Proc Natl Acad Sci USA* **92**(12):5258–5265 (1995).
49. Willcox JK, Ash SL, Catignani GL. Antioxidants and prevention of chronic disease. *Crit Rev Food Sci Nutr* **44**(4):275–295 (2004).
50. Conklin KA. Cancer chemotherapy and antioxidants. *J Nutr* **134**(11):3201S–3204S (2004).
51. D'Andrea GM. Use of antioxidants during chemotherapy and radiotherapy should be avoided. *CA Cancer J Clin* **55**(5): 319–321 (2005).
52. Block KI, Koch AC, Mead MN, *et al*. Impact of antioxidant supplementation on chemotherapeutic toxicity: a systematic review of the evidence from randomized controlled trials. *Int J Cancer* **123**(6):1227–1239 (2008).
53. Moss RW. Do antioxidants interfere with radiation therapy for cancer? *Integr Cancer Ther* **6**(3):281–292 (2007).

54. Sasse AD, Clark LG, Sasse EC, *et al*. Amifostine reduces side effects and improves complete response rate during radiotherapy: results of a meta-analysis. *Int J Radiat Oncol Biol Phys* **64**(3):784–791 (2006).
55. Greenlee H, Gammon MD, Abrahamson PE, *et al*. Prevalence and predictors of antioxidant supplement use during breast cancer treatment: the Long Island Breast Cancer Study Project. *Cancer* **115**(14):3271–3282 (2009).
56. Dennert G, Horneber M. Selenium for alleviating the side effects of chemotherapy, radiotherapy and surgery in cancer patients. *Cochrane Database Syst Rev* **3**:CD005037 (2006).
57. Tabassum A, Bristow RG, Venkateswaran V. Ingestion of selenium and other antioxidants during prostate cancer radiotherapy: a good thing? *Cancer Treat Rev* **36**(3):230–234 (2010).
58. Haseen F, Cantwell MM, O'Sullivan JM, *et al*. Is there a benefit from lycopene supplementation in men with prostate cancer? A systematic review. *Prostate Cancer Prostatic Dis* **12**(4):325–332 (2009).
59. Roffe L, Schmidt K, Ernst E. Efficacy of coenzyme Q10 for improved tolerability of cancer treatments: a systematic review. *J Clin Oncol* **22**(21):4418–4424 (2004).
60. Ladas EJ, Jacobson JS, Kennedy DD, *et al*. Antioxidants and cancer therapy: a systematic review. *J Clin Oncol* **22**(3): 517–528 (2004).
61. Lawenda BD, Kelly KM, Ladas EJ, *et al*. Should supplemental antioxidant administration be avoided during chemotherapy and radiation therapy? *J Natl Cancer Inst* **100**(11):773–783 (2008).
62. Block KI, Koch AC, Mead MN, *et al*. Impact of antioxidant supplementation on chemotherapeutic efficacy: a systematic review of the evidence from randomized controlled trials. *Cancer Treat Rev* **33**(5):407–418 (2007).
63. Mell LK, Malik R, Komaki R, *et al*. Effect of amifostine on response rates in locally advanced non-small-cell lung cancer patients treated on randomized controlled trials: a meta-analysis. *Int J Radiat Oncol Biol Phys* **68**(1):111–118 (2007).
64. Coulter ID, Hardy ML, Morton SC, *et al*. Antioxidants vitamin C and vitamin E for the prevention and treatment of cancer. *J Gen Intern Med* **21**(7):735–744 (2006).
65. Mills E, Wu P, Seely D, *et al*. Melatonin in the treatment of cancer: a systematic review of randomized controlled trials and meta-analysis. *J Pineal Res* **39**(4):360–366 (2005).

66. Myung SK, Kim Y, Ju W, *et al*. Effects of antioxidant supplements on cancer prevention: meta-analysis of randomized controlled trials. *Ann Oncol* **21**(1):166–179 (2010).
67. Bardia A, Tleyjeh IM, Cerhan JR, *et al*. Efficacy of antioxidant supplementation in reducing primary cancer incidence and mortality: systematic review and meta-analysis. *Mayo Clin Proc* **83**(1):23–34 (2008).
68. Papaioannou D, Cooper K, Carroll CC, *et al*. Antioxidants in the chemoprevention of colorectal cancer and colorectal adenomas in the general population: a systematic review and meta-analysis. *Colorectal Dis* (in press).
69. Bjelakovic B, Nikolova D, Simonetti RG, *et al*. Systematic review: primary and secondary prevention of gastrointestinal cancers with antioxidant supplements. *Aliment Pharmacol Ther* **28**(6): 689–703 (2008).
70. Alkhenizan A, Hafez K. The role of vitamin E in the prevention of cancer: a meta-analysis of randomized controlled trials. *Ann Saudi Med* **27**(6):409–414 (2007).
71. Pham DQ, Plakogiannis R. Vitamin E supplementation in cardiovascular disease and cancer prevention: part 1. *Ann Pharmacother* **39**(11):1870–1878 (2005).
72. Cho E, Hunter DJ, Spiegelman D, *et al*. Intakes of vitamins A, C and E and folate and multivitamins and lung cancer: a pooled analysis of 8 prospective studies. *Int J Cancer* **118**(4): 970–978 (2006).
73. Gallicchio L, Boyd K, Matanoski G, *et al*. Carotenoids and the risk of developing lung cancer: a systematic review. *Am J Clin Nutr* **88**(2):372–383 (2008).
74. Hathcock JN, Azzi A, Blumberg J, *et al*. Vitamins E and C are safe across a broad range of intakes. *Am J Clin Nutr* **81**(4):736–745 (2005).
75. World Cancer Research Fund and American Institute for Cancer Research (AICR). *Food, Nutrition, Physical Activity, and the Prevention of Cancer: A Global Perspective*, AICR, Washington DC (2007).
76. Avula CPR, Lawrence RA, Jolly CA, *et al*. Role of n-3 polyunsaturated fatty acids (PUFA) in autoimmunity, inflammation, carcinogenesis, and apoptosis. *Recent Res Dev Lipids* **4**(2):303–319 (2000).
77. Johnson IT. Anticarcinogenic effects of diet-related apoptosis in the colorectal mucosa. *Food Chem Toxicol* **40**(8):1171–1178 (2002).

78. Dewey A, Baughan C, Dean T, *et al.* Eicosapentaenoic acid (EPA, an omega-3 fatty acid from fish oils) for the treatment of cancer cachexia. *Cochrane Database Syst Rev* **24**(1):CD004597 (2007).
79. Colomer R, Moreno-Nogueira JM, García-Luna PP, *et al.* N-3 fatty acids, cancer and cachexia: a systematic review of the literature. *Br J Nutr* **97**(5):823–831 (2007).
80. MacLean CH, Newberry SJ, Mojica WA, *et al.* Effects of omega-3 fatty acids on cancer risk: a systematic review. *JAMA* **295**(4):403–415 (2006).
81. Carayol M, Grosclaude P, Delpierre C. Prospective studies of dietary alpha-linolenic acid intake and prostate cancer risk: a meta-analysis. *Cancer Causes Control* **21**(3):347–355 (2010).
82. Simon JA, Chen YH, Bent S. The relation of alpha-linolenic acid to the risk of prostate cancer: a systematic review and meta-analysis. *Am J Clin Nutr* **89**(5):1558S–1564S (2009).
83. Brouwer IA. Omega-3 PUFA: good or bad for prostate cancer. *Prostaglandins Leukot Essent Fatty Acids* **79**(3–5):97–99 (2008).
84. Mathews J. Media feeds frenzy over shark cartilage as cancer treatment. *J Natl Cancer Inst* **85**(15):1190–1191 (1993).
85. Lane IW, Comac L. *Sharks Don't Get Cancer*, Avery Publishing, New York (1992).
86. Ostrander GK, Cheng KC, Wolf JC, *et al.* Shark cartilage, cancer and the growing threat of pseudoscience. *Cancer Res* **64**(23):8485–8491 (2004).
87. Miller DR, Anderson GT, Stark JJ, *et al.* Phase I/II trial of the safety and efficacy of shark cartilage in the treatment of advanced cancer. *J Clin Oncol* **16**(11):3649–3655 (1998).
88. Gingras D, Renaud A, Mousseau N, *et al.* Shark cartilage extracts as antiangiogenic agents: smart drinks or bitter pills? *Cancer Metastasis Rev* **19**(1–2):83–86 (2000).
89. Pauli BU, Memoli VA, Kuettner KE. Regulation of tumor invasion by cartilage-derived anti-invasion factor in vitro. *J Natl Cancer Inst* **67**:65–73 (1981).
90. Kuettner KE, Pauli BU. Inhibition of tumor invasion by tissue-derived proteinase inhibitors. *Monogr Pathol* **27**:1711–1782 (1986).
91. Loprinzi CL, Levitt R, Barton DL, *et al.* Evaluation of shark cartilage in patients with advanced cancer: a North Central Cancer Treatment Group trial. *Cancer* **104**(1):176–182 (2005).
92. Lu C, Lee JJ, Komaki R, *et al.* Chemoradiotherapy with or without AE-941 in stage III non-small cell lung cancer: a randomized phase III trial. *J Natl Cancer Inst* **102**(12):859–865 (2010).

93. AEterna Zentaris. AEterna Laboratories reports phase III trial results in renal cell carcinoma with Neovastat. http://www.aeternazentaris.com/en/page.php?p=60&q=46 [Accessed 22 June 2010].
94. Fukuda T, Ito H, Mukainaka T, *et al.* Anti-tumor promoting effect of glycosides from Prunus persica seeds. *Biol Pharm Bull* **26**(2):271–273 (2003).
95. Milazzo S, Lejeune S, Ernst E. Laetrile for cancer: a systematic review of the clinical evidence. *Support Care Cancer* **15**(6):583–595 (2007).
96. Moertel CG, Fleming TR, Rubin J, *et al.* A clinical trial of amygdalin (Laetrile) in the treatment of human cancer. *N Engl J Med* **306**(4): 201–206 (1982).
97. Syrigos KN, Rowlinson-Busza G, Epenetos AA. In vitro cytotoxicity following specific activation of amygdalin by beta-glucosidase conjugated to a bladder cancer-associated monoclonal antibody. *Int J Cancer* **78**(6):712–719 (1998).
98. Chiu J, Yau T, Epstein RJ. Complications of traditional Chinese/herbal medicines (TCM): a guide for perplexed oncologists and other cancer caregivers. *Support Care Cancer* **17**(3):231–240 (2009).
99. Li GQ, Duke CC, Roufogalis BD. The quality and safety of traditional Chinese medicines. *Aust Prescr* **26**:128–130 (2003).
100. Wu T, Munro AJ, Guanjian L, *et al.* Chinese medical herbs for chemotherapy side effects in colorectal cancer patients. *Cochrane Database Syst Rev* **1**: CD004540 (2005).
101. Wei H, Sun R, Xiao W, *et al.* Traditional Chinese medicine Astragalus reverses predominance of Th2 cytokines and their up-stream transcript factors in lung cancer patients. *Oncol Rep* **10**(5):1507–1512 (2003).
102. Zwickey H, Brush J, Iacullo CM, *et al.* The effect of Echinacea purpurea, Astragalus membranaceus and Glycyrrhiza glabra on CD25 expression in humans: a pilot study. *Phytother Res* **21**(11):1109–1112 (2007).
103. McCulloch M, See C, Shu XJ, *et al.* Astragalus-based Chinese herbs and platinum-based chemotherapy for advanced non-small-cell lung cancer: meta-analysis of randomized trials. *J Clin Oncol* **24**(3):419–430 (2006).
104. Wu T, Munro AJ, Guanjian L, *et al.* Chinese medical herbs for chemotherapy side effects in colorectal cancer patients. *Cochrane Database Syst Rev* **1**:CD004540 (2005).

105. Ma WH, Duan KN, Feng M, *et al.* Aidi injection as an adjunct therapy for non-small cell lung cancer: a systematic review. *Zhong Xi Yi Jie He Xue Bao* **7**:315–324 (2009).
106. Cassileth BR, Rizvi N, Deng G, *et al.* Safety and pharmacokinetic trial of docetaxel plus an Astragalus-based herbal formula for non-small cell lung cancer patients. *Cancer Chemother Pharmacol* **65**(1):67–71 (2009).
107. Lee JJ, Lee JJ. A phase II study of an herbal decoction that includes Astragali radix for cancer-associated anorexia in patients with advanced cancer. *Integr Cancer Ther* **9**(1):24–31 (2010).
108. Shi Y, Li M, Xu F. A review of the study on swainsonine — toxic elements of locoweed. *Zhong Yao Cai* **22**(1):47–49 (1999).
109. Jia L, Zhao Y, Liang XJ. Current evaluation of the millennium phytomedicine — ginseng (II): collected chemical entities, modern pharmacology, and clinical applications emanated from traditional Chinese medicine. *Curr Med Chem* **16**(22):2924–2942 (2009).
110. Wu P, Dugoua JJ, Eyawo O, *et al.* Traditional Chinese medicines in the treatment of hepatocellular cancers: a systematic review and meta-analysis. *J Exp Clin Cancer Res* **28**: 112 (2009).
111. Block KI, Mead MN. Immune system effects of echinacea, ginseng, and astragalus: a review. *Integr Cancer Ther* **2**(3):247–267 (2003).
112. Coon JT, Ernst E. Panax ginseng: a systematic review of adverse effects and drug interactions. *Drug Saf* **25**(5):323–344 (2002).
113. Kumar NB, Allen B, Bell H. Perioperative herbal supplement use in cancer patients: potential implications and recommendations for presurgical screening. *Cancer Control* **12**(3):149–157 (2005).
114. Izzo AA, Ernst E. Interactions between herbal medicines and prescribed drugs: an updated systematic review. *Drugs* **69**(13): 1777–1798 (2009).
115. Smith M, Boon HS. Counseling cancer patients about herbal medicine. *Patient Educ Couns* **38**(2):109–120 (1999).
116. Liu J, Burdette JE, Xu H, *et al.* Evaluation of estrogenic activity of plant extracts for the potential treatment of menopausal symptoms. *J Agric Food Chem* **49**(5):2472–2479 (2001).
117. Chaiyakunapruk N, Kitikannakorn N, Nathisuwan S, *et al.* The efficacy of ginger for the prevention of postoperative nausea and vomiting: a meta-analysis. *Am J Obstet Gynecol* **194**(1):95–99 (2006).

118. Zick SM, Ruffin MT, Lee J, *et al.* Phase II trial of encapsulated ginger as a treatment for chemotherapy-induced nausea and vomiting. *Support Care Cancer* **17**(5):563–572 (2009).
119. Yang AK, He SM, Liu L, *et al.* Herbal interactions with anticancer drugs: mechanistic and clinical considerations. *Curr Med Chem* **17**(16):1635–1678 (2010).
120. Mahajna J, Dotan N, Zaidman BZ, *et al.* Pharmacological values of medicinal mushrooms for prostate cancer therapy: the case of Ganoderma lucidum. *Nutr Cancer* **61**(1):16–26 (2009).
121. Cassileth B. Complementary therapies, herbs, and other OTC agents: reishi mushroom. *Oncology (Williston Park)* **23**(8):728 (2009).
122. Wachtel-Galor S, Tomlinson B, Benzie IF. *Ganoderma lucidum* ("Lingzhi"), a Chinese medicinal mushroom: biomarker responses in a controlled human supplementation study. *Br J Nutr* **91**(2):263–269 (2004).
123. Shord SS, Shah K, Lukose A. Drug-botanical interactions: a review of the laboratory, animal, and human data for 8 common botanicals. *Integr Cancer Ther* **8**(3):208–227 (2009).
124. Food and Drug Administration (FDA). Letter responding to health claim petition dated January 27, 2004: green tea and reduced risk of cancer health claim (docket number 2004Q-0083). http://www.fda.gov/Food/LabelingNutrition/LabelClaims/QualifiedHealthClaims/ucm072774.htm [Accessed 1 May 2010].
125. Sturgeon JJ, Williams M, van Servellen G. Efficacy of green tea in the prevention of cancers. *Nurs Health Sci* **11**(4):436–446 (2009).
126. Liu J, Xing J, Fei Y. Green tea (Camellia sinensis) and cancer prevention: a systematic review of randomized trials and epidemiological studies. *Chin Med* **3**:12 (2008).
127. Pisters KM, Newman RA, Coldman B, *et al.* Phase I trial of oral green tea extract in adult patients with solid tumors. *J Clin Oncol* **19**(6):1830–1838 (2001).
128. Laurie SA, Miller VA, Grant SC, *et al.* Phase I study of green tea extract in patients with advanced lung cancer. *Cancer Chemother Pharmacol* **55**(1):33–38 (2005).
129. Golden EB, Lam PY, Kardosh A, *et al.* Green tea polyphenols block the anticancer effects of bortezomib and other boronic acid-based proteasome inhibitors. *Blood* **113**(23):5927–5937 (2009).
130. Mahadevan S, Park Y. Multifaceted therapeutic benefits of Ginkgo biloba L.: chemistry, efficacy, safety, and uses. *J Food Sci* **73**(1):R14–R19 (2008).

131. Linde K, Berner MM, Kriston L. St John's wort for major depression. *Cochrane Database Syst Rev* **4**: CD000448 (2008).
132. Borrelli F, Izzo AA. Herb-drug interactions with St John's wort (Hypericum perforatum): an update on clinical observations. *AAPSJ* **11**(4):710–727 (2009).
133. Ariga T, Seki T. Antithrombotic and anticancer effects of garlic-derived sulfur compounds: a review. *Biofactors* **26**(2):93–103 (2006).
134. Iciek M, Kwiecień I, Włodek L. Biological properties of garlic and garlic-derived organosulfur compounds. *Environ Mol Mutagen* **50**(3):247–265 (2009).
135. Fleischauer AT, Poole C, Arab L. Garlic consumption and cancer prevention: meta-analyses of colorectal and stomach cancers. *Am J Clin Nutr* **72**(4):1047–1052 (2000).
136. Ngo SN, Williams DB, Cobiac L, *et al*. Does garlic reduce risk of colorectal cancer? A systematic review. *J Nutr* **137**(10):2264–2269 (2007).
137. You WC, Brown LM, Zhang L, *et al*. Randomized double-blind factorial trial of three treatments to reduce the prevalence of precancerous gastric lesions. *J Natl Cancer Inst* **98**(14):974–983 (2006).
138. Borrelli F, Capasso R, Izzo AA. Garlic (Allium sativum L.): adverse effects and drug interactions in humans. *Mol Nutr Food Res* **51**(11):1386–1397 (2007).
139. Gurley BJ, Gardner SF, Hubbard MA, *et al*. Cytochrome P450 phenotypic ratios for predicting herb-drug interactions in humans, *Clin Pharmacol Ther*. **72**(3):276–287 (2002).
140. Markowitz JS, Devane CL, Chavin KD, et al. Effects of garlic (Allium sativum L.) supplementation on cytochrome P450 2D6 and 3A4 activity in healthy volunteers. *Clin Pharmacol Ther* **74**(2):170–177 (2003).
141. Sparreboom A, Cox MC, Acharya MR, *et al*. Herbal remedies in the United States: potential adverse interactions with anticancer agents. *J Clin Oncol*. **22**(12):2489–2503 (2004).
142. Saw JT, Bahari MB, Ang HH, *et al*. Potential drug-herb interaction with antiplatelet/anticoagulant drugs. *Complement Ther Clin Pract* **12**(4):236–241 (2006).
143. Singh YN. Potential for interaction of kava and St. John's wort with drugs. *J Ethnopharmacol* **100**(1–2):108–113 (2005).
144. Pittler MH, Ernst E. Kava extract versus placebo for treating anxiety. *Cochrane Database Syst Rev* **1**:CD003383 (2003).

145. Mathews JD, Riley MD, Fejo L, *et al*. Effects of the heavy usage of kava on physical health: summary of a pilot survey in an aboriginal community. *Med J Aust* **148**(11):548–555 (1988).
146. Robinson V, Bergfeld WF, Belsito DV, *et al*. Final report on the safety assessment of Piper Methysticum leaf/root/stem extract and Piper Methysticum root extract. *Int J Toxicol* **28**(6S):175S–188S (2009).
147. Fernández-San-Martín MI, Masa-Font R, Palacios-Soler L, *et al*. Effectiveness of valerian on insomnia: a meta-analysis of randomized placebo-controlled trials. *Sleep Med* **11**(6):505–511 (2010).
148. Garges HP, Varia I, Doraiswamy PM. Cardiac complications and delirium associated with valerian root withdrawal. *JAMA* **280**(18): 1566–1567 (1998).
149. Miyasaka LS, Atallah AN, Soares BG. Valerian for anxiety disorders. *Cochrane Database Syst Rev* **4**:CD004515 (2006).
150. Taibi DM, Landis CA, Petry H, *et al*. A systematic review of valerian as a sleep aid: safe but not effective. *Sleep Med Rev* **11**(3):209–230 (2007).
151. Bayles B, Usatine R. Evening primrose oil. *Am Fam Physician* **80**(12):1405–1408 (2009).
152. Adelson KB, Loprinzi CL, Hershman DL. Treatment of hot flushes in breast and prostate cancer. *Expert Opin Pharmacother* **6**(7):1095–1106 (2005).
153. Rossouw JE, Anderson GL, Prentice RL, *et al*. Risks and benefits of estrogen plus progestin in healthy postmenopausal women: principal results from the women's health initiative randomized controlled trial. *JAMA* **288**(3):321–333 (2002).
154. Cheema D, Coomarasamy A, El-Toukhy T. Non-hormonal therapy of post-menopausal vasomotor symptoms: a structured evidence-based review. *Arch Gynecol Obstet* **276**(5):463–469 (2007).
155. Rock E, DeMichele A. Nutritional approaches to late toxicities of adjuvant chemotherapy in breast cancer survivors. *J Nutr* **133**(11 suppl 1):3785S–3793S (2003).
156. Seibel MM. Treating hot flushes without hormone replacement therapy. *J Fam Pract* **52**:291–296 (2003).
157. Shams T, Setia MS, Hemmings R, *et al*. Efficacy of black cohosh-containing preparations on menopausal symptoms: a meta-analysis. *Altern Ther Health Med* **16**(1):36–44 (2010).

158. Palacio C, Masri G, Mooradian AD. Black cohosh for the management of menopausal symptoms: a systematic review of clinical trials. *Drugs Aging* **26**(1):23–36 (2009).
159. Walji R, Boon H, Guns E, *et al.* Black cohosh (Cimicifuga racemosa [L.] Nutt.): safety and efficacy for cancer patients. *Support Care Cancer* **15**(8):913–921 (2007).
160. Kennelly EJ, Baggett S, Nuntanakorn P, *et al.* Analysis of thirteen populations of black cohosh for formononetin. *Phytomedicine* **9**(5):461–467 (2002).
161. Huntley A. The safety of black cohosh (Actaea racemosa, Cimicifuga racemosa). *Expert Opin Drug Saf* **3**(6):615–623 (2004).
162. Huntley AL, Thompson Coon J, Ernst E. The safety of herbal medicinal products derived from Echinacea species: a systematic review. *Drug Saf* **28**(5):387–400 (2005).
163. Basch E, Ulbricht C, Basch S, *et al.* An evidence-based systemic review Echinacea E. angustifolia DC, E. pallida, E. purpurea by the Natural Standard Research Collaboration. *J Herb Pharmacother* **5**:57–88 (2005).
164. Freeman C, Spelman K. A critical evaluation of drug interactions with Echinacea spp. *Mol Nutr Food Res* **52**(7):789–798 (2008).
165. Tamayo C, Diamond S. Review of clinical trials evaluating safety and efficacy of milk thistle (Silybum marianum [L.] Gaertn.). *Integr Cancer Ther* **6**(2):146–157 (2007).
166. Sagar SM. Future directions for research on Silybum marianum for cancer patients. *Integr Cancer Ther* **6**(2):166–173 (2007).
167. Floyd J, Mirza I, Sachs B, *et al.* Hepatotoxicity of chemotherapy. *Semin Oncol* **33**:50–67 (2006).
168. Rambaldi A, Jacobs BP, Gluud C. Milk thistle for alcoholic and/or hepatitis B or C virus liver diseases. *Cochrane Database Syst Rev* **4**:CD003620 (2007).
169. Greenlee H, Abascal K, Yarnell E, *et al.* Clinical applications of Silybum marianum in oncology. *Integr Cancer Ther* **6**(2):158–165 (2007).
170. Ladas EJ, Kelly KM. Milk thistle: is there a role for its use as an adjunct therapy in patients with cancer? *J Altern Complement Med* **9**(3):411–416 (2003).
171. Jacobs BP, Dennehy C, Ramirez G, *et al.* Milk thistle for the treatment of liver disease: a systematic review and meta-analysis. *Am J Med* **113**(6):506–515 (2002).

172. Mulrow C, Lawrence V, Jacobs B, *et al.* Milk thistle: effects on liver disease and cirrhosis and clinical adverse effects. *Evid Rep Technol Assess (Summ)* **21**:1–3 (2000).
173. Flaig TW, Gustafson DL, Su LJ, *et al.* A phase I and pharmacokinetic study of silybin-phytosome in prostate cancer patients. *Invest New Drugs* **25**(2):139–146 (2007).
174. Kienle S, Kiene H, Albonico HU. *Anthroposophic Medicine: Effectiveness, Utility, Costs, Safety*, Schattauer Verlag, Stuttgart (2006).
175. Hajto T, Hostanska K, Berki T, *et al.* Oncopharmacological perspectives of a plant lectin (Viscum album agglutinin-I): overview of recent results from in vitro experiments and in vivo animal models, and their possible relevance for clinical applications. *Evid Based Complement Altern Med* **2**:59–67 (2005).
176. Ernst E, Schmidt K, Steuer-Vogt MK. Mistletoe for cancer? A systematic review of randomised clinical trials. *Int J Cancer* **107**(2):262–267 (2003).
177. Kienle GS, Berrino F, Büssing A, *et al.* Mistletoe in cancer — a systematic review on controlled clinical trials. *Eur J Med Res* **8**(3):109–119 (2003).
178. Kienle GS, Kiene H. Complementary cancer therapy: a systematic review of prospective clinical trials on anthroposophic mistletoe extracts. *Eur J Med Res* **12**(3):103–119 (2007).
179. Horneber MA, Bueschel G, Huber R, *et al.* Mistletoe therapy in oncology. *Cochrane Database Syst Rev* **2**:CD003297 (2008).
180. Melzer J, Iten F, Hostanska K, *et al.* Efficacy and safety of mistletoe preparations (Viscum album) for patients with cancer diseases. A systematic review. *Forsch Komplementmed* **16**(4):217–226 (2009).
181. Kienle GS, Kiene H. Influence of Viscum album L (European mistletoe) extracts on quality of life in cancer patients: a systematic review of controlled clinical studies. *Integr Cancer Ther* **9**(2):142–157 (2010).
182. Saller R, Kramer S, Iten F, *et al.* Unerwünschte wirkungen der misteltherapie bei tumorpatienten — eine systematische übersicht. In Scheer R, Bauer H, Becker V, *et al.* (eds), *Fortschritte in der Misteltherapie. Aktueller Stand der Forschung und klinische Anwendung*, KVC, Essen, pp. 367–403 (2005).
183. Büssing A, Stumpf C, Tröger W, *et al.* Course of mitogen-stimulated T lymphocytes in cancer patients treated with Viscum album extracts. *Anticancer Res* **27**(4C):2903–2910 (2007).

184. National Center for Complementary and Alternative Medicine (NCCAM). Manipulative and body-based practices: an overview (NCCAM Publication No. D238). http://www.fvpt.com/manipulative.pdf [Accessed 15 June 2010].
185. Ernst E. The safety of massage therapy. *Rheumatology (Oxford)* **42**(9):1101–1106 (2003).
186. Corbin L. Safety and efficacy of massage therapy for patients with cancer. *Cancer Control* **12(3)**:158–164 (2005).
187. Maddocks-Jennings W, Wilkinson JM. Aromatherapy practice in nursing: literature review. *J Adv Nurs* **48**(1):93–103 (2004).
188. Fellowes D, Barnes K, Wilkinson S. Aromatherapy and massage for symptom relief in patients with cancer. *Cochrane Database Syst Rev* **2**:CD002287 (2004).
189. Ernst E. Massage therapy for cancer palliation and supportive care: a systematic review of randomised clinical trials. *Support Care Cancer* **17**(4):333–337 (2009).
190. Chao LF, Zhang AL, Liu HE, *et al*. The efficacy of acupoint stimulation for the management of therapy-related adverse events in patients with breast cancer: a systematic review. *Breast Cancer Res Treat* **118**(2):255–267 (2009).
191. Melchart D, Weidenhammer W, Streng A, *et al*. Prospective investigation of adverse effects of acupuncture in 97 733 patients. *Arch Intern Med* **164**(1):104–105 (2004).
192. Lee H, Schmidt K, Ernst E. Acupuncture for the relief of cancer-related pain — a systematic review. *Eur J Pain* **9**(4):437–444 (2005).
193. Robb KA, Bennett MI, Johnson MI, *et al*. Transcutaneous electric nerve stimulation (TENS) for cancer pain in adults. *Cochrane Database Syst Rev* **3**:CD006276 (2008).
194. Lee MS, Kim KH, Choi SM, *et al*. Acupuncture for treating hot flashes in breast cancer patients: a systematic review. *Breast Cancer Res Treat* **115**(3):497–503 (2009).
195. Lee MS, Kim KH, Shin BC, *et al*. Acupuncture for treating hot flushes in men with prostate cancer: a systematic review. *Support Care Cancer* **17**(7):763–770 (2009).
196. Ezzo JM, Richardson MA, Vickers A, *et al*. Acupuncture-point stimulation for chemotherapy-induced nausea or vomiting, *Cochrane Database Syst Rev* **2**:CD002285 (2006).

197. Lu W, Hu D, Dean-Clower E, *et al*. Acupuncture for chemotherapy-induced leukopenia: exploratory meta-analysis of randomized controlled trials. *J Soc Integr Oncol* **5**(1):1–10 (2007).
198. Cho JH, Chung WK, Kang W, *et al*. Manual acupuncture improved quality of life in cancer patients with radiation-induced xerostomia. *J Altern Complement Med* **14**(5):523–526 (2008).
199. Garcia MK, Chiang JS, Cohen L, *et al*. Acupuncture for radiation-induced xerostomia in patients with cancer: a pilot study. *Head Neck* **31**(10):1360–1368 (2009).
200. Newton RU, Galvão DA. Exercise in prevention and management of cancer. *Curr Treat Options Oncol* **9**(2–3):135–146 (2008).
201. Hayes SC, Spence RR, Galvão DA, *et al*. Australian association for exercise and sport science position stand: optimising cancer outcomes through exercise. *J Sci Med Sport* **12**:428–434 (2009).
202. Morey MC, Snyder DC, Sloane R, *et al*. Effects of home-based diet and exercise on functional outcomes among older, overweight long-term cancer survivors: RENEW: a randomized controlled trial. *JAMA* **301**(18):1883–1891 (2009).
203. De Backer IC, Schep G, Backx FJ, *et al*. Resistance training in cancer survivors: a systematic review. *Int J Sports Med* **30**(10):703–712 (2009).
204. Cheema B, Gaul CA, Lane K, *et al*. Progressive resistance training in breast cancer: a systematic review of clinical trials. *Breast Cancer Res Treat* **109**(1):9–26 (2008).
205. Speck RM, Courneya KS, Mâsse LC, *et al*. An update of controlled physical activity trials in cancer survivors: a systematic review and meta-analysis. *J Cancer Surviv* **4**(2):87–100 (2010).
206. Jacobsen PB, Donovan KA, Vadaparampil ST, *et al*. Systematic review and meta-analysis of psychological and activity-based interventions for cancer-related fatigue. *Health Psychol* **26**(6):660–667 (2007).
207. Cramp F, Daniel J. Exercise for the management of cancer-related fatigue in adults. *Cochrane Database Syst Rev* **2**:CD006145 (2008).
208. Velthuis MJ, Agasi-Idenburg SC, Aufdemkampe G, *et al*. The effect of physical exercise on cancer-related fatigue during cancer treatment: a meta-analysis of randomised controlled trials. *Clin Oncol (R Coll Radiol)* **22**(3):208–221 (2010).

209. Conn VS, Hafdahl AR, Porock DC, *et al.* A meta-analysis of exercise interventions among people treated for cancer. *Support Care Cancer* **14**(7):699–712 (2006).
210. Beaton R, Pagdin-Friesen W, Robertson C, *et al.* Effects of exercise intervention on persons with metastatic cancer: a systematic review. *Physiother Can* **61**(3):141–153 (2009).
211. Markes M, Brockow T, Resch KL. Exercise for women receiving adjuvant therapy for breast cancer. *Cochrane Database Syst Rev* **4**: CD005001 (2006).
212. Duijts SF, Faber MM, Oldenburg HS, *et al.* Effectiveness of behavioral techniques and physical exercise on psychosocial functioning and health-related quality of life in breast cancer patients and survivors — a meta-analysis. *Psychooncology* **20**(2):115–126 (2011).
213. Vallbona C, Richards T. Evolution of magnetic therapy from alternative to traditional medicine. *Phys Med Rehabil Clin N Am* **10**(3):729–775 (1999).
214. National Center for Complementary and Alternative Medicine (NCCAM). *Energy Medicine: An Overview* (NCCAM Publication No. D235). http://www.umbwellness.org/PDF_files/energymed.pdf [Accessed 15 June 2010].
215. Hintz KJ, Yount GL, Kadar I, *et al.* Bioenergy definitions and research guidelines. *Altern Ther Health Med* **9**(suppl 3):A13–A30 (2003).
216. So PS, Jiang Y, Qin Y. Touch therapies for pain relief in adults. *Cochrane Database Syst Rev* **4**:CD006535 (2008).
217. Ng B. Qigong-induced mental disorders: a review. *ANZ J Psychiatry* **33**:197–206 (1999).
218. Shan HH. Culture-bound psychiatric disorders associated with Qigong practice in China. *Hong Kong J Psychiatry* **10**(3):12–14 (2000).
219. Ulbricht C, Bent S, Chao W, *et al.* An evidence-based review of Qi Gong by the Natural Standard Research Collaboration. *Natural Med J* **2**(5):7–15 (2010).
220. Lee S. Cultures in psychiatric nosology: the CCMD-2-R and international classification of mental disorders. *Cult Med Psychiatry* **20**:421–472 (1996).
221. Zhang TL, Xu TH. *Correcting Deviations from the Path of Qigong*, Publishing House of People's Health, Beijing (1997).
222. Han CM, Ji WJ. Qigong induced mental disorders. *Chinese Qigong* **1**:37–38 (1997).

223. Ryu H, Mo HY, Mo GD, *et al.* Delayed cutaneous hypersensitivity reactions in Qigong (chun do sun bup) trainees by multitest cell mediated immunity, *Am J Chin Med.* **23**(2):139–144 (1995).
224. Chen K, Yeung R. Exploratory studies of Qigong therapy for cancer in China. *Integr Cancer Ther* **1**(4):345–370 (2002).
225. Lee MS, Chen KW, Sancier KM, *et al.* Qigong for cancer treatment: a systematic review of controlled clinical trials. *Acta Oncol* **46**(6):717–722 (2007).
226. Jain S, Mills PJ. Biofield therapies: helpful or full of hype? A best evidence synthesis. *Int J Behav Med* **17**(1):1–16 (2010).
227. University of New South Wales Department of Physics. *The Electromagnetic Spectrum.* Available at http://www.phys.unsw.edu.au/~jw/EMspectrum.html [Accessed 16 June 2010].
228. Review Committee on Microwave Cancer Therapy and National Health and Medical Research Council. *Review of the Use of Microwave Therapy for the Treatment of Patients with Cancer.* http://www.nhmrc.gov.au/_files_nhmrc/file/publications/synopses/nh67.pdf [Accessed 16 June 2010].
229. Wust P, Gellermann J, Harder C, *et al.* Rationale for using invasive thermometry for regional hyperthermia of pelvic tumors. *Int J Radiat Oncol Biol Phys* **41**:1129–1137 (1998).
230. Lowenthal RM. Integrative oncology in Australia. *J Soc Integr Oncol* **4**(2):82–85 (2006).

4

The Regulation of Complementary and Alternative Medicine

Ken Harvey

ABSTRACT

Government regulation and registration of health practitioners aims to ensure a minimal level of education and training, appropriate standards of professional behaviour and effective and efficient complaint-handling mechanisms. Although medical practitioners, pharmacists, nurses and some other categories of health practitioners are registered by government, most have received little or no training in complementary and alternative medicine (CAM). Some doctors who practise "integrative medicine" are an exception. CAM practitioners such as naturopaths, herbalists and homeopaths have not yet achieved national registration, in part because of division in their ranks, but also because of their extremely varied training.

Unlike conventional medicines, the Australian Therapeutic Goods Administration does not evaluate complementary medicines for efficacy. They do ensure that AUST L-labelled products contain "relatively safe" ingredients and are manufactured according to Good Manufacturing Practice. However, claims made for complementary medicines are often far in advance of the scientific evidence available, whereas information about possible adverse effects, including interaction with conventional medicines, is often lacking. A similar situation exists for diagnostic and therapeutic devices used by CAM practitioners. The majority are regarded as "low risk" by the regulator and are not assessed to see if they work. A complaint system exists, but it is underresourced, overloaded and lacks effective sanctions. As a consequence, numerous claims that have been proven to breach the Therapeutic Goods Advertising Code continue to be made about CAM medicines and devices. The government has acknowledged these problems and several working groups are currently discussing possible regulatory reform. Meanwhile, caveat emptor applies (let the buyer beware).

Keywords: CAM; Complementary Medicine; Integrative Medicine; Regulation.

INTRODUCTION

Australia is a multi-cultural society with an indigenous and immigrant population encompassing many cultural, ethnic, linguistic and religious traditions. Around one in four Australians were born overseas. This raises the question of how to ensure that a diverse population has access to their own (and other) traditional medicines, while at the same time protecting them from the dangers of unregulated practitioners and products.

DEFINITIONS

Complementary and alternative medicine (CAM) is an inclusive term, incorporating complementary therapies, alternative medical systems and complementary medicines. The term is also abbreviated to complementary medicine (without an "s") and used as a synonym for alternative medicine, natural medicine and traditional medicine. Integrative medicine is a term used when combining conventional and complementary medicine with reasonable evidence of safety and effectiveness.

Complementary therapies include massage, meditation, yoga and tai chi, aromatherapy, reflexology, iridology, reiki and other biofield therapies.

Alternative medical systems developed in Western cultures include chiropractic, naturopathy and homeopathy, whereas traditional Chinese medicine and ayurveda are examples of systems developed in Eastern cultures.

Complementary medicines are defined (and regulated) by the Therapeutic Goods Administration (TGA) as medicinal products containing vitamins, minerals, herbs, homeopathic medicines, traditional Chinese medicines, ayurvedic (Indian) medicines and Australian indigenous medicines.[1]

A medical device is defined (and regulated by the TGA) as any instrument, apparatus, appliance or other article (whether used alone or in combination, and including the software necessary for its proper application) intended to be used on human beings for the prevention, diagnosis, cure or alleviation of a disease, ailment, defect or injury.[2] A range of controversial diagnostic and therapeutic devices are used by CAM practitioners, including bioelectronic machines such as VEGA and MORA, bioimpedance analysis and haemaview blood screening.

THE REGULATION OF PRACTITIONERS

Government regulation and registration of health practitioners aims to ensure a minimal level of education and training, appropriate standards of professional behaviour and effective and efficient complaint-handling mechanisms. Medical practitioners, nurses (including midwives), dentists (including dental hygienists, dental prosthetists and dental therapists), optometrists, osteopaths, chiropractors, pharmacists, physiotherapists, podiatrists and psychologists are currently registered in all Australian States and Territories. A single national registration and accreditation system was established for the above professions on 1 July 2010.[3] However, despite registration, Australian doctors, pharmacists and nurses have usually received little or no training in CAM, although this situation is now improving. In addition, a number of post-graduate courses and a professional society are available for doctors interested in integrative medicine.[4] The latter can assist consumers to choose an appropriately trained integrative practitioner.

Chinese traditional medicine practitioners and acupuncturists are registered in Victoria, but not in other States. Naturopaths, homeopaths and other CAM practitioners have not yet achieved national registration status, in part because of division in their ranks, but also because of their varied training. An Australian Register of naturopaths and herbalists is in the process of being established, in the hope that this will encourage the standards necessary for national registration.[5] Other categories of CAM practitioners may be members of professional associations; this can assist their patients in obtaining GST-free services and private health insurance rebates, but it does not necessarily ensure evidence-based practice, continuing professional education or good complaint-handling processes.

THE REGULATION OF PRODUCTS

Complementary medicines and medical devices (as defined above) are regulated by the TGA. The legislative basis is the *Therapeutic Goods Act 1989* and the *Therapeutic Goods Regulations 1990*, as amended by the *Therapeutic Goods Amendment (Medical Devices) Bill 2002* and the *Therapeutic Goods (Medical Devices) Regulations 2002*. All therapeutic goods that are imported into, supplied in or exported from Australia must be included on the Australian Register of Therapeutic Goods (ARTG) prior to supply. The aim is to ensure the quality, safety and efficacy of therapeutic goods. A two-tiered regulatory system is based on risk assessment.[6]

Most complementary medicines are regulated as "Listed" (low-risk) products by the TGA. They are identified by an AUST L number on the product label. Product efficacy is not evaluated. Sponsors self-enter details of their product on the ARTG using a web-based electronic listing facility. The only routine checks made are that the ingredients are on the TGA's "relatively low-risk" list. Listed medicines are restricted to indication and claims relating to health maintenance, health enhancement or non-serious, self-limiting conditions. Sponsors must certify that they hold evidence supporting the claims made about their product (evidence of "traditional use" is acceptable), but their product information and promotional material are rarely reviewed. The listing system provides rapid market entry at minimal cost.

By contrast, conventional medicines ("Registered" products) are thoroughly evaluated by the TGA for safety, quality and efficacy before they are allowed onto the market. They are identified by an AUST R number on the product label. Generic versions of clinically proven products must demonstrate therapeutic equivalence. Sponsors of both innovator and generic products must negotiate approved product information with the TGA and also provide consistent consumer medicine information and promotion. Registration fees are substantial and the time taken for evaluation can be protracted.

Medical devices are classified according to their intended use, the level of risk and their degree of invasiveness in the human body. Certification by the TGA or an overseas notified body is required for higher risk devices. Most Class I (low-risk) devices do not need a TGA conformity assessment certificate. However, the manufacturer must declare to the TGA that "the device is suitable for the intended purpose".[2]

All medicines and medical devices are required to be produced in accordance with Good Manufacturing Practice (GMP) and all are subjected to post-marketing surveillance, prioritised according to risk. The latter includes monitoring reported adverse reactions and random and targeted audits of GMP and testing for conformity with the regulations.

The promotion of therapeutic goods in Australia is subject to a complex system of co-regulation, underpinned by the *Therapeutic Goods Act 1989* and the *Trade Practices Act 1974*. The Therapeutic Goods Advertising Code provides the standard for all advertising directed to consumers.[7] In addition, there are relevant industry codes of practice. In general, promotional claims should be accurate (capable of *substantiation* from the scientific literature), balanced (taking into account all of the evidence available and including both benefits and risks) and up-to-date. There are substantial differences in the timeliness, transparency and the sanctions applied by the different systems to complaints about the promotion of therapeutic goods, especially complementary medicines compared with conventional medicines.

Although the Australian regulation of medicines and devices used in CAM is far more rigorous than that of many other countries, a number of problems have emerged.[8,9]

CURRENT CONTROVERSIES AND PROBLEMS

Product Claims, Names and Warnings

Research on complementary medicines used for weight loss showed that some sponsors self-entered indications and/or claims on the ARTG that could not be substantiated. These were then used in promotional material. Other sponsors made conservative claims on the ARTG, but then made very different claims in promotional campaigns. In addition, product names such as "Fat Magnet", "Weight Loss Accelerate" and "Slim-Me" appear equally misleading and deceptive. Device sponsors use similar strategies, such as "Accent FatBlaster Radio Frequency Device".

In 2007, the TGA was asked to review the efficacy of all ingredients used in weight-loss products, in the hope that upstream evaluation would reduce the need for downstream complaints. What ultimately resulted was a "Draft Guideline for Levels and Kinds of Evidence for Listed Medicines with Indications and Claims for Weight Loss"; this document has yet to be finalised 3 years later.[10]

The problem of unsubstantiated claims is not limited to CAM weight-loss products. Some recent examples submitted to the Complaint Resolution Panel (CRP) include "All adults should take vitamins to prevent chronic disease", "Homeopathic immunisation is a safe and effective way to protect you and your family against childhood and other epidemic diseases", "Biosun Hopi Ear Candles are a truly safe and natural product" and "there are no reports in the literature of an interaction between glucosamine and warfarin". None of these statements are in accordance with the scientific literature and the last one also contradicts warnings by the Australian Adverse Drug Reaction Advisory Committee. Currently, the only way to correct such inaccuracies is by submitting complaints. However, the CRP is underresourced, overloaded and lacks effective sanctions. It even lacks resources to follow-up its own determinations, which make them easily ignored. It can take multiple complaints before non-compliance with a CRP determination is passed to the TGA. That organisation, citing "commercial-in-confidence" considerations, currently tells complainants nothing and publicises nothing. A recent Parliamentary Secretary for Health in Australia with responsibility for the TGA,

Mark Butler, has agreed that the current situation is "deeply unsatisfactory" and has asked his Department to prepare a public discussion paper of policy options.[11]

Research by the Australian National Prescribing System (NPS) showed a major disconnect between consumers' perception of complementary medicines as "natural" and "risk-free" and the reality that they contain pharmacologically active substances capable of producing drug–drug interactions and adverse effects.[12] My own analysis of advertisements for complementary medicines suggests that this perception is created and/or maintained by extensive promotion that emphasises the word "natural" and the use of associated imagery and colour.

Warnings about serious drug side-effects and drug–drug interactions are currently communicated to health professionals by Australian Prescriber.[13] In addition, the TGA may require sponsors to add key warnings to the medicine label for consumers. The following is a recent example "Warning: In very rare cases, black cohosh has been associated with liver failure". However, there are now numerous Australian Internet sites from which consumers can purchase complementary medicines without having the opportunity to read a product label; there is no requirement that important safety information should be communicated on these websites and there is variable implementation of such warnings.

Similarly, the perception that complementary medicines are part of a "holistic" approach to "maintaining good health" ignores the reality that many of these products are devised and marketed (in isolation) to take advantage of consumer anxieties and concerns. For example, although there is good evidence that some formulations of Hawthorn extract can be an effective treatment for heart failure, its common promotion for "heart health" would appear to be the complementary medicine version of "disease-mongering".

Product Efficacy

Traditional use has revealed many useful herbal products, such as *Artemisia annua* for the treatment of malaria and St. John's wort for the management of mild to moderate depression. But traditional therapies have also proved to be harmful; the bloodletting that was performed for centuries by the medical profession is a classic example. When clinical trials were conducted, bloodletting was shown to kill patients, not cure them. Scientific study is required.

Herbal products are comprised of a complex mix of ingredients; just as all red wine is not of Bordeaux quality, different products containing the same herb are not necessarily chemically or therapeutically equivalent. Variability can be caused by the use of different species or subspecies, growth conditions, methods of cultivation, the time of year and stage of growth cycle harvested, extraction methods, and formulation and storage of the finished product. Even glucosamine (used for arthritis) is available as several salts: glucosamine sulphate, glucosamine hydrochloride, and also as *N*-acetyl glucosamine, in many different formulations and with varied evidence of efficacy from clinical trials.[14]

The TGA does not require clinical trial data to support the efficacy of listed herbal medicines, or evidence of therapeutic equivalence with proven products. As a result, there is no certainty that all formulations of complementary medicines on the Australian market are efficacious. Nor does the TGA require evidence of efficacy for CAM devices that they regard as "low risk".

Adulterated and Substandard Products

The TGA has detected dangerous adulteration of some complementary medicines, such as the Herbal Health International products "Excite" for women and "Ultimates" for men, found to contain an analogue of sildenafil (Viagra).[15] These products have been taken off the market.

Other types of adulteration do not concern safety, but rather truth in labelling and product integrity. For example, products containing *Ginkgo biloba* in the USA have been shown to be frequently adulterated or "spiked" with less expensive sources of flavonol glycosides, such as rutin (from buckwheat), that can trick routine testing to make a product with little or no real ginkgo appear to be the real thing. When the TGA investigated similar products in Australia, six of 20 randomly sampled products had results consistent with adulteration.[16] The TGA now requires sponsors to test for such adulteration. Substandard products containing low levels of active ingredients (e.g. *Echinacea*) have also been found in Australia by Choice, emphasising the need for targeted audits of GMP and testing of product ingredients.[17]

Harm

Although complementary medicines are regarded as "relatively low-risk" products, they are not without adverse effects and interactions with conventional drugs. For example, *Echinacea* can cause allergic reactions, black cohosh has been associated with rare cases of liver failure requiring liver transplantation and St. John's wort interacts with a wide range of conventional drugs, including oral contraceptives.[18] In addition, when a number of "relatively low-risk" ingredients are combined, unexpected adverse effects may result.[19] Recognition of such problems can be difficult, because many patients do not tell their doctors that they are taking complementary medicines and doctors often do not ask. As a result, adverse effects of complementary medicines are almost certainly underrecognised. In addition, ineffective complementary medicines have a significant adverse effect on consumers' hip pockets (or purses) and, more importantly, they can delay or prevent the use of more evidence-based therapy.

Independent Information

Unlike conventional medicines, complementary medicines lack TGA-approved product information and consumer medicine information. NPS research also showed that GPs and pharmacists believed that they did not have enough access to evidence-based information about complementary medicines. As a result they were not confident in discussing these medicines with their patients. Many GPs and pharmacists were unaware of the side-effects of some commonly used complementary medicines and their potential interactions with conventional medicines. More than 80% of GPs and community pharmacists felt that complementary medicines needed more scientific testing.[12]

The NPS has identified and recommended several sources of good independent information about complementary medicines, but these require payment and are not widely used. In addition, generic information about an ingredient does not necessarily apply to specific Australian formulations. The ARTG does provide public summaries of product information, but this is compiled by the sponsor, rarely reviewed by the TGA and often contains information that lacks an evidence base. The Canadian Natural Health Products Ingredients Database is more helpful, as it contains referenced information on indications and risks.[20] The American National Center for Complementary and Alternative Medicines (NCCAM) is a reliable source of information about CAM including information about specific complementary therapies and medicines.[21] Questionable CAM diagnostic and therapeutic devices can be found at Device Watch.[22]

Research

From an industry perspective, difficulties in protecting the intellectual property of complementary medicines significantly inhibit investment in research. Once an ingredient or herbal extract is characterised, it can be used by any sponsor and the claims made are not usually restricted by regulators to specific formulations that have shown clinical efficacy.

In 2007–08, in recognition of the need to strengthen the evidence supporting complementary medicines, the Australian government announced more that $7 million in research grants. Funding of $1.74 million was awarded to establish three National Institute of Complementary Medicine Collaborative Centres and a further $5.3 million for 13 projects funded by the National Health and Medical Research Council.[23] The NCCAM has also invested substantial research funds to improve the evidence base.[24]

CONCLUSION

The Australian regulatory system for medicines and devices used in CAM is regarded as the world's best practice. In addition, most health professionals and consumers accept that evidence-based CAM has a place in health-care. Despite this, dubious products with unethical claims have proliferated and it is difficult for individual consumers or health practitioners to distinguish efficacious products from those of uncertain quality and efficacy.

There is also no agreed content for educating health professionals about complementary medicines and devices. Pressure is being brought to bear by health professionals and consumer organisations to improve the regulatory and educational systems but, not surprisingly, some vested interests wish to preserve the status quo. The government has provided welcome funds for CAM research and has acknowledged problems with advertising and complaint systems and has set up several working groups to formulate policy options for regulatory reform.

REFERENCES

1. Therapeutic Goods Administration. The regulation of complementary medicines in Australia — an overview. Australian Government, Department of Health and Ageing, Therapeutic Goods Administration, April 2006. http://www.tga.gov.au/cm/cmreg-aust.htm. [Accessed 14 February 2010].
2. Therapeutic Goods Administration. Australian medical devices guidelines: 1. An overview of the new medical devices regulatory system. Australian Government, Department of Health and Ageing, Therapeutic Goods Administration. http://www.tga.gov.au/docs/html/devguid1.htm. [Accessed February 2010].
3. Australia's Health Workforce Online. National Registration and Accreditation Scheme. National Health Workforce Taskforce. http://www.nhwt.gov.au/natreg.asp. [Accessed 19 February 2010].
4. Australasian Integrative Medicine Association. About AIMA. http://www.aima.net.au/about_aima.html. [Accessed 7 February 2010].
5. The Australian Register of Naturopaths and Herbalists. National Register to Make Complementary Medicine Safer. ARONAH Steering Committee. http://www.aronah.org/news.html. [Accessed 19 February 2010].
6. Therapeutic Goods Administration. Regulation of therapeutic goods in Australia, April 2005. Australian Government, Department of Health and Ageing, Therapeutic Goods Administration. http://www.tga.gov.au/docs/html/tga/tgaginfo.htm. [Accessed 7 February 2010].
7. Therapeutic Goods Advertising Code Council. Overview of Therapeutic Goods Advertising: The Code. Therapeutic Goods

Advertising Code Council. http://www.tgacc.com.au/codeList.cfm?CFID=37358754. [Accessed 28 February 2010].

8. Harvey KJ, Korczak VS, Marron LJ, *et al.* Commercialism, choice and consumer protection: regulation of complementary medicines in Australia. *MJA* **188**(1):21–25 (2008). http://www.mja.com.au/public/issues/188_01_070108/har10522_fm.html. [Accessed 14 February 2010].
9. Harvey K. A review of proposals to reform the regulation of complementary medicines. *Aust Health Rev* **33**(2):279–285 (2009).
10. Therapeutic Goods Administration. Guideline for Levels and Kinds of Evidence for Listed Medicines with Indications and Claims for Weight Loss. Consultation draft. Australian Government, Department of Health and Ageing, Therapeutic Goods Administration, February 2009. http://www.tga.gov.au/cm/consult/drweightloss.pdf. [Accessed 19 February 2010].
11. Australian Broadcasting Commission Radio. National Interest: The Medicines Regulation Headache Transcript, 25 September 2009. http://www.abc.net.au/rn/nationalinterest/stories/2009/2696989.htm. [Accessed 19 February 2010].
12. National Prescribing Service. Complementary Medicines Research Project. National Prescribing Service, 2008. http://www.nps.org.au/research_and_evaluation/research/current_research/complementary_medicines. [Accessed 19 February 2010].
13. National Prescribing Service. Australian Prescriber. Canberra. http://www.australianprescriber.com. [Accessed 14 February 2010].
14. Vlad SC, LaValley MP, McAlindon TE, *et al.* Glucosamine for pain in osteoarthritis: why do trial results differ? *Arthritis Rheum* **56**: 2267–2277 (2007).
15. Therapeutic Goods Administration. Excite for Women, Ultimates for Men. Medicine Recall. Australian Government, Department of Health and Ageing, Therapeutic Goods Administration, 20 April 2007. http://www.tga.gov.au/recalls/2007/excite.htm. [Accessed 1 February 2010].
16. Therapeutic Goods Administration. Composition of Ginkgo biloba products. Australian Government, Department of Health and Ageing, Therapeutic Goods Administration. 2 October 2009. http://www.tga.gov.au/alerts/medicines/gingko.htm. [Accessed 1 February 2010].

17. *Choice. Test: Echinacea. Low Levels of Active Ingredients*? Australian Consumer's Association (2005).
18. Braun L, Cohen M. *Herbs and Natural Supplements. An Evidence-Based Guide*, 2nd edn., Elsevier Mosby, Sydney (2007).
19. Rashid NN, Grant J. Hydroxycut hepatotoxicity. *MJA* **192**(3):173–174 (2010). http://www.mja.com.au/public/issues/192_03_010210/letters_010210_fm-4.html. [Accessed 19 February 2010].
20. Canadian Natural Products Directorate. Natural Health Products Ingredients Database. Health Canada, 2010. http://www.hc-sc.gc.ca/dhp-mps/prodnatur/applications/online-enligne/nhpid-bipsn-eng.php. [Accessed 19 February 2010].
21. National Institutes of Health. National Center for Complementary and Alternative Medicines (NCCAM). Department of Health and Human Services, USA. http://nccam.nih.gov. [Accessed 28 February 2010].
22. Barrett S. Device watch. http://www.devicewatch.org/. [Accessed 15 February 2010].
23. McLucas J. Complementary medicine gets a boost. Australian Government, Department of Health and Ageing, Media Release. 30 March 2008. http://www.health.gov.au/internet/ministers/publishing.nsf/Content/mr-yr08-jm-jm002.htm. [Accessed 15 February 2010].
24. National Institutes of Health. National Center for Complementary and Alternative Medicines (NCCAM). Funding Strategy: Fiscal Year 2010. Department of Health and Human Services, USA. http://nccam.nih.gov/grants/strategy/2010.htm. [Accessed 15 February 2010].

5

Perspective on Chinese Medicine in Complementary and Alternative Medicine

James Flowers

ABSTRACT

The rapidly globalising field of Chinese medicine is becoming known to a wide audience. Less understood are the historical and philosophical underpinnings of this field of therapy, based as they are on theories such as *qi, yin yang* and the five phases. The central and canonical text, the *Yellow Emperor's Inner Canon*, compiled some thousands of years ago, remains the basis for this unique way of understanding this type of contextual thinking, in which everything that exists in the world and its phenomena are connected as a totality. This way of thought can be described as correlative and also applies to the human body, shaping an approach that seeks to diagnose and treat the whole person rather than a disease. Contemporary practitioners receive training in university degree courses, while being trained in basic biomedical principles for at least 4 years. Practitioners are normally trained to administer Chinese herbal therapy, acupuncture and medical techniques such as massage. These therapies are normally gentle in effect yet profound in healing strength. The rationale in classical Chinese medicine is to strengthen the capacity of the patient to heal, repair and invigorate. This is in line with the principle of seeking balance and harmony, key tenets of Confucian thought. In China and Korea, Chinese medicine is very much a part of these respective countries' national health systems. Moving outside its heartland in East Asia, Chinese medicine is likely to play a more significant role in health systems across the world.

Keywords: Acupuncture; Chinese Medicine; Herbs; Massage.

INTRODUCTION

This chapter provides an introduction to Chinese medicine. Most people's exposure to this field of practical knowledge may be with some experience of acupuncture, herbal medication, Chinese massage or perhaps some therapeutic exercise like *taiji* or *qigong*. I suggest that, although these forms of therapy are indeed concrete manifestations of Chinese medicine, they are merely superficial phenomena without an appreciation that these practices are but the outward expression of a complex and profound long process of refinement of Chinese philosophy infused with a unique view of the world. This way of understanding assumes that everything is connected and that correlative thinking is the norm. I have not attempted a technical outline of Chinese medicine, as this would have run the risk of repeating the work of many others.[1–7] Rather, this is a perusal of some perspectives pertinent to the area of Chinese medicine.

The questions in the mind of most readers would typically range from 'How does it work?' to 'What diseases can it treat'? To start, I suggest that an appreciation of this field would be inadequate without at least a rudimentary grasp of pre-modern Chinese thought. Modern interpretations, aiming to fit into the biomedical model, miss the point. An open-minded appreciation of Chinese medicine that allows for an understanding on its own terms need not preclude analytical frameworks shaped by modern methods of analysis. Chinese medicine is necessarily characterised by multiple perspectives.

Despite the vast literature, many of the key ideas can be found in one seminal text, the *Yellow Emperor's Inner Canon* or *Huang Di*

Nei Jing.[8–11] Rather than merely being a medical text of past historical interest, compiled more than 2,000 years ago, it still provides the theoretical ballast for Chinese medicine today.[12] It is of relevance that this compilation also remains the text that contains the ideas that have most shaped Chinese thinking about the world, ranging across all fields of human endeavour.

While noting that the history of Chinese medicine is long and varied, necessarily encompassing many diverse streams and currents, it is important to know that the form of Chinese medicine that is practised most widely today has been coloured by perspectives of modern biomedicine.[13] For the sake of distinction, this chapter will discuss the form of Chinese medicine untouched by scientific biomedicine, without delving into a reality shaped by modernity. This approach may help the lay reader to ponder on its unique approaches.

Scholars have shown that historically, in China, most medical consultations have been with folk-healers or religious healers.[14] For the purpose of distinction, it is important to know that the medicine known as Chinese medicine today derives from the practices of the literate and scholarly elites of pre-modern China.[15] If it is accepted that China's civilisation was characterised by a thirst for bookish learning and rigorous education, then an appreciation may be gleaned that this form of medicine is not one stuck in the realm of mystical speculation, but rather in empirical evidence building and in massive volumes of literary medical writings. The fact that practitioners of this form of medicine insist on applying the nationalist epithet of 'Chinese' provides an obvious clue to the inextricable links with Chinese cultural approaches in general and to Chinese philosophical perspectives in particular, Chinese medicine only assuming the title of 'Chinese' in the 20th century.[16] This renaming was in response to the challenge of the newly introduced biomedicine from the West.

Despite the seeming distractions from the pragmatic applications of Chinese medicine, I argue that this is not an alien realm of knowledge. If it can be accepted that there are diverse ways of knowing the world, then Chinese medicine, even outside its original homeland, becomes very much a component of the global human project to seek ways to prevent and treat disease. Chinese medicine can be learned, regardless of culture or background.

In this regard, people from very different backgrounds are studying Chinese medicine, either for interest or as a career path. As the influence of Chinese civilisation and its concomitant thought patterns grows alongside its economic development, it seems inexorable that its medicine will play an increasingly important role. The development of a new cultural nationalism in China is married with an increased interest in China's past, in which medicine can be included.[17] Of significance in this regard is that in 2012 the Australian government will begin the implementation of national statutory registration of practitioners of Chinese medicine.[18] This will occur largely as a response to the use of Chinese medicine therapy by a growing and substantial number of patients.

From a Western perspective, China is the ultimate other, it being possible to regard Chinese medicine as perhaps the epitome of this ultimate other, with its ineffable descriptions of *qi* and its vague allusions to *yin* and *yang* and five phase theory.[19] Efforts continue to validate Chinese medicine in scientific terms. These, so far, have defied a comprehensive scientific explanation. On its own terms, it is not a mysterious esoteric field, but a discipline that can be learned with enough effort and application. The contemporary solution offered is to attempt to subject Chinese medicine to standardisation. That this has not been achieved testifies to the innate diversity of the field. As part of this effort, quite significant steps towards standardisation have been taken by incorporating Chinese medicine into university education, where it now sits.

In the following section I will summarise the practices of Chinese medicine. The subsequent section will look at the theoretical philosophy.

APPLICATIONS OF CHINESE MEDICINE

While acknowledging the caveat of the complexity of Chinese medicine, it may be useful for the purposes of this chapter to briefly outline the training that students in the university system receive. In Australia, they spend 4 years in a bachelor course in which they are trained in major theoretical concepts in assessing human health, imbalance and disease. They are trained in the major diagnostic techniques of Chinese medicine and are then trained to assess patients for suitable therapeutic strategies. They are trained to prescribe herbal remedies, administer acupuncture and be aware of some lifestyle and dietary issues. They also spend a large part of these 4 years being trained in anatomy, physiology, pathology and diagnosis in the area of scientific biomedicine. The rationale for receiving training in this discipline is that practitioners in the field should have broad medical knowledge and be aware of the diagnoses and treatment regimes that patients receive from GPs in clinics and doctors in hospitals.

One factor that precipitates diversity in the field is that practitioners commonly undertake further training in a large variety of techniques and variations in approach. These range from exploration of various schools, lineages and masters to an emphasis on a large variety of different diagnostic methods, to methods incorporating Chinese astrology, and to variations influenced by certain Japanese and Korean styles. This is even before we take into account geographical variations, such as the incorporation of European or Australian herbs and the reality whereby some practitioners combine their therapies with modalities such as Bach flower remedies and homeopathy.

Contrary to the reality of a diversity in the field, most modern research in Chinese medicine accepts that it is simply the medication that is important. This runs counter to the historical development of medicine in China, where the skill of the practitioner was considered paramount. At the heart of this was the project of self-cultivation. Related to this was the idea of compassion and social skills. A key point made in the *Inner Canon* was that one's spirit or state of mind is central to a person's being and intimately related to good health. The more one is in harmony with self and the mind calm, the more potent will be the *qi* (or energy) of that person.

Diversity is also allowed to flourish because the vast majority of practitioners in a country like Australia remain outside the official hospital system. In a typical privately-run small clinic, a practitioner may specialise in acupuncture, herbs or, as is often the case, offer a combination of both services. Acupuncture and herbs represent different approaches to achieving treatment results, while sharing pivotal theories, such as those discussed in the *Inner Canon*.

Herbs

The Chinese herbal *materia medica* contains thousands of substances, but the average practitioner would use not more than three or four hundred of the more common of these substances, along with their preferred favourites.[20] The reference to the medicines being herbal is not strictly accurate. Although the majority of substances used are of plant origin, a small proportion is of mineral and animal origin.

There is variation in the approach of practitioners prescribing herbs, related to style and more commonly related to the method of preparation of the herbs. According to the diagnosis, each patient would be prescribed an individualised prescription. This is commonly a mixture of up to 20 substances. It is common for the prescription to contain 10–12 ingredients, with an average of about 6–12 s for each substance. There is a range of methods of taking the herbal medication. The traditional and most common method has been to prescribe a mixture of dried substances, such as dried leaves, barks, seeds and roots. These should be boiled in water, with the remaining liquid acting as the medicine. In most cases, this would then be drunk, but sometimes they are applied externally to the skin. This is the classical method and most closely linked to what could be described as elite medicine, designed to deal with the most complex of cases. These could range from mixtures to cure a common cold to more severe diseases ranging from high blood pressure to diseases of the major organs.

Alongside this method is the more pragmatic use of single herbs for a simple and usually less severe case. A common example is the use of ginseng as a herb to strengthen body and mind.

In more recent times, an industry has developed, whereby herbs are taken in the form of pills, powders or granules that can be dissolved in hot water. In some countries an industry has developed of prepared bottles of liquid drink, although this is not the practice in Australia.

One Chinese herb that has been used for centuries in various scenarios is artemisia. In recent times its extract has been used in biomedicine to treat malaria.[21] It must be said that this approach is far removed from the classical Chinese approach of complex individualised prescriptions. In ancient China this prescription could even be changed daily, but normally every few days. In a contemporary setting it would be the norm to pay a visit to the practitioner about once a week, where the complex prescription would usually be altered slightly or drastically, according to the situation.

The herbs are adjusted to fit the intricate and highly individualised state of the patient. The aim is usually to balance *yin* and *yang*. There are herbs that perform particular functions, such as boosting *qi*, harmonising *qi*, reinforcing blood, reinforcing *yang*, nourishing *yin*, invigorating the flow of blood or stopping bleeding. Some others promote urination, or regulate digestion and other organic functions. Herbs can be warming, cooling or neutral. This is not a reference to actual temperature, but rather a reference to the nature of the *qi* of the herb that will be imparted into the human body upon consumption. Likewise, all foods are said to have a certain nature, not limited to hot or cold. For example, ginger is said to be warm in nature, while being able to play a role in expelling externally contracted pathogens, this being consistent with its acrid nature. Gypsum, however, is an example of a medicinal substance that is cold in nature.

Chinese medicine is not just a way of curing disease, but a method to aid in the prevention of disease and in building up *qi* and supporting a healthy psychological state. Complex herbal mixtures are tailored to the individual and to the particular circumstance, while embracing the concept that everything is in a constant state of flux and change. By enabling the *qi* to be strong and flowing smoothly, the aim is not only to rectify existing disease, but also to assist the body to ward off sickness or not to succumb to pathogenic factors.

One notices that many of the ingredients in the *materia medica* are also food substances, whereas other herbs stray into the area where much caution and expertise are required before any internal consumption. A typical example of a herb that is also commonly used for culinary purposes is ginger. In Chinese medicine it is rare to take it as a single substance. Rather, in both cooking and healing, it is the complex mixture or the symphony of a number of ingredients in a mixture that holds the key to benefit. That is why the idea of trialling fixed medicines is problematic. It is not a one-size-fits-all approach, but a highly tailored approach akin to the finest bespoke maker of suits in Savile Row.

Acupuncture

More commonly known in Western countries than Chinese herbs, acupuncture relies on the use of fine stainless steel needles inserted into the body at various points.[22] Although it may sound particularly gruesome to the uninitiated, the trained practitioner is able to insert the needle safely and with a minimum of discomfort. Based on the same theoretical principles as Chinese herbal medicine, the idea of the needle insertion is to direct, guide or stimulate the *qi* of the patient, in order to enhance the healing process or to strengthen the workings of the human body. The number of needles inserted in a patient in one session varies, ranging from one to dozens of needles. It is common to insert about ten needles, although there is no fixed number. Again, this depends on the particular permutations in the case presented by each individual patient.

The accepted conceptualisation is that channels run throughout the body, these being the main paths through which *qi* travels and spreads throughout the entire body. There are 14 major channels, 12 of them being related to a particular organ. Along each channel are situated particular points, the major ones numbering well over 300. Like the prescribing of herbs, there are a vast number of possibilities of combinations of points suited to the particular context and the particular condition of the patient. It needs to be said that the time of day and time of year and the weather are important factors in deciding which combination of points to select.

Students necessarily spend years learning the endless intricate subtleties of acupuncture before mastering this art. Dexterity of manual technique is of course of vital importance, skills that need to be practised for years. On top of this, if one believes in the existence of *qi*, many eminent scholars in the field have, especially in the past, emphasised the mental state of the practitioner as being an indispensable factor in the healing process.[23] The Chinese conceptualisation of *qi* rests on the assumption that we all embody a personal type of *qi*. Chinese philosophy's key tenet is that we are all connected in a real sense. If this is true, then the *qi* of the practitioner has a particular effect on the patient and vice versa. There is not enough space to elaborate here, but this *qi* could consciously be influenced by the act of the lifelong habit of practising self-cultivation.

Moxibustion is a therapeutic technique closely related to acupuncture, in the sense that it involves some kind of external physical stimulus to the body. Unlike acupuncture, there is no penetration of the body. This therapy involves the burning of a herb called mugwort or moxa, which burns slowly, something like tobacco. In various forms, such as rolls or cones or applied to the end of the acupuncture needles, not only is some warmth generated, which is said to enter the channels, but the therapeutic effect of the herb helps to stimulate healing or regeneration. It is usually placed strategically near the skin, so that it may provide the patient with an obvious feeling of warmth.

In the Chinese language, acupuncture and moxibustion are usually referred to together, there being no single word for acupuncture alone. Like Chinese herbs, acupuncture and moxibustion can work well in treating many diseases successfully, as well as in disease prevention and rejuvenation.

Manual Therapy

There is a large range of manual techniques in the repertoire of Chinese medicine, ranging from strenuous manipulations to gentle soothing techniques. Although in practical terms these techniques are in the main for problems of the musculoskeletal system, as known in the modern sense, they are also often used to promote healing for many organic conditions ranging from hypertension to diarrhoea. The rationale is that, by using manual application to affect the channels and associated points, a stimulus is activated in the body. Many readers may be familiar with reflexology and its idea of stimulating particular parts of the sole of the foot to seek therapeutic effect. Reflection on this approach may help us to understand the reasoning behind massage and manipulation techniques in Chinese medicine.

Dietary Advice and Yangsheng

A very broad aspect of Chinese medicine, and one that is by no means insignificant, is that of *yangsheng*, or preserving life. This diverse area may be said to include dietary advice with its emphasis being related to regulation of lifestyle.[24] In this field there are endless permutations with relation to health, vitality and healing. These include guidelines on approaches to sleep and rest, and include the area of countless types of exercise routines. Many followers of these techniques incorporate such exercise routines into their daily lives. As an example we may look at the exercise regime of the 18th century emperor of China, Qianlong. The palace records list his exercise regime as including knocking the upper and lower teeth together, swallowing his saliva and plucking his ears. Rubbing of his nose, rolling of his eyes and kneading his feet followed these routines. Finally he would stretch his limbs and raise his arms.[25] These exercises are not remarkable in themselves, but rather show a fairly standard routine practised by Chinese people for thousands of years. Millions of Chinese people still do these exercises on a daily basis.

Many may be familiar with other exercises such as *taiji*, which follows the principles of *qi* and *yin yang*. A related area, meditation, very much a part of the Chinese tradition, brings us into areas associated with an awareness of realms of consciousness.

To summarise, there is a large variety of styles and a veritable panoply of tools in the kitbag of Chinese medicine. A practitioner may tend towards one technique or tend towards diversity and use a range of therapies all at once. Whatever the case, in classical Chinese medicine the aim is to balance the person and to ensure a healthy flow of *qi*. All of this has as its aim to restore and to invigorate the natural healing properties of the body. Approaches in technique may differ, but the rationale will normally be just that. The classical approach is not to cure disease as such, but to enable the body to heal and to right what is wrong. By righting what is wrong or by restoring balance, diseases are cured, but that is secondary to the primary aim to restore the wholeness of the person. By this logic, Chinese medical therapies not only cure disease, but also enhance wellness.

A final caveat is that, even if this sounds simplistic, the ability to practise well requires the skills of highly trained practitioners with many years of intensive learning. For this reason, self-prescribing or looking up remedies in books or on the Internet is never recommended.

The 20th century saw a trend towards increased specialisation in many areas of endeavour and especially in the professions and in natural science. One writer has described this trend as the hardening of the categories.[26] The area of Chinese thought was characterised by the fervent desire to be a generalist. In this spirit, I argue that a general education remains a foundation in grasping the subtle and intricate complexities of Chinese medical theory.

A HERETICAL THOUGHT — THE POWER OF GOD WITHOUT GOD

If readers at this point are hoping for a scientific explanation of Chinese medicine, they may be disappointed. Genuine scientific explanation still eludes Chinese medicine. Scientific trials continue apace, while numbers of people work feverishly in laboratories to attempt to prove the existence of an identifiable physical entity such as *qi*.

It is fairly clear that the over-riding characteristic of Chinese thought and the application thereof is the ability to see the whole picture, with the idea that any object or any phenomenon is intimately tied to and influenced by every other thing or phenomenon. The only difference is in the degree of connectedness. The giant and extremely influential philosopher Wang Yangming argued that to know the essence of existence is to know the essence of every object or phenomena.[27] What he was alluding to was an understanding of *qi*. Furthermore, he showed that introspection could not solve everything, but that one gained understanding by being active and by engaging in the world.

This may sound obtuse, but the relevance to Chinese medicine is that the core of classical Chinese medicine rests on the idea that the body is an integrated whole, akin to a symphony orchestra. This idea of a whole means that each and every minor symptom is included in any diagnosis and must necessarily be understood by the practitioner as part of a larger and general pattern. To do otherwise is not to practise classical Chinese medicine, but a truncated version. These symptoms include every single minor and major physical ache, pain, discomfort or unusual feeling, not in isolation but in relation to each other, with little distinction made between objective and subjective feelings. Most importantly, the psyche or the mind is not separated from the physical body. Any subjective feelings, whether conscious or not, are taken into account in any assessment of a patient. Any emotion — whether it is happiness, sadness, anger or whatever — is believed to have a direct, concrete impact on the physical body. Any imbalance in the physical body, likewise, is said to impact on the emotional state of a person. The two are as one.

Furthermore, if it is acknowledged that everything that exists is connected, one accepts that the external, physical environment affects humans. It is for this reason that much attention is paid to the weather and the climate by practitioners of classical Chinese medicine. In pre-modern China, this attention to the external environment extended to detailed observation of geography, geology and the stars, all of which were believed to have an influence on human health.

Concepts of interconnectedness alone are inadequate in portrayals of Chinese medicine, as numerous other cultures are also shaped by similar ideas identifying humans as being part of a singular mosaic of existence. Only in very recent years have some contemporary thinkers begun to show that the philosophical pillar that has given a distinctive character to the practice of classical Chinese medicine has been the general range of ideas known as Confucianism. Many in the West perceive the field of thought of Confucianism as being a prescriptive, restricting and stultifying force. Rather, in the Confucian tradition, implicit is the idea that self-cultivation or self-improvement enables a balance and a deep connection with the world that ultimately is the key to good health, both physical and psychological. The Jesuits trained spiritual warriors who identified themselves as servants of God above all. The Confucians trained spiritual adepts who identified themselves as servants principally of improving the human lot. This idea bypassed God. The significance of this way of thinking for understanding Chinese medicine is the idea that humans are not just hapless victims of whatever God decides to do with us, but that we can determine, or at least play a significant role in, our own health. Health largely depends on our own action and thoughts, while obviously not excluding unavoidable factors like genetics and unavoidable accidents. In other words, we have a say in the matter. This is the nub of it. The patient is not just a passive recipient, but also a key active agent in the healing process, this also being contingent upon how one relates to the external environment, and most importantly the human environment.

Buddhism's impact on medical thought in China has also been of huge significance.[28] This area of thought with its notions of mindfulness reinforces the idea that humans are active and significant agents in determining health, whether by lifestyle or by discipline of the mind.

Many of the ideas implicit in the practice of Chinese medicine are not discussed in texts of Chinese medicine. This is because most of the ideas were unspoken assumptions embedded in a general Chinese view of the world and its phenomena. In more contemporary times, this omission of key concepts in texts can be attributed to the categorisation of medicine as somehow separate from everyday life and phenomena.

The key ideas in Chinese medicine derive from the *Yellow Emperor's Inner Canon*. A key concept therein, *yin yang*, cannot be understood without some understanding of many aspects of Chinese philosophy such as Confucianism and Daoism. Most germane in this regard is correlative and contextual thinking.

Qi is often translated into English as some type of energy force or power. This does not quite capture the meaning of *qi*. The idea of energy approaches the meaning but does not capture the universality and ubiquity of *qi*. It also does not capture the infinitesimal variety in permutations of *qi*. Yet others, especially eminent philosophers in Chinese history, described *qi* as a moral force.[29] *Qi* can only be understood in context. The description of *qi* as the power of God without God may be approaching heresy, but is one way of attempting to understand this concept. *Qi* is everything with all phenomena depending on *qi*. Key is the idea of understanding the configuration of the universe as one whole with the health of the individual intimately tied to that whole.

Yin yang theory has guided Chinese thought for millennia and remains a bedrock idea in Chinese medicine, as much as it ever was. It contains the idea of seeking balance and harmony in everything. Rather than describing a duality in things, it is a way of seeing multiple possibilities in one entity. It enables an entry point into balancing the human body. In the spirit of Ockham's razor, some patients will be said to have too much heat, causing, in turn, discomfort or disease. Simply put, regardless of the label attached to the medical condition, treatment whether by herbs or acupuncture will aim to cool the patient down. This is not to refer to body temperature in the commonly understood sense, but rather a subjective feeling of heat caused by an imbalance of *qi*. This cooling may be done by prescribing directly cooling herbs, or by herbs that harmonise imbalance, there not being just one available strategy.

Immediately prior to the onset of pedagogical modernity in China, every child who received an education started with a primer known as the *San Zi Jing*. This primer served to instil the idea of generalist knowledge as the key to understanding any particularity. Its premise leaves us with the plea that one must first know the nature of the world before one can understand the Chinese conceptualisation of health and medicine. To compartmentalise or to categorise is to miss the essence of a problem, based as it is in totality.

It also needs to be mentioned that as part of *Inner Canon* thinking there was the concept of *wu xing* — with its idea of analysing the world with reference to five phases or elements: wood, fire, earth, metal and water. These alignments, while never being fixed, relate to various aspects of the body and mind. Earth, for example, is said to be related to the spleen and the colour yellow among a host of other correspondences.

While the *Inner Canon* provided bedrock ideas, Chinese medicine has evolved during many centuries of change and development. Despite the transformations wrought by time and experience, a feature of contemporary practice is that many books written centuries ago are still referred to as valuable reference material. One text that is constantly referred to and that is used as a guide by many in the field is *Shang Han Lun* or *On Cold Damage* written by Zhang Zhongjing nearly two millennia ago.[30] Zhang built on the *Inner Canon* to devise a more elaborate and complex system to treat many difficult diseases. Dozens of his formulations are still used routinely by many practitioners on a daily basis.

In the 18th century and onwards another complex approach to treatment, known as *Wen Bing*, was devised by a number of doctors.[31] As in the legacy of Zhang Zhongjing, these formulations are commonly used today. Many of these formulas are used to treat complex cases, both chronic and acute. It is not widely known that

Chinese medicine was the most efficacious form of medicine during the SARS crisis of 2003 and that formulas such as those from the *Wen Bing* were the most popular.

DIAGNOSTIC TECHNIQUES

The diagnostic techniques commonly used by contemporary practitioners are described as looking, listening/smelling, asking and touching. Employing the senses, the practitioner makes an assessment of the patient's condition according to a comprehensive picture of the person as a whole. Probably key among these diagnostic methods are observing the face of the patient and feeling of the pulse. Assessing the pulse employs a complex system that requires years of learning and experience. The radial pulse is felt at the wrist crease to assess the state of the patient's *qi*. Three positions are felt on each arm, each position representing a different part of the body. The pulse is then felt at different depths after applying pressure with the three fingers. By assessing the state of a person's *qi* the well-trained practitioner may identify disease or imbalance of *qi* and *yin yang* well before disease manifests. In this regard, Chinese medicine places great emphasis on preventative medicine, in addition to curing disease.

CONCLUSION

Chinese medicine is growing in popularity on a global scale. In the hands of trained practitioners it is a safe, effective and powerful medicine. Derived as it is from Chinese thought, it is representative of a profound philosophical approach based on empirical evidence.

In China and Korea it is very much a part of the respective national health systems. Outside its heartland in East Asia it is becoming integrated into various health systems. As an example, the Davidoff Comprehensive Cancer Centre in Beilinson Hospital in Tel Aviv, Israel, operates an Integrative Medicine Unit for cancer patients.[32] This unit includes a team of practitioners of Chinese medicine who provide herbal and acupuncture treatment alongside the more conventional medical treatment. Could this be the seed of other such units across the world? Evidence points to the likelihood of this. This could be said to be part of the quest for gentleness and balance in medical treatment.

ACKNOWLEDGEMENTS

I would like to thank Professor Ian Olver for his support and assistance while I prepared this text.

REFERENCES

1. Kaptchuk TJ. *Chinese Medicine: The Web That Has No Weaver,* 2nd edn, Contemporary Books, New York (2000).
2. Ellis A, Wiseman N, Boss K. *Fundamentals of Chinese Acupuncture,* Paradigm Publications, Brookline (1991).
3. Maciocia G. *The Foundations of Chinese Medicine: A Comprehensive Text for Acupuncturists and Herbalists,* 2nd edn, Churchill Livingstone, Oxford (2005).
4. Beinfeld H, Korngold E. *Between Heaven and Earth: A Guide to Chinese Medicine,* Ballantine Books, New York (1992).
5. Ross J. *Zang Fu: The Organ Systems of Traditional Medicine,* 2nd edn, Churchill Livingstone, Oxford (1986).
6. Liu Y. *The Essential Book of Traditional Chinese Medicine,* 2nd edn, Columbia University Press, New York (1995).
7. Porkert M. *Theoretical Foundations of Chinese Medicine,* MIT Press, Cambridge (1978).
8. Wu. *Yellow Emperor's Canon Internal Medicine* (translated), China Science and Technology Press, Beijing (2005).
9. Ni M. *The Yellow Emperor's Classic of Medicine* (translated), Shambhala, Boston (1995).
10. Li Z, Liu X. *Yellow Emperor's Canon of Medicine: Plain Conversation,* World Books Publishing, Beijing (2005).
11. Lu H. *A Complete Translation of the Yellow Emperor's Classic of Internal Medicine and the Difficult Classic,* 2nd edn, International College of Traditional Chinese Medicine, Vancouver (2009).
12. Sivin N. Drawing insights from Chinese medicine. In Lai K (ed), *New Interdisciplinary Perspectives in Chinese Philosophy,* no. 34, pp. 43–55 (2007).

13. Scheid V. *Chinese Medicine in Contemporary China: Plurality and Synthesis,* Duke University Press, Durham (2002).
14. Lloyd GE, Sivin N. *The Way and the Word: Science and Medicine in Early China and Greece,* Yale University Press, New Haven (2002).
15. Scheid V. *Currents of Tradition in Chinese Medicine 1626–2006,* Eastland Press, Seattle (2007).
16. Wang J. *A Life History of Ren Yingqiu; Historical Problems, Mythology, Continuity, Difference in Chinese Medical Modernity,* University of North Carolina, Chapel Hill (2003).
17. Guo Y. *Cultural Nationalism in Contemporary China,* Routledge Curzon, London (2004).
18. *Australia's Health Workforce Online* [Accessed 4 January 2010]. http://www.nhwt.gov.au/natreg.asp.
19. Ryckmans P. The Chinese attitude towards the past. In *China Heritage Quarterly,* no. 14 (2008). <http://www.chinaheritagequarterly.org/articles.php?searchterm=014_chineseAttitude.inc&issue=014> [Accessed 22 August 2009].
20. Bensky D, Clavey S, Stoger E. *Materia Medica: Chinese Herbal Medicine,* 3rd edn, Eastland Press, Seattle (2004).
21. Lei SH. From Changshan to a new anti-malarial drug: re-networking Chinese drugs and excluding Chinese doctors. In *The Social Studies of Science,* Vol. 29, no. 3, pp. 323–358 (1999).
22. Deadman P, Baker K, Al-Khafaji M. *A Manual of Acupuncture,* Journal of Chinese Medicine, London (1998).
23. Rossi E. *Shen, Psycho-Emotional Aspects of Chinese Medicine,* Churchill Livingstone, Oxford (2007).
24. Lu HC. *Chinese System of Food Cures: Prevention and Remedies,* Sterling, Chalvey (1986).
25. Keji C. From emperors to fisheyes: a conversation about Chinese medicine with Dr Chen Keji, in *Heaven Earth, The Chinese Art of Living,* Vol. 2, no. 1 (1992).
26. Hall DL, Ames RT. *Anticipating China,* State University of New York Press, Albany (1995).
27. Cua AS. *The Unity of Knowledge and Action: A Study in Wang Yang-ming's Moral Psychology,* University of Hawaii Press, Honolulu (1982).
28. Unschuld P. *Medicine in China A History of Ideas,* University of California Press, Berkeley, pp. 132–148 (1985).

29. Flowers J. What is Qi? In *Evidence-Based Complementary and Alternative Medicine*, Vol. 4, no. 3 (2006). *http://ecam.oxfordjournals.org/cgi/content/full/3/4/551* [Accessed 21 August 2009].
30. Mitchell C, Ye F, Wiseman N. *Shang Han Lun on Cold Damage*, Paradigm Publications, Brookline (1999).
31. Liu G. *Warm Diseases A Clinical Guide*, Eastland Press, Seattle (2001).
32. *Rabin Medical Centre*. http://www.clalit.org.il/rabin/Content/Content.asp?CID=618&u=2501 [Accessed 4 February 2010].

6

Disentangling the Evidence: The Efficacy of Meditation in People with Cancer

**Deborah Black,
Leigh Wilson and
Ramesh Manocha**

ABSTRACT

Meditation is often used as an adjunct to medical therapies by people who have cancer. There has long been a debate in both the medical and lay communities about the therapeutic use of meditation, and whether its use has any impact on quality of life, pain relief and long-term survival in people who have cancer. This chapter examines, in detail, the scientific research investigating the effects of meditation in people who have cancer. Also reported are the experiences of health practitioners and cancer survivors who use meditation as part of cancer therapy. In conclusion, the chapter makes recommendations for future research strategies, based on the current available evidence.

Keywords: Meditation; Cancer; Quality of Life; Pain.

INTRODUCTION

Increasingly, complementary therapies that focus on mind–body medicine are used alongside traditional medical therapies in people who have cancer.[1] In spite of the increase in popularity of complementary therapies, there has long been a debate about their efficacy in the management of cancer symptoms, effect on quality of life and possible relationship to long-term survival and/or cancer recurrence.[2] Included in the mind–body medicine group are many complementary therapies including: yoga, tai chi, biofeedback, hypnosis, guided imagery, art therapy, light therapy and others.[3]

One of the most commonly used complementary therapies is meditation — an ancient practice used in some parts of the world for more than 5000 years.[4] The word meditation is derived from the Latin *meditari*, which means 'to engage in contemplation or reflection'.[5]

WHAT IS MEDITATION?

The scientific literature characterises meditation in a number of different ways, and there is no clear consensus on a definition of meditation. Of the many taxonomies proposed by various scholars, we use the following for the purposes of discussion in this chapter. We broadly categorise meditation into two main types: (1) "narrow focus" meditation, where practitioners focus on regulation of the breath, mental stillness or some other factor as a method of obtaining a deep state of calm and mental quiet and (2) "broad focus" meditation such as in mindfulness, where practitioners direct their attention at a broad field of sensory input. Simultaneously, practitioners attempt to minimise mental or emotional reactions to those sensory inputs.

Narrow focus meditation can include techniques such as: (1) transcendental meditation (TM)[6,7] and (2) the relaxation response. The relaxation response can be understood as a modern adaptation of a simple yogic breathing technique; however, Benson, who developed the method, emphasises that it is a universal phenomenon embedded in many different religious and cultural traditions. Proponents claim that they facilitate positive transformation of human consciousness.[8,9] Although meditation and relaxation are commonly grouped together, there are researchers who highlight the differences between the mental silence of meditation and the somatic arousal reduction effects of relaxation.[9] Benson's theory of the relaxation response arose from initial studies of TM practitioners. He later realised that the same physiological and psychological phenomena could be elicited by simple relaxation methods.[10] He found that associated with meditation and relaxation were a range of physiological changes to the body including: decreased oxygen consumption, heart rate, respiratory rate, arterial blood lactate and an increase in the frequency and intensity of alpha and theta brain waves. Benson proposed that this decreased sympathetic nervous system activity acted to antagonise the flight-or-fight response, and therefore reduced overall body stress.[10]

Mindfulness meditation has gained prominence in Western medicine over the past decade. It is most frequently associated with the Mindfulness-Based Stress Reduction (MBSR) programmes developed by Jon Kabat-Zinn.[3,11] The earliest MBSR programmes were in oncology settings at the Massachusetts Cancer Treatment Centre. They are a multimodal strategy involving not only meditation, but also conventional strategies for reducing stress, as well as general advice on how to experience life more fully, being in touch with emotions.[2,12] Mindfulness meditation is primarily concerned with the concept of non-judgemental, non-reactive acceptance, broad focus attention and controlling one's responses to stressful situations.[13] Unlike TM or relaxation-based meditation, the primary aim of the mindfulness technique is not relaxation, although a relaxed state may result.[2]

Meditation has been studied in a range of medical conditions — most commonly hypertension, heart disease, depression and irritable bowel syndrome. The number of randomised controlled trials is limited, particularly in the field of adjuvant cancer therapy.[14] The lack of high-level medical evidence has resulted in a vigorous debate that continues around the efficacy and usefulness of meditation-based therapies in people who have cancer.[5,15]

THE MEDITATION RESEARCH DEBATE

Conducting research into meditation in any chronic illness brings with it many challenges and limitations.[5,16] The challenges in conducting randomised controlled trials of meditation use are highlighted by the difficulties associated with allocation concealment, double blinding and allocation to a technique that is prevalent in popular culture, available in most cities and discussed widely in the media.[5,15] This is particularly the case in people with cancer, where evidence suggests that this group (particularly women), are more likely to use complementary therapies such as meditation to try to cure or increase cancer survival, or to relieve symptoms of the disease and the associated treatments.[16–20] In view of the difficulties associated with conducting research that provides high-level evidence, the majority of studies investigating meditation are neither randomised nor experimental, and are more likely to be case-control studies, observational studies or case reports.[5,15,18,19]

The most comprehensive and recent review of research into meditation was published in 2007 by a team from the University of Alberta's (Canada) Evidence-Based Practice Center.[5] This review investigated over 800 studies of meditation used in a range of medical conditions, and highlighted the heterogeneity of study participants, the diverse methods of recruitment and the variety of outcome measures studied, particularly in people with cancer.[5,15] One of the challenges in investigating research into the effects of meditation in people with cancer is the confusion with regard to how to precisely define the independent variable 'meditation'.[9] In some studies, meditation refers to traditional Eastern-type concentration meditation and in others, the mindfulness-based stress reduction approach or a combination of the two methods. The differences in definition and research methods probably account for much of the inconsistency in the results of the research undertaken in meditation and mindfulness programmes.[5,9,18]

Breast, prostate, colorectal and lung cancers are currently the leading cause of cancer deaths in Australia and around the world.[20] The majority of studies into meditation used by people with cancer have been undertaken in two main groups; (1) those with clearly defined breast or prostate cancers and (2) those with a primary cancer of unknown origin.[17] Evidence suggests that many patients wish to take control of their cancer management.[17,21] The type of management strategies (for disease progression and symptom relief) used by people with cancer differs depending on a range of factors including: type of cancer, prognosis, personality traits, educational and socio-economic status, physical ability and lifestyle choices.[2,13,22] These factors, in conjunction with the use of multiple and often overlapping complementary therapies, differences in outcome measurement and inconsistencies in definitions of meditation, make well-defined, accurate and reliable research almost impossible. Teasing out the factors that influence a person with cancer to use meditation is also an extremely difficult task in view of these interacting variables.

THE AUSTRALIAN EXPERIENCE

One of the earliest practitioners of meditation in Australia was Dr Ainslie Meares, a psychiatrist who used meditation and hypnosis in a range of chronic conditions. In 1976, he reported a case of cancer regression that he attributed to intensive meditation in the *Medical Journal of Australia*.[23] At 30-year follow-up, the patient was still alive and in remission.[24] Meares' method of meditation did not include mental imagery, but focused purely on mental relaxation, stillness and quiet.

In Australia, practitioners such as Ian Gawler and Petrea King (both cancer survivors) have designed programmes focusing on the positive effects of living healthily and using meditation as a positive aid to living with cancer.[25,26] In a personal interview with the founder of the Quest for Life Foundation, Petrea King stresses that meditation is not a way of avoiding death or curing cancer, but a technique that enables people with cancer to quieten the mind, disentangle thoughts and live life in a more conscious and aware state.[25] Programmes run by the Quest for Life Foundation use meditation to quieten the mind, enabling participants to focus on four key aspects of dealing with cancer. In brief, these are: (1) responding, rather than reacting, to a diagnosis of cancer; (2) finding peace in the present moment — thereby making a commitment to living, and communicating effectively with self and others; (3) identifying and taking on the challenge in life that gives life purpose and meaning; and (4) developing a sense of connectedness — to self, community, friends and spirit.[25] Although there has been no research into the survival outcomes associated with the Quest for Life Foundation programme, King stated that many people with cancer who participate in these programmes live far longer than either predicted at diagnosis, or anticipated by clinicians based on clinical evidence.[25] Although these claims have not been tested in clinical trials, there is no doubt that many cancer sufferers appear to find comfort and support in such programmes. Similar results have been noted in programmes conducted by the Gawler Foundation in Melbourne. Founder and cancer survivor Ian Gawler uses meditation as a major component of the programmes run by the Gawler Foundation, and focuses on the strength of the mind–body connection. In a personal interview, Gawler comments on the three key areas of cancer therapy, defining them as: conventional (medical and surgical), complementary and lifestyle therapies.[26] In his view, meditation is a lifestyle choice rather than a complementary therapy, as it is able to be integrated into daily life, along with exercise, diet and other health behaviours.[26]

Research into the effects of meditation in people with cancer in an Australian context is limited. Case reports of remarkable survival in people experiencing advanced cancer were published in Australia as early as 1976.[23,27] Recent Australian studies have focused on the experience of women with breast cancer, and participants in the Gawler Foundation intervention programme for people with cancer.[28,29] These studies reported conflicting results when investigating the effects of mind–body lifestyle interventions, thereby continuing the debate around the efficacy of psychosocial interventions including meditation, particularly with regard to increased survival.

THE EXTANT EVIDENCE

Notwithstanding the issues impacting on the quality and reliability of the available evidence, the effects of meditation on quality of life, symptom relief and survival in people with cancer offer clinicians and researchers some insights that may be useful. MBSR programmes are more likely to be subject to rigorous investigation as compared with less Westernised methods. There is, however, considerable overlap in the types of mind–body interventions used and reported in both randomised and non-randomised trials.[5,22] Table 1 outlines the four randomised controlled studies found in our literature search.[30–33] Other studies in people with cancer are presented in Table 2.[29,34–40]

Table 1. RCT studies of meditation in people with cancer.

Author/ group	Population	Cancer type	Number of participants	Inclusion criteria	Study type	Meditation type	Outcome measure	Results	Comments	Ethics
RCT										
Monti *et al.*[30] ERA Level B	Hospital patients receiving treatment. Women aged 26–82.	Mixed: breast, gynaecological, haematological, neurological, rectal, others.	n = 111. 93 provided 8 week data. 45 in intervention group and 48 in control arm.	Receiving active treatment (chemotherapy, radiation, Tamoxifen) or for side-effects or other cancer-related procedures.	RCT	MBAT (8 weekly sessions, 2.5 h session).	Psychological distress, QoL (SCL-90, SF36 mental health component).	Subjects in MBAT intervention group had statistically significant reduction in distress, mental health, general health and vitality.	Cannot be generalised long-term.	Yes
Shapiro *et al.*[33] ERA Level A	Female, English-speaking hospital outpatients. Recruited from medical oncologist practices in Tucson, USA (38–77 years old).	Stage II breast cancer in remission	n = 63. 31 in MBSR group. 32 in free-choice control group.	Females, English-speaking with Stage II breast cancer in remission and within 2 years post-treatment.	RCT	MBSR programme weekly 2 h sessions for 6 weeks plus 6 h silent retreat.	Sleep diary. Pre- and post-POMS, BDI, FACIT-B and others.	No significant relationship between sleep and MBSR practice.	Randomisation methods unclear–part of larger study, not blinded, 12% controls and 16% treatment group lost to follow-up.	Yes

(*Continued*)

Table 1. *(Continued).*

Author/group	Population	Cancer type	Number of participants	Inclusion criteria	Study type	Meditation type	Outcome measure	Results	Comments	Ethics
Hebert *et al.*[32] ERA Level A	Hospital patients receiving treatment. Enrolled from four hospital sites.	Breast cancer stage I or II.	n = 172. 51 enrolled in meditation arm. 50 enrolled in dietary arm. 56 in usual care arm.	Ages between 20 and 65, diagnosed within the previous 2 years. Receiving active treatment (chemotherapy, radiation, Tamoxifen).	RCT	University of Massachusetts Stress Reduction Clinic Programme. 15 week sessions.	Body mass, 7DDR dietary fat, complex carbohydrates, fibre, self-esteem, mood.	Increases in self-esteem and self-efficacy. Weight loss in the dietary arm of the study and also meditation group.	Confounded by the dietary aspect of the study. Participants with weight issues experience other emotional factors.	Yes
Speca *et al.*[31] ERA Level A	Convenience sample — referred by clinicians and self through advertisements.	Breast, ovarian, prostate, NHL, melanoma, endometrial, colon, cervical, others.	n = 109 (90 completed, 73 women, 17 men). 53 treatment. 37 controls on waiting list (hospital outpatients).	Any patient having received a confirmed diagnosis of cancer at any time was eligible.	RCT	MBSR programme 7 weekly sessions plus home practice.	POMS and SOSI. Mood and stress.	No significant difference between treatment group and controls in levels of mood and stress.	Beneficial overall in general health and coping skills. Higher than average stress patients may seek out programmes of this type.	Consent gained, ethics not mentioned.

ERA: Excellence in research Australia journal ranking.
POMS: Profile of mood state.
SCL-90: Symptom check list (90 components).
SOSI: Symptoms of stress inventory.
FACIT-B: Functional assessment of chronic illness therapy–breast.
BDI: Beck depression inventory.
7DDR: 7 day dietary recall.
MBAT: Mindfulness-based at therapy.

Table 2. Non-RCT studies of meditation in people with cancer.

Author/group	Population	Cancer type	Number of participants	Inclusion criteria	Study type	Meditation type	Outcome measure	Results	Comments	Ethics
Non-RCT										
Carlson *et al.*[34] after Speca *et al.*[31] ERA Level C	Uncontrolled outcomes study of follow-up to Speca *et al.*[31] Convenience sample.	Breast, ovarian, prostate, NHL, melanoma endometrial, colon, cervical, others.	n = 54 (all had undergone intervention). 10 men 44 women.	As in Speca *et al.*	rCT follow-up.	MBSR programme practice follow-up.	POMS and SOSI mood and stress.	Mean POMS score decreased from 17.4 to 10.7. Small but non-significant decreases were observed in SOSI scores.	Other concomitant therapies not recorded or considered.	Informed consent, ethics not mentioned.
Saxe *et al.*[35] ERA Level A	Men with prostate cancer and their partners — recruitment by referral from oncologists.	Prostate	n = 10 men and their partners. Participants acted as own control before and after.	Diagnosed adenocarcinoma of the prostate, postprostatectomy, and increasing levels of PSA on >2 tests.	Longitudinal pre- and post-test.	MBSR programme 12 weekly classes of 3–4 h duration. Participants also followed plant-based diet.	Pre- and post-measures of diet, weight, physical activity and PSA levels.	PSA levels decreased in 8 participants. Mean doubling time of PSA increased from 6.5 to 17.7 months.	Uncontrolled. Diet precludes evaluation for effectiveness of meditation programme.	Not mentioned.

(*Continued*)

Table 2. (Continued).

Author/ group	Population	Cancer type	Number of participants	Inclusion criteria	Study type	Meditation type	Outcome measure	Results	Comments	Ethics
Majumdar *et al.*[36] ERA Level A	All with chronic illness (some had cancer). Aged 22–62 years. No controls.	NHL, breast (others had other chronic conditions not cancer).	$n = 21$. 17 women 4 men.	Open to all unless they were suicidal or currently psychotic.	Exploratory study longitudinal pre- and post-test.	MBSR programme 8 weekly sessions for 2.5 h plus 7 h silent retreat. Audio tapes provided.	Five questionnaires for physical symptoms, QoL and wellbeing. Post-intervention telephone interviews and questionnaire.	Statistically significant changes in emotional, general and physical wellbeing ($P \leq 0.001$ to $P \leq 0.047$) and QoL ($P \leq 0.001$ to $P \leq 0.002$).	Small sample size. Participants paid for the course themselves, compliance unknown.	Ethics committee approval not mentioned.
Carlson *et al.*[37] ERA Level B	Breast or prostate cancer sufferers, aged >18 and 3 months post-surgery. Volunteers and by invitation. No controls.	Breast, prostate.	$n = 59$ outpatients. Age range not stated — mean age 54.5 years.	Stage 0, I or II breast cancer or localised prostate cancer.	Longitudinal pre- and post-test.	MBSR programme 90 min weekly group sessions for 8 weeks plus 3 h silent retreat. Audio tapes provided.	POMS, SOSI, EORTC, QLQ-30. Health behaviour questionnaire including sleep and sleep quality. Blood and saliva samples for DHEAS and melatonin.	Significant improvement in QoL ($t = -2.23$, $P < 0.05$), stress ($t = 3.23$, $P < 0.01$) and sleep quality. No significant improvements in mood or immuno-stimulation.	No controls, no long-term follow-up.	Not mentioned.

(Continued)

Table 2. (Continued).

Author/group	Population	Cancer type	Number of participants	Inclusion criteria	Study type	Meditation type	Outcome measure	Results	Comments	Ethics
Garland *et al.*[38] ERA Level C	Self-selected patients over 18 years who spoke English and had a cancer diagnosis.	Breast, prostate, colorectal, lung, ear, nose/throat, brain, skin, lymphatic, others.	n = 60	Not specified.	Longitudinal pre- and post-test.	MBSR programme 8 weekly sessions each 1.5 h plus 3 h silent retreat.	PSQI, SOSI, POMS and physical health components.	Also investigated healing arts to MBSR, not randomised, significant improvement in spirituality and mood disturbance in MBSR group.	Waiting list control group, low rates of questionnaire completion, attrition from pre- to post-intervention and small sample size.	Yes
Carlson *et al.*[39] ERA Level B	Convenience sample — referred by clinicians and self through advertisements.	Breast, prostate, ovarian, NHL.	n = 63	Not specified.	Longitudinal pre- and post-test.	MBSR programme 8 weekly sessions each 90 min plus a 3 h silent retreat at week 6.	SOSI, FACIT-Sp (spirituality), POMS, physical health components.	Improvements in sleep quality, stress, mood and apparent fatigue levels in those with cancer.	No assessment of fatigue and no follow-up.	Informed consent but no ethics approval.

(*Continued*)

Table 2. *(Continued)*.

Author/ group	Population	Cancer type	Number of participants	Inclusion criteria	Study type	Meditation type	Outcome measure	Results	Comments	Ethics
Tacon *et al.*[13] ERA Level C	Hospital patients and medical practices and cancer support groups — self-selected. Aged 30–75 years.	Breast	n = 27.	In active treatment.	Longitudinal pre- and post-test.	MBSR programme for 8 weeks, 90 min session.	Mental adjustment (MAC) and health locus of control (MHLC).	Significant reduction in stress and anxiety scores after the 8 week programme.	No controls.	Consent but no ethics approval.
Reavely *et al.*[29] ERA Level A	Participants in the Gawler Foundation programme. Age range 23–78 mean age 51.3.	Mixed cancers — 60% had metastatic disease.	n = 112. 75 women 37 men.	6.3% never had active treatment. 38.4% undergoing active treatment. 47.3% currently no treatment.	Longitudinal cohort study.	10 day residential programme with follow-up at 3, 6 and 12 months.	POMS, Mini-MAC, FACIT-Sp.	Mini Mac scores showed improved coping skills post-intervention. Improved QoL in those who had low QoL at outset.	No control group with which to compare.	Yes

ERA: Excellence in research Australia journal ranking.
POMS: Profile of mood state.
SOSI: Symptoms of stress inventory.

Effects of Meditation on Quality of Life and Wellbeing

Quality of life and/or wellbeing are outcomes measured in almost all randomised and non-randomised controlled studies of meditation in cancer reported in the literature.[5] In almost all of the studies in our review, research undertaken in people with prostate and breast cancer showed that participants have a significant reduction in stress levels associated with cancer, improvements in quality of life and sleep, and a decrease in distress levels correlating to the amount of time spent in meditation daily.[29,31–34,37,40] Mindfulness meditation has been specifically shown to relieve anxiety, stress, fatigue, sleep disturbance and general mood disorders, thereby improving overall quality of life.[1,22] In a study investigating participants in the Gawler Foundation programme, Reavley and colleagues found that participation in the programme significantly improved mood, coping skills and quality of life in patients with cancer.[29] This was particularly the case in participants whose emotional wellbeing and quality of life were low on entry into the programmes, and is proposed to be due to the effects of meditation in reducing anxiety and improving wellbeing. A limitation of many of the studies undertaken in people with cancer was that they did not have a control group, thereby limiting the reliability of the response shift over time.[5,29,35]

Effects of Meditation on Cancer Pain

Pain, fatigue and sleep disturbance are amongst the most common symptoms experienced by people with cancer.[41,42] Approximately 59% of people receiving treatment for cancers and 64% of people undergoing treatment for advanced, metastatic or terminal disease experience pain.[41] Pain, stress and difficulties in coping were the key reasons that medical practitioners originally focused research into meditation and mindfulness.[43] Although there are many studies investigating the effects of meditation (especially MBSR) on pain in chronic illness, the research in patients with cancer is limited.[5,14,44] Ludwig suggests that a reduction in pain through meditation practice could be related to a decrease in perception of pain, or an increased ability to tolerate pain.[43] In other chronic pain studies, mindfulness meditation has been shown to reduce the perception of pain by as much as 50% compared with a control group.[11] In a systematic review of the literature investigating the pain–fatigue–sleep disturbance clustering of symptoms in people with cancer, Kwekkeboom and colleagues found that meditation and relaxation therapies may offer benefit to patients suffering pain in association with fatigue and sleep disturbances.[42] The benefits of these therapies are that most people are able to undertake them, as they require little physical effort. On a more negative note, people who are very ill or experiencing a high degree of pain may not be able to sustain the concentration required to effectively carry out concentration-type meditation exercises and may derive more benefit from mindfulness and relaxation approaches.[2]

Practising Meditation and Cancer Survival

Many of the early studies into meditation and cancer report small-scale, correlational and anecdotal studies where patients participating in mind–body medicine such as meditation experienced improved survival or remission.[24,27] In an early study of meditation and psychosocial support, Spiegel found that patients with cancer who undertook their intervention lived longer than those who did not.[45] Other early case reports described remarkable survival in patients who displayed particular psychological characteristics, such as: a fighting spirit, acceptance of their cancer and engagement and authentic living.[46–48] Attempts to replicate these findings in subsequent studies failed to generate the same outcomes. In the 1980s a number of randomly controlled trials (RCTs) investigated the use of meditation associated with psychosocial support, such as support groups and group therapy, with mixed results.[49–51] There are no studies that definitively link meditation, relaxation or MBSR with an increased survival in people with cancer, although some studies do conclude by suggesting that there is potential for increased longevity in certain patients, based on the type of cancer, psychological status and amount of meditation undertaken daily. Monti and colleagues propose the potential role of mind–body therapies in cancer survivorship by highlighting the increasing numbers of cancer survivors who use complementary medicine, particularly in the post-treatment phase.[52] In separate interviews, both Petrea King and Ian Gawler cite numerous case studies of people with cancer far outliving their expected lifespan, and/or experiencing complete remission from cancer as a result of mind–body medicine programmes that include meditation.[25,26] Gawler Foundation senior therapist Paul Bedson states that meditation and other healthy lifestyle choices contribute to a renewed body balance, enabling the patient to think clearly and consciously about their approach to life, dealing with cancer and living each day to the best of their ability.[53] It should be noted that these hypotheses have not been tested with rigorous scientific studies.

The Burden of Guilt Associated with Non-Treatment

All patients have the choice whether to use complementary therapies (including meditation) as part of their cancer therapy. Although a large number of patients do try at least some complementary therapies, others choose not to undertake any treatment.[45] Spiegel suggests that this may be for a number of reasons, including the feelings of personal guilt associated with the non-efficacy of treatment and re-emergence of cancer or fear of the side-effects associated with treatment.[45] Quest for Life Foundation founder Petrea King comments that a person's decision not to undertake treatment (whether conventional medical treatment or complementary) is often more difficult on the family and relatives than the person themselves.[25] Deciding to forego treatment can place additional stress on the person with cancer if their family react negatively to this decision. In this instance, the patient is made to feel guilty for not embarking on any treatment that in the eyes of the family may 'make them better'.[25]

The Medical Profession and Meditation Therapy

Following the published research of Kabat-Zinn and others at major cancer treatment centres in the USA, support for MBSR programmes and broader-based meditation practice to assist people with cancer has increased in the medical profession worldwide. Initially sceptical of the impact and efficacy of many complementary therapies, medical practitioners would dissuade patients from undertaking therapies considered alternative. Medical practitioners probably feel less threatened by the concept of meditation because it is non-invasive, non-pharmacological and does not conflict with mainstream treatments. Although many medical practitioners now perceive meditation as mainstream and acceptable as a health-care strategy, it is still a poorly understood discipline.[9,54] Many oncologists experience difficulty in discussing options for alternative therapies that patients may find useful. This is particularly the case for meditation, where research evidence is limited. Cancer survivors Petrea King and Ian Gawler each suggest that meditation should be viewed as a lifestyle choice, rather like exercise or diet, and should not be viewed as complementary therapy (which suggests taking herbal therapy or pills).[25,26] This approach may make it easier for people with cancer and their treating physicians to discuss a range of positive health choices that may assist the patient to manage their disease with a sense of empowerment.

CONCLUSION

Although there is a dearth of quantitative research into meditation as an adjunct therapy in cancer treatment, there are a number of studies that provide reasonable evidence that levels of distress are reduced and quality of life, sleep and general wellbeing are improved by the use of meditation.[29,30,32,40] There remains limited evidence on the effect of meditation on levels of pain in people with cancer and the effect of meditation on long-term survival and health outcomes.[5,55] One of the most difficult aspects of conducting research into meditation in people with cancer is the inability to conduct double-blind randomised controlled trials in a group of patients with identical characteristics.[18,19] In the absence of definitive evidence for benefit, withholding treatment such as meditation in a randomised controlled trial in the case of cancer may be ethically questionable. The recent increase in the number of research grants for studies investigating mind–body medicine in a range of chronic conditions, and the increased number of studies into meditation, highlights the research commitment in this area. A search of the peer-reviewed literature using the terms 'cancer' and 'meditation' combined highlights the increase in research articles over time (Fig. 1). Although there is an increase in research, the results of the effects of meditation on cancer outcomes are still equivocal.

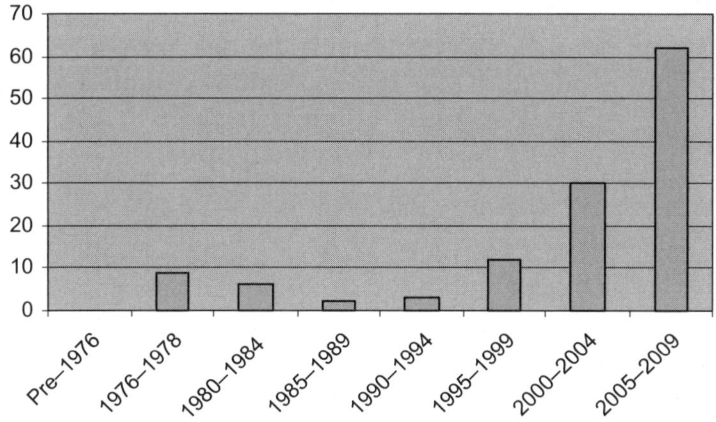

Fig. 1. Number of research articles using search term 'cancer and meditation' published in peer-reviewed literature 1976–2009.

Future researchers examining the efficacy of meditation for people with cancer will find it almost impossible to isolate the effects of meditation in cancer patients for two main reasons. Firstly, in a recent as yet unpublished thesis, Manocha provides evidence that, in long-term practitioners of meditation, the *number* of times that one meditates does not provide the same effect as the depth or quality of the experience.[54] The association between quality meditation (described more accurately as 'thoughtlessness awareness') was clearly demonstrated in Manocha's study and was measured using the SF36. The frequency of thoughtlessness awareness had a significant positive impact on a number of the SF36 subscales relating to mental health. Therefore, the outward practice of meditation may not have the same impact as the inner experience, particularly if the meditation does not provide a high degree of thoughtlessness awareness.[54] Secondly, if, as Gawler suggests, meditation is a lifestyle choice rather than a complementary therapy, cancer survivors who undertake meditation are very likely to undertake other positive lifestyle choices such as good diet, exercise and not smoking. Results of research in this group are therefore likely to be affected by these confounders.

There is a need, and a recommendation, for future research that compares cases of specific cancers to a clearly defined and well-matched control group. A study of this type must have sufficient power to detect a difference in any possible effect of meditation on long-term survival or remission and should incorporate any potential confounding variables, such as other complementary therapies, which may be used by study participants. The ethical dilemma of asking study participants with cancer not to try other therapies that may give them hope, or pain relief, while part of a study is very real and is partially the reason why there are so many studies that are longitudinal, uncontrolled and have a poorly defined study population.

REFERENCES

1. Bonnadonna R. Meditation's impact on chronic illness. *Hol Nurs Pract* **17**:309–319 (2003).
2. Ott MJ, *et al.* Mindfulness meditation for oncology patients: a discussion and critical review. *Integr Cancer Ther* **5**:98–108 (2006).
3. Barrows KA, Jacobs BP. Mind–body medicine: an introduction and review of the literature. *Med Clin North Am* **86**:11–31 (2002).
4. Walters JD. *The Art and Science of Raja Yoga: Fourteen Steps to Higher Awareness*, Motilal Banarsidass (2002).
5. University of Alberta Evidence-Based Practice Center. *Meditation Practices for Health: State of the Research*, University of Alberta, Edmonton, Alberta, Canada (2007).
6. National Cancer Institute Cancer Statistics Branch. U.S. Department of Health and Human Services. National Cancer Institute Cancer Incidence–Surveillance Evaluation and End Results (SEER) Registries Limited Use (2008).
7. Kornfield J. *A Path with Heart: A Guide Through the Perils and Promises of Spiritual Life*, Bantam Books (1993).
8. Kornfield J. *Buddhist Meditation and Consciousness Research*, Basic Books (1992).
9. Manocha R. Why meditation? *Aust Fam Physician* **29**:1135–1138 (2000).
10. Benson H, Beary JF, Carol MP. The relaxation response. *Psychiatry* **37**:37–46 (1974).
11. Kabat-Zinn JMA, Kristeller J, Peterson LG, *et al.* Effectiveness of a meditation-based stress reduction program in the treatment of anxiety disorders. *Am J Psych* **149**:936–943 (1992).

12. Kabat-Zinn J. An outpatient program in behavioural medicine for chronic pain patients based on the practice of mindfulness meditation: theoretical considerations and preliminary results. *Gen Hosp Psychiatry* **4**:33–47 (1982).
13. Tacon AM. Meditation as a complementary therapy in cancer. *Fam Comm Health* **26**:64–73 (2003).
14. Orme-Johnson DW. Commentary on the AHRQ Report on Research on Meditation Practices in Health. *J Altern Complement Med* **14**:1215–1221 (2008).
15. Shannahoff-Khalsa D. The complications of meditation trials and research: issues raised by the Robinson, Mathews and Witek-Janusek paper — "Psycho-endocrine-immune response to mindfulness based stress reduction in individuals infected with the human immunodeficiency virus: a quasiexperimental study". *J Altern Complement Med* **9**:603–605 (2003).
16. Rees RW, Feigel I, Vickers A, *et al.* Prevalence of complementary therapy use by women with breast cancer: a population based survey. *Eur J Cancer* **36**:1359–1364 (2000).
17. Smith JE, *et al.* Mindfulness-based stress reduction as supportive therapy in cancer care: systematic review [erratum appears in *J Adv Nurs* **53**(5):618 (2006)]. *J Adv Nurs* **52**:315–327 (2005).
18. Bottomley A. To randomise or not to randomise: methodological pitfalls of the RCT design in psychosocial intervention studies. *Eur J Cancer Care* **6**:222–230 (1997).
19. Efficace F, Bottomley A, Vanvoorden V, *et al.* Methodological issues in assessing health-related quality of life of colorectal cancer patients in randomised controlled trials. *Eur J Cancer* **40**:187–197 (2004).
20. Australian Institute for Health and Welfare. *Australia's People*, Canberra (2006).
21. Cassileth B, Chapman C. Alternative and complementary cancer therapies. *Cancer* **77**:1026–1034 (1996).
22. Ledesma D, Kumano H, Ledesma D, *et al.* Mindfulness-based stress reduction and cancer: a meta-analysis. *Psychooncology* **18**:571–579 (2009).
23. Meares A. Regression of osteogenic sarcoma metastases associated with intensive meditation. *Med J Aust* **2**:433 (1978).
24. Jelinek GA, Gawler RH. Thirty-year follow-up at pneumonectomy of a 58 year old survivor of dissiminated osteosarcoma. *Med J Aust* **189**:663–665 (2008).

25. King P. *Meditation and Cancer: An Interview with Petrea King*, Sydney (2010).
26. Gawler I. *Meditation and Cancer: An Interview with Ian Gawler*, Sydney (2010).
27. Meares A. What can a patient expect from intensive meditation? *Aust Fam Physician* **9**:322–325 (1980).
28. Phillips KA, *et al*. Psychosocial factors and survival of young women with breast cancer: a population-based prospective cohort study. *J Clin Oncol* **26**:4666–4671 (2008).
29. Reavley N, *et al*. Evaluation of the effects of a psychosocial intervention on mood, coping, and quality of life in cancer patients. *Integr Cancer Ther* **8**:47–55 (2009).
30. Monti D, Peterson C, Shakin Kunkel EJ, *et al*. A randomized controlled trial of mindfulness based art therapy (MBAT) for women with cancer. *Psychooncology* **15**:363–373 (2006).
31. Speca M, Carlson LE, Goodey E, *et al*. A randomized, wait-list controlled clinical trial: the effect of a mindfulness meditation-based stress reduction program on mood and symptoms of stress in cancer outpatients. *Psychosom Med* **62**:613–622 (2000).
32. Hebert J, Ebbeling CB, Olendzki BC, *et al*. Change in women's diet and body mass following intensive intervention for early stage breast cancer. *J Am Diet Assoc* **101**:421–431 (2001).
33. Shapiro S, Bootzin RR, Figueredo AJ, *et al*. The efficacy of mindfulness-based stress reduction in the treatment of sleep disturbance in women with breast cancer: an exploratory study. *J Psychosom Res* **54**:85–91 (2003).
34. Carlson LE, Ursuliak Z, Goodey E, *et al*. The effects of a mindfulness meditation-based stress reduction program on mood and symptoms of stress in cancer outpatients: 6-month follow-up. *Support Care Cancer* **9**:112–123 (2001).
35. Saxe GA, Hebert JA, Carmody JF, *et al*. Can diet in conjunction with stress reduction affect the rate of increase in prostate specific antigen after biochemical recurrence of prostate cancer? *J Urol* **166**:2202–2207 (2001).
36. Majumdar M, Grossman P, Dietz-Washkowski B, *et al*. Does mindfulness meditation contribute to health? Outcome evaluation of a German sample. *J Altern Complement Med* **8**:719–730 (2002).
37. Carlson LE, *et al*. Mindfulness-based stress reduction in relation to quality of life, mood, symptoms of stress and levels of cortisol,

dehydroepiandrosterone sulfate (DHEAS) and melatonin in breast and prostate cancer outpatients. *Psychoneuroendocrinology* **29**:448–474 (2004).

38. Garland SN, Carlson LE, Cook S, *et al.* A non-randomised comparison of mindfulness based stress reduction and healing arts programs for facilitating post-traumatic growth and spirituality in cancer outpatients. *Support Cancer Care* **15**:949–961 (2007).
39. Carlson LE, Garland SN, Carlson LE, *et al.* Impact of mindfulness-based stress reduction (MBSR) on sleep, mood, stress and fatigue symptoms in cancer outpatients. *Int J Behav Med* **12**:278–285 (2005).
40. Tacon A, Caldera YM, Ronaghan C. Mindfulness-based stress reduction in women with breast cancer. *Fam Syst Health* **22**:193–203 (2004).
41. van den Beuken-van Everdingen MHJ, de Rijke JM, Kessels AG, *et al.* Prevalence of pain in patients with cancer: a systematic review of the last 40 years. *Ann Oncol* **18**:1437–1449 (2007).
42. Kwekkeboom K, Cherwin CH, Lee JW, *et al.* Mind-body treatments for the pain-fatigue-sleep disturbance symptom cluster in persons with cancer. *J Pain Symptom Manage* **39**:126–138 (2010).
43. Ludwig DS, Kabat-Zinn J. Mindfulness in medicine. *JAMA* **300**:1350–1352 (2008).
44. Deng G, Cassileth BR, Deng G, *et al.* Integrative oncology: complementary therapies for pain, anxiety, and mood disturbance. *CA: Cancer J Clin* **55**:109–116 (2005).
45. Spiegel D. Can psychotherapy prolong cancer survival? *Psychosomatics* **31**:361–366 (1990).
46. Hubscher R. Spontaneous remission: an example of health promotion. *Nurs Pract Forum* **3**:228–235 (1992).
47. Roud PC. Psychosocial variables associated with the exceptional survival of patients with advanced malignant disease. *Int J Psychiatry Med* **16**:113–122 (1986).
48. Berland W. Can the self affect the course of cancer? *Mind-Body Med* **2**:5–19 (1995).
49. Cunningham AJ, Edmonds CVI, Jenkins GP, *et al.* Randomized controlled trial of the effects of group psychological therapy on survival in women with metastatic breast cancer. *Psychooncology* **7**:508–517 (1998).
50. Stephen JE, Rahn M, Verhoef M. What is the state of evidence on the mind-cancer survival question, and where do we go from here? A point of view. *Support Care Cancer* **15**:923–930 (2007).

51. Creagan ET. Attitude and disposition: do they make a difference in cancer survival? *J Prosthet Dentistry* **82**:52–55 (1999).
52. Monti DA, *et al*. Potential role of mind-body therapies in cancer survivorship. *Cancer* **112**:2607–2616 (2008).
53. Bedson P. *Meditation and Cancer Therapies: An Interview with Dr Paul Bedson*, The Gawler Foundation, Sydney (2010).
54. Manocha R. *Does Meditation Have a Specific Effect? A Systematic Investigation Into the Effects of the Mental Silence Experience*, PhD thesis, University of NSW (2009).
55. Monti D, Sufian M, Peterson C. Potential role of mind-body therapies in cancer survivorship. *Cancer* **112**(11 suppl):2607–2615 (2008).

7

Should Spirituality and Prayer be Part of Complementary Therapies?

Ian N. Olver

ABSTRACT

Although mind–body medicine is considered part of complementary therapies, the inclusion of prayer is more controversial. If counted as such, it certainly results in inflated figures of overall complementary therapy use. Spirituality must be differentiated from religiosity and validated scales of spiritual well-being have been developed. The Functional Assessment of Chronic Illness Therapy–Spiritual Well-Being scale has three domains of peace, meaning and faith. Using such a scale, research groups have found that spiritual well-being is a unique predictor of quality of life. In studies of the impact of intercessory prayer on health outcomes, Cochrane reviews of the randomised studies have resulted in equivocal findings. Many methodological issues have arisen about study design, and even whether procedures such as randomisation and blinding are appropriate for studies of metaphysical phenomena, where the mechanism is unknown. The use of clinical endpoints has been questioned and this makes comparisons between studies difficult. A randomised controlled trial of intercessory prayer is described, where the endpoint was to determine whether there was an improvement in spiritual well-being. It was a large study with 999 patients. The outcome was that a statistically significant improvement in spiritual well-being was found but with a small effect size. The result raises questions about the way forward.

Keywords: Blinding; Complementary Therapy; Intercessory Prayer; Randomisation; Spirituality.

Most classifications of complementary and alternative medicine (CAM) include a group of healing practices often grouped under the title of mind–body medicine.[1] The suggestion is that a cognitive process with the mind will alter the body's function. This group usually includes various forms of meditation, prayer and therapies allowing creative expression through music or art.

Although the mechanism may not be clear, some of the psychological techniques that were classified under CAMs are now part of conventional medicine, where group therapy in patient support groups, cognitive behavioural therapy or mindfulness meditation is now considered mainstream.[2,3] The field of psychoneuroimmunology has suggested that links may exist between psychological states and immune function.[4]

Prayer can be more controversial in a discussion on CAMs. In a US study of the use of complementary medicines by patients with cancer during their treatment, it was found that 91% used at least one form of CAMs and the most frequent CAMs were prayer, relaxation and exercise.[5] Similarly, in a study in Nigeria, prayer accounted for 49.4% of the CAMs usage, second only to the use of herbs.[6] A study in Brazil, which aimed to see whether the CAMs use in the West was reflected amongst the poor in that country, showed a high rate of CAMs use, but what needed comparing with the West was the use of herbal medicines, and prayer had to be excluded because it was inflating what was actually a low indigenous CAMs use in Brazil.[7] This issue was highlighted in a socio-demographic study of CAM usage in the US that showed that different types of CAM were used by different groups. In general, whites used more CAM than non-whites, except in the case of prayer, and overall CAM users were better educated, except in the use of prayer. The authors concluded that these different use patterns are hidden when the heterogeneous practices encompassed in CAMs are all grouped together in analyses.[8] Prayer, therefore, should probably be considered a specific subgroup of CAMs, with those who pray having different characteristics to other users of CAMs.

SPIRITUAL WELL-BEING

Spirituality is often defined as the search for meaning to one's life.[9] This should be distinguished from religiosity, which is just one manifestation of spirituality. Religiosity is defined by participation in the practices of particular religious groups.

The Behavioural Research Centre of the American Cancer Society has published a study examining the association between spiritual well-being and CAMs use in over 4000 cancer survivors.[10] They used the Functional Assessment of Chronic Illness Therapy–Spiritual Well-Being (FACIT-Sp) scale, which in addition to general quality of life (QOL) questions, includes specific questions exploring the three domains of spiritual well-being: faith, peace and meaning.[9,11,12] They studied 19 CAMs in five domains; of particular relevance to this discussion, mind–body methods were divided into religious/spiritual (R/S) and non-R/S. They found that the meaning and faith subscales were associated with greater use of CAMs, but the peace subscale was associated with less use of R/S CAMs, but not less use of non-R/S CAMs. As above, the prevalence of CAMs use dropped overall if R/S CAMs were excluded. As part of their conclusions, the authors suggest that R/S CAMs should be thought of as a separate category of CAMs.

After the development of the FACIT-Sp, Brady and co-workers explored the relationship between spiritual well-being and a QOL assessment in 1610 patients with cancer from four sites in the US and two sites in Puerto Rico.[13] They found a significant positive association between spiritual well-being and general QOL, and the subscales measuring emotional, physical and social/family well-being, beyond what could be expected from the association with demographic and disease variables. Spiritual well-being in this study was a unique predictor of QOL beyond those subscales. Those patients reporting high levels of spiritual well-being seemed able to enjoy life despite symptoms such as pain and fatigue, which was not the case with patients whose spiritual well-being was measured as low.

Cotton and colleagues examined the relationship between the FACT-B scale for breast cancer and spiritual well-being, QOL and psychological adjustment to cancer in 142 patients.[14] Again, they reported that spiritual well-being was positively correlated with

QOL but also that it was positively correlated with the coping styles of fighting spirit and fatalism, and negatively correlated with hopelessness/helplessness, anxious preoccupation and avoidance on the Mini-Mental Adjustment to Cancer (mini-MAC) scale.[15] These results seemed anomalous, as fighting spirit and avoidance were previously shown to prolong disease-free survival and fatalism did not. The authors contend, however, that in this case fatalism, rather than being stoic resignation, as it is commonly interpreted, simply indicated an acceptance of the illness.

My research team has had a chance to look at the association between spiritual well-being and QOL in an Australian population.[16] We were conducting a study of the impact of intercessory prayer, where at baseline patients completed both the FACIT-Sp and the full version of the MAC scales. Similar to Brady and colleagues, we sought to establish the relationship between QOL and spiritual well-being and to examine the relationship with coping styles after the Cotton study. We initially studied 449 patients. At the time of the study, the FACIT-Sp was analysed in two rather than three subsets; faith and peace/meaning.

We found, like Brady and colleagues, that spiritual well-being was strongly positively associated with general QOL and its physical, social/family, emotional and functional subscales. It has been argued that spiritual well-being may be just another expression of emotional well-being; however, that spiritual well-being as measured by the FACIT-Sp was an independent predictor of QOL.[17] Further, our results support the outcomes of a recent meta-analysis that included 51 studies.[18]

Not all of the subscales have the same relationships with QOL. We found that compared with faith, the meaning/peace component showed a strong positive relationship with QOL. Faith was less likely to affect the patients' experiences of cancer. Unlike Brady we did not find that improved spiritual well-being improved the enjoyment of life in the face of chronic symptoms of pain or fatigue.

PRAYER

The perspective on spirituality and CAMs that I wish to share comes from my experience of trying to investigate whether the impact of intercessory prayer could be measured. I was faced with three preliminary questions: Why do a study of prayer? Should you do such a study? How do you do such a study?

Many complementary practices have eventually been subjected to formal scientific study because they are in widespread use and there builds up a large series of anecdotal reports of the treatment's efficacy. Prayer, as we have shown, is one of the most common interventions outside physical medicine.[19] In the US a survey of patients reported that 43% prayed for themselves and 24.4% were aware of being prayed for by others. The association with improved QOL needs further exploration.[20,21]

Moreover, there have been many attempts to formally study intercessory prayer, that is prayer for others, where those who pray are often remote from the patient and believe that they are interceding by praying to God. The Cochrane Collaboration has reviewed the studies of intercessory prayer for the alleviation of illness. Such reviews were published in 2000, 2004 and 2009.[22–24] The latest review identified 10 randomised studies that involved 7646 patients. There are some positive studies, but many are not, and the reviewers suggested that the evidence did not enable a recommendation to be made for the use of prayer for healing, but neither were there any adverse effects found. Because of the large number of studies yielding such an equivocal result, they further suggested that time and effort were better directed to other fields of research. For most of the studies published, there are letters to the editors of the journals criticising the methodology and any assumptions made. However, the number of anecdotal reports, some randomised studies that have reported positive results, and an equivocal conclusion from Cochrane answer the first question as to why there is a reason for studying prayer. Meditative prayer for oneself has also been characterised as a coping mechanism, which is one suggested reason for patients who pray feeling better.[20,21]

The question of whether studies of the impact of prayer should be done, however, goes beyond the Cochrane argument, which seems to be one of what is the best use of resources. There are theological considerations. Halperin has criticised studies of intercessory prayer on the religious grounds of being interpreted as testing God, which he deems as inappropriate from a Biblical viewpoint (Deuteronomy 6:16, Matthew 4:7).[25] However, Chibnall and colleagues also suggest that such studies are not appropriate on

Biblical grounds and that scientific processes such as randomisation and blinding are inappropriate for studying metaphysical phenomena. They do not accept the construct validity of prayer as an intervention because its mechanism is unknown. Also they question those studies that have blinded the intercessors as this would preclude other possible mechanisms such as telepathy, and the use of such a design suggests that the investigator only believes that the effect is from God. They therefore see randomisation in prayer studies as an attempt to assess God.[26] In a response to their paper Harris *et al.* rejected this and countered with the Biblical story of Elijah who conducted a controlled experiment challenging 450 prophets of Baal to offer a sacrifice to their God while he did so to his God (1 Kings 18:19–40).[27] The specified endpoint was to be the God who answered with fire. As the story goes, the God of the Israelites did just that, thereby showing, according to Harris, a willingness to be involved in a trial!

Arguments of that nature aside, intriguing theologically as they may be, are beyond the scope of this chapter. It is often asked, however, why people who pray think that they would be needed to intercede to an all-knowing god. In the Christian tradition it is a considered a command from God, an act of faith and a privilege as part of the relationship between the prayer and God, which also benefits the person who prays. Also it is believed that God granted free will to his creation, which would in turn necessitate us to intercede if we wanted God's intervention.

As investigators, I believe that we were not testing God, but simply trying to see if we can measure, on a formal scale of spiritual well-being, the impact of prayer over a controlled population, in order to further investigate the anecdotal reports of its efficacy. On the questions of mechanism of action, the explanations for the mechanism of remote prayer have ranged from having faith in the power of God, or a god, to non-local phenomena in quantum mechanics. The studies in the medical literature do not address the mechanism of the effect, and this has been a point of criticism. However, many treatments have been tested in randomised controlled trials before their mechanisms of action are known, and particularly in cancer where both chemotherapy and radiotherapy are prime examples. It will help to focus on the difficulties of investigating CAMs, particularly where the mechanisms are unknown, if we address the question of how to design a study of intercessory prayer. The Cochrane analysis identified methodological problems with intercessory prayer studies that included many different endpoints. Interpretation can vary. In the studies that assessed survival, the meta-analysis did not reach statistical significance and had a wide confidence interval (CI) (95% CI 0.38–1.38). Equivocal results were recorded in all studies except one, which was strongly positive.[28] However if the data are analysed using a fixed-effects model instead of a random-effects model the meta-analysis becomes statistically significant (RR 0.73, CI 0.59–0.91).

One of the initial large randomised studies that focussed attention on the study of intercessory prayer was by Randolph Byrd. After gaining their consent, he randomised 393 patients, being admitted to coronary care, to being prayed for daily by selected Christian intercessors outside the hospital, or not being prayed for.[29] There were 57 patients who refused to participate. Both patients and clinicians were blinded to which group the patients belonged. The endpoints were the complications experienced. These were both compiled into a severity score and subjected to multivariate analysis. Both of these techniques yielded a significant difference favouring the group who had received the prayer.

A decade later Harris and colleagues attempted to replicate these results.[30] There were significant differences between the Harris and Byrd studies. Harris performed a blinded randomised trial with 990 patients, who did not know the nature of the trial, and were randomly allocated to being prayed for by Christian intercessors or being part of a control group. Their endpoint was a score summarising coronary care complications. These differed from those clinical endpoints used by Byrd, making the studies difficult to compare. Harris reported a statistically significant difference in the complication scores favouring the group that had been prayed for ($P = 0.04$), but there was no difference in the length of stay. However, others have reanalysed the data, correcting for multiple comparisons or revising which complications are to be considered and the significant difference between the groups is no longer apparent.[31,32]

Other intercessory prayer studies have included children with leukaemia,[33] adults with arthritis[34] or AIDS,[35] and patients with alcohol addiction.[36] There have also been commentaries and letters about these trials that criticise the aims of such studies or the methodologies used.[31,32,37]

In 2001 an intriguing article appeared in the *British Medical Journal* written by Leonard Leibovici.[38] He studied 3393 adult patients who had been diagnosed as suffering from septicaemia in a hospital between 1990 and 1996. In a double-blind, parallel-group, randomised controlled trial he studied a retroactive intervention by having the active group prayed for in 2001. His stated reasoning was to extend the observations of the Harris and Byrd studies and assume that time was not necessarily linear and that God was certainly not constrained by time. He used as his endpoint mortality in hospital, length of stay in hospital and duration of the fever. Although there was no statistically significant difference in mortality, the length of stay in hospital and duration of fever were significantly shorter in the intervention group than in the control group ($P = 0.01$ and $P = 0.04$).

The endpoints were clinical and arbitrarily selected. It is difficult to know whether this study is presented as a serious trial in its own right, or whether the author wished to make a point that statistically significant results can occur in a well-designed randomised study in selected endpoints by chance. That would mean that they were not clinically meaningful, but could not be dismissed just because of not being able to demonstrate a mechanism of action. Alternatively, he could have been engaging in whimsy for the Christmas edition of the journal.

DESIGNING STUDIES OF PRAYER

Our group accepted the challenge of designing a study of intercessory prayer.

We consulted with a theologian and at least decided that such an enquiry was not "testing God" but trying to see if we could measure in a population the contribution of the widespread practice of praying for others to their well-being, in patients with cancer.

We took into account the methodological discussion above, and the recommendation of the Cochrane review that future randomised studies should follow the CONSORT (Consolidated Standards of Reporting Trials) guidelines for reporting results and methodology. These ask for details of every aspect of the trial, such as the method of randomisation, determination of sample size, reason for dropout, pre-determined endpoints and statistical methods.[39]

Our first and most significant design decision was the choice of a validated objective endpoint, the change on a scale of spiritual well-being. This seemed to us to be the most likely measurable parameter to change as a result of prayer for others, and avoided using multiple clinical endpoints. We chose the FACIT-Sp scale of spiritual well-being, which has been previously described.

The second issue was to treat prayer as a "black box". We were not designing a study to investigate mechanisms and so it was more important that the intercessors were genuinely praying for those randomised to prayer. Prayer groups don't necessarily pray in any pattern but from their viewpoint "as the Spirit leads them". We also told the prayer group that they were part of a study and we wanted them to pray for a number of patients. Prayer groups often pray for people that they don't know; friends and relatives of others, for example. The group wanted enough information about the patients to be able to focus upon them to pray and they were satisfied with first name, marital status, age, occupation and type of cancer. We were satisfied that the patients' confidentiality was protected, as individuals could not be identified by those doing the praying, who were remote from the hospital.

The study was a conventional randomised double-blind parallel-group study. The randomisation schedule paralleled the Harris study where the actual sequence was whether the unit record number was odd or even, but only the data manager assigning the groups knew that. The blinding was maintained until after the data were analysed. The patients were told that we wished to study QOL and spiritual well-being and how it changed over time and gave consent to this. The nature of the randomisation was not revealed to them, to eliminate any placebo effect. The ethics committee accepted this "deception" design as it is standard in the psychological literature and acceptable if the information cannot be obtained in any other way, and the intervention is very unlikely to cause harm. We could not control for contamination of the control group by others praying for them, but in a large trial this is likely to have less impact.

The patient population were patients newly enrolled in one of the cancer units at an Australian teaching hospital. They had to be over 18 and speak English, as they were required to complete both QOL and spiritual well-being scales at study entry and then 6 months later.

The numbers required in the trial were based on the numbers used in the Harris study of cardiology patients.[27] To determine whether groups significantly differed in well-being scores over time, mixed between–within subject analyses of variance were used. Exact *P*-values were reported but, in addition, effect sizes, to show the magnitude of the difference, were also reported [partial eta squared (η^2) values]. As some results were clearly hypothesised and all analyses were pre-determined, Bonferroni adjustments for multiple testing were not considered necessary.[40]

A further design issue, which we did not consider initially, was raised by Benor in a letter to *Alternative Therapies in Health and Medicine*.[41] He suggested that the expectations of the researchers themselves may impact on the outcome of the studies, even if blinded. This type of suggestion also occurs in Chinese medicine where it is believed that qi or universal energy binds all people together. There is actually a fascinating study by Solfvin where, in an experiment with animals, the expectation of the animal handlers did correlate with the outcome of their experiments.[42] Benor suggests that at least the expectations of the researchers should be reported, even if a mechanism for how they would influence the outcome is unclear. In our study of intercessory prayer we had investigators with a whole spectrum of beliefs, so there was no consistency in the direction of expectation.

RESULTS OF A STUDY OF INTERCESSORY PRAYER

I have already alluded to an initial report from our study of intercessory prayer that demonstrated, from the baseline characteristics, that spiritual well-being was an independent contributor to QOL.[16] In a randomised controlled double-blind study of intercessory prayer we accrued 999 patients (509 in the intervention and 490 in the control group) and 665 of them completed the FACIT-Sp at both time-points. There were no significant differences in demographic characteristics between the two groups.

To summarise the outcome, we did find a statistically significant difference in spiritual well-being in the group who had been prayed for ($P = 0.03$). However, the size of the effect was small (partial $\eta^2 = 0.2$). Also, there was a corresponding improvement in emotional well-being, showing a moderate degree of change.[43]

This is an intriguing result. What does it mean? What impact could it have clinically, if there is only a small change? Are there further methodological issues to tackle? Is the scale of spiritual well-being sufficiently sensitive to detect outcomes that are spiritually based? What, if anything, should we do next? Should intercessory prayer be considered a part of complementary and alternative therapies?

REFERENCES

1. National Centre for Complementary and Alternate Medicine. What is CAM? http://nccam.nih.gov/health/whatiscam/overview.htm#what [Accessed 14 April 2010].
2. Bottomley A. Group cognitive behavioural therapy interventions with cancer patients: a review of the literature. *Eur J Cancer Care (Engl)* **5**:143–146 (1996).
3. Matchim Y, Armer JM. Measuring the psychological impact of mindfulness mediation on health among patients with cancer: a literature review. *Oncol Nurs Forum* **34**:1059–1066 (2007).
4. McCain NL. Psychoneuroimmunology, spirituality, and cancer. *Gynecol Oncol* **99**(3 suppl 1):S121 (2005).
5. Yates JS, Mustian KM, Morrow GR, *et al*. Prevalence of complementary and alternative medicine use in cancer patients during treatment. *Support Care Cancer* **13**:806–811 (2005).
6. Ezeome ER, Anarado AN. Use of complementary medicine by cancer patients at the University of Nigeria Teaching Hospital, Enugu, Nigeria. *BMC Complement Altern Med* **7**:28 (2006).
7. Tovey P, de Barros NF, Hoehne EL, *et al*. Use of traditional medicine and globalized complementary and alternative medicine among low-income cancer service users in Brazil. *Integr Cancer Ther* **5**:232–235 (2006).
8. Conboy L, Patel S, Kaptchuk TJ, *et al*. Sociodemographic determinants of the utilization of specific types of complementary and alternative medicine: an analysis based on a nationally representative survey sample. *J Altern Complement Med* **11**:977–994 (2005).

9. Peterman AH, Fitchett G, Brady MJ, *et al.* Measuring spiritual well-being in people with cancer: the functional assessment of chronic illness therapy — spiritual well-being scale (FACIT-Sp). *Ann Behav Med* **24**:49–58 (2002).
10. Crammer C, Kaw C, Gansler T, *et al.* Cancer survivors' spiritual well-being and use of complementary methods: a report from the American Cancer Society's studies of cancer survivors. *J Relig Health* **50**:92–107 (2010).
11. Cella DF, Tulsky DS, Gray G, *et al.* The Functional Assessment of Cancer Therapy (FACT) scale: development and validation of the general measure. *J Clin Oncol* **11**:570–579 (1993).
12. Canada AL, Murphy PE, Fitchett G, *et al.* A 3-factor model for the FACIT-Sp. *Psycho-Oncology* **17**:908–916 (2008).
13. Brady MJ, Peterman AH, Fitchett G, *et al.* A case for including spirituality in quality of life measurement in oncology. *Psycho-Oncology* **8**:417–428 (1999).
14. Cotton SP, Levine EG, Fitzpatrick CM, *et al.* Exploring the relationships among spiritual wellbeing, quality of life, and psychological adjustment in women with breast cancer. *Psycho-Oncology* **8**:429–438 (1999).
15. Watson M, Greer S, Bliss JM. *Mental Adjustment to Cancer (MAC) Scale. User's Manual.* CRC Psychological Medicine Research Group, Royal Marsden Hospital, Sutton, Surrey, UK (1989).
16. Whitford HS, Olver IN, Peterson MJ. Spirituality as a core domain in the assessment of quality of life in oncology. *Psycho-Oncology* **17:**1121–1128 (2008).
17. Cella DF. Quality of life: the concept. *J Palliat Care,* **8**:8–13 (1992).
18. Sawatzky R, Ratner PA, Chiu L. A meta-analysis of the relationship between spirituality and quality of life. *Soc Indic Res* **72**:153–188 (2005).
19. McCaffrey AM, Eisenberg DM, Legedza AT, *et al.* Prayer for health concerns: results of a national survey on prevalence and patterns of use. *Arch Intern Med* **164**:858–862 (2004).
20. Büssing A, Fischer J, Ostermann T, *et al.* Reliance on God's help as a measure of intrinsic religiosity in healthy elderly and patients with chronic diseases. Correlations with health-related quality of life? *Appl Res Qual Life* **4**:77–90 (2009).
21. Masters KS, Spielmans GI. Prayer and health: review, meta-analysis, and research agenda. *J Behav Med* **30**:329–338 (2007).

22. Roberts L, Ahmed I, Hall S. Intercessory prayer for the alleviation of ill health. *Cochrane Database Syst Rev* (2):CD000368. Review (2000).
23. Roberts L, Ahmed I, Hall S. Intercessory prayer for the alleviation of ill health. *Cochrane Database Syst Rev* Jan 24;(1):CD000368. Review (2007).
24. Roberts L, Ahmed I, Hall S, *et al.* Intercessory prayer for the alleviation of ill health. *Cochrane Database Syst Rev* Apr 15;(2):CD000368. Review (2009).
25. Halperin EC. Should academic medical centres conduct clinical trials of the efficacy of intercessory prayer? *Acad Med* **76**:791–797 (2001).
26. Chibnall JT. Experiments on distant intercessory prayer. Commentary. *Arch Intern Med* **161**:2529–2536 (2001).
27. Harris WS, Isley WL. Massah and mechanisms. *Arch Intern Med* **162**:1420 (2002).
28. Aviles JM, Whelan E, Hernke DA, *et al.* Intercessory prayer and cardiovascular disease progression in a coronary care unit population: a randomized controlled trial. *Mayo Clin Proc* **76**:1192–1198 (2001).
29. Byrd RC. Positive therapeutic effects of intercessory prayer in a coronary care unit population. *Southern Med J* **81**:826–829 (1988).
30. Harris W, Gowda M, Kolb J, *et al.* A randomized, controlled trial of the effects of remote, intercessory prayer on outcomes in patients admitted to the coronary care unit. *Arch Intern Med* **159**:2273–2278 (1999).
31. Van der Does W. A randomised, controlled trial of prayer? *Arch Intern Med* **160**:1871–1872 (2000).
32. Price JM. Does prayer really set one apart? *Arch Intern Med* **160**:1873 (2000).
33. Collipp PJ. The efficacy of prayer: a triple-blind study. *Med Times* **97**:201–204 (1969).
34. Joyce CRB, Welldon RMC. The objective efficacy of prayer. *J Chron Disord* **18**:367–377 (1965).
35. Astin JA, Stone J, Abrams DI, *et al.* The efficacy of distant healing for human immunodeficiency virus–results of a randomized trial. *Altern Ther Health Med* **12**:36–41 (2006).
36. Walker SR, Tonigan JS, Miller W, *et al.* Intercessory prayer in the treatment of alcohol abuse and independence: a pilot investigation. *Altern Ther Health Med* **3**:79–86 (1997).
37. Kavanagh BD. Clinical trials of intercessory prayers? *Acad Med* **77**:109 (2002).

38. Leibovici L. Effects of remote, retroactive intercessory prayer on outcomes in patients with bloodstream infection: randomised controlled trial. *BMJ* **323**:1450–1451 (2001).
39. Moher D, Hopewell S, Schulz KF, *et al.* CONSORT 2010 explanation and elaboration: updated guidelines for reporting parallel group randomised trials. *J Clin Epidemol* **63**:e1–37 (2010).
40. Perneger TV. What's wrong with Bonferroni adjustments? *BMJ* **316**:1236–1238 (1998).
41. Benor DJ. Prayer study: what about expectancy effects among the researchers themselves? Letter. *Altern Ther Health Med* **8**:20–21 (2002).
42. Solfvin J. Experimenter expectancy: prayer study. Letter. *Altern Ther Health Med* **8**:18–19 (2002).
43. Olver IN, Whitford H. Prayer improves spiritual wellbeing in a randomized controlled trial in patients with cancer. *Asia Pacific J Clin Oncol* **5**: Abs 145, A172 (2009).

8

From Traditional Medicines to Drug Discovery

Monica C. Robotin

ABSTRACT

Of the estimated 300,000 higher plants available today, more than one in ten have a documented medical use, but the pharmacological properties of few of them have been thoroughly investigated. Botanical products are used as traditional medicine in many cultures, where plants are customarily used as plant mixtures, which pose challenges to the identification of active compounds and in ensuring the consistency and quality control of these products. Although the evidence of effectiveness of herbal medicines used by traditional medical systems such as traditional Chinese medicine or ayurveda is often anecdotal, rather than derived from rigorous clinical trials, studies confirmed a biological basis for the effect of many of these traditional herbal preparations. This chapter will discuss the various contexts in which ethno-pharmacological information has led to drug discovery, the different modalities in which plants contributed to drug discovery, as well as some of the challenges arising in designing botanical studies. Since the Industrial Revolution, the process of drug discovery has utilized both traditional methods derived from medicinal plants and combinatorial synthesis. Natural products are likely to remain significant contributors to drug discovery, as the chemical structures found in nature greatly exceed the synthetic capabilities of medicinal chemistry. Even in the context of ready access to purified human enzymes and receptors, 65% of drugs approved for marketing in the last decade of the last century were based on natural products. It may be possible that treating cancer in the future will involve a combined approach, in which Western medicine will be used to destroy the tumour, whereas other treatments, such as traditional Chinese medicine will address the entire "unhealthy" condition, bringing about a change in the body environment that could further facilitate cure.

Keywords: Combinatorial Synthesis; Drug Discovery; Ethnopharmacology; Medicinal Plants; Traditional Medical Systems.

BACKGROUND

Human cultures have been using botanical products for medicinal purposes since the dawn of civilization, as illustrated in some of the earliest written documents discovered in China, Sumeria and Egypt.[1–3] The herbal knowledge of early civilizations has subsequently extended to Europe and the Middle East and by the 1800s, in addition to indigenous herbs, European countries also had a thriving trade in exotic medicinal plants from all over the globe.[2]

Of the estimated 300,000 higher plants available today, about 1% are used as foods and 10–15% have a documented medical use.[4] Approximately 80% of the world population lives in the developing world, where plants represent the primary source of medicine and it is estimated that more than 60% of the world's population still relies primarily on traditional medicines for their health-care needs.[5,6] The World Health Organization estimates that some 20,000 species of higher plants are being used for medicinal purposes throughout the world,[7] yet only a small percentage of these plants have been thoroughly investigated in terms of their pharmacological properties.[8]

Botanical products are used in various forms: the entire plant (or parts of it), as herbal materials (plant oils, juices or resins) or as herbal preparations (where purified or extracted compounds are mixed with other ingredients to make pills, powders or topical preparations).[9] Unlike orthodox medicine, which uses drugs generally as single chemical entities, traditional medicine commonly uses plants as mixtures, where the different elements act in different ways and on different parts of the body to produce their desired effect. The complexity of these mixtures poses significant challenges to the identification of active compounds and in ensuring the consistency and quality control of these products.[1]

The major traditional medical systems [traditional Chinese medicine (TCM), ayurveda and unani] share some common features, which include a long history of written documentation, a theoretical base, a periodical review of their body of knowledge and teaching through a formalized educational system.[6]

The millennia-old TCM remains in use by the Chinese medical system of today and is recognized in many other East Asian countries. TCM is based upon a philosophy that provides the underpinning of a holistic system of medicine, using natural products of plant, animal or mineral origin.[10,11] Its cornerstone is a belief that health is the product of a balance of energy forces throughout body systems,[12] so that illness can be effectively treated by a combination of natural products and taking into account the patient's general condition.[11] The search for active medicinal compounds from plants goes back to Chinese ancient history, when the Chinese doctor Shen Nong is reputed to have tested hundreds of plants for possible medicinal effects.[4] Although all TCMs are of natural origin, some 80% of them derive from plants, with the remainder being of animal or mineral origin.[13] The first written documentation of TCM dates back to the second century AD and has entries for each day of the year: 252 botanical entries, 67 of animal origin and 45 mineral entries.[10] To date, over 12,000 medicinal preparations from natural sources have been recorded and over 5000 validated as folk medicines in the Chinese traditional medical system.[4]

Although TCM occasionally uses single herbs (such as ginseng, gingko, ephedra and liquorice), more often the prescription involves multi-component herbal preparations, some in use since antiquity.[13] In instances where the isolation and characterization of active compounds was carried out successfully, the observed effects often validated their use in traditional medicine and in some cases it could be demonstrated that different compounds worked synergistically to achieve desired therapeutic effects.[1]

Studies of Chinese medicinal herbs confirmed a biological basis for their effect, with some inducing apoptosis, immunomodulation, or inhibiting telomerase activity or the growth of tumours,[11,14] although the evidence about the effectiveness of Chinese herbs is often anecdotal, rather than derived from Western-style, rigorous clinical trials.[14]

A recent literature search by Molassiotis *et al.* identified 49 studies of randomized controlled trial (RCT) design, or having a comparison group that examined the clinical effects of Chinese herbs in cancer treatment.[14] With one exception,[15] the study quality was low, but the overall impression was that Chinese herbs could prevent or alleviate the effects of conventional chemotherapy, with many studies reporting significant improvements in participants' quality of life.[14] The significant number of studies reporting positive findings suggests that Chinese herbs should remain the subject of rigorous study in cancer therapeutics.[14]

Ayurvedic medicine describes "nourishing and rejuvenation drugs" used for longevity, memory preservation and immunomodulation, with effects mediated via the neuroendocrine axis.[16] Some of the plants used have complex activities, e.g. *Glycyrrhyza glabra* root (liquorice), commonly used for minor throat infections also has antioxidant, chemoprotective and antimicrobial activities, whereas *Withania somnifera* (Ashwagandha/Indian ginseng/winter cherry) has immunomodulatory, antitumour, cytoprotective and antioxidant properties.[17]

Unfortunately the knowledge base of indigenous plant use is slowly being eroded, with Western-dominated culture and education superseding many of the local traditions.[1,18] Until the 1980s there was little interest in the Western world in preserving indigenous knowledge of plants and minimal effort expended in assisting communities to preserve this knowledge.[19] There remains an imperative to catalogue the actual use of medical plants and develop research programmes in traditional medicines, and increasingly Western research organizations appreciate the value of this information.[18,19] The loss of habitat, particularly in the tropical forests, may lead to many of the plants in use today becoming extinct in the near future, so there is an acute need to ensure species and habitat preservation and, to the extent possible, to preferentially use cultivated plants in preference to harvesting them from the wild.[1,20]

PLANTS IN WESTERN MEDICINE — THE ROLE OF ETHNOPHARMACOLOGY

Ethnopharmacology is a sophisticated approach to drug discovery involving botany, chemistry, pharmacology as well as many other scientific disciplines.[21] Its beginnings are credited to two French pharmacists, Pierre-Joseph Pelletier and Joseph Bienaimé Caventou, who in 1820 extracted the active principle from the bark of several species of *Cinchona* and promoted the use of quinine for the treatment of malaria, thus marking the inception of a new scientific discipline.[22,23]

Historically, ethno-pharmacological information led to drug discovery in various contexts:

1. The use of unmodified plant products where their ethnomedical use suggested efficacy for specific medical conditions, i.e. foxglove for the treatment of heart failure.
2. The use of products where the unmodified natural product gave a remote indication of their usefulness (i.e. vincristine, used by indigenous cultures for the treatment of diabetes, but subsequently found to be an effective anticancer agent).[24,25]
3. The use of modified natural or synthetic products, based upon natural products used in folk medicine (e.g. aspirin).[8,24]

The development of organic chemistry can be traced back to the Industrial Revolution, which marked a preference for synthetic products for the treatment of disease; as pure compounds could be readily obtained, the conventional wisdom was that structural modifications required to produce more active and safer drugs would be readily available and supersede the use of herbs. This was occurring in the context of pharmaceutical company expansion and was viewed as the "way of the future", whereas the drugs sourced from natural products were seen as remedies employed by poorly educated or lower income people, or tied up with religious superstitions, with no real pharmacological value.[8]

With the advent of synthetic organic chemistry in the 1940s and 1950s, compound synthesis became an increasingly popular method of drug discovery,[6] as high-throughput biochemical screening technologies (which are ill-suited for the screening of natural products) became pre-eminent.[26] Meanwhile many old botanical drugs were removed from officinal compendia.[27]

Interest in natural medicines as a source of new drugs seems to be a cyclical process, with a resurgence of interest occurring in the 1970s, when many pharmaceutical companies developed active research programmes into natural substances as a source of potential new drugs.[1,28] During the 1960s and 1970s, the emphasis of research shifted from being compound-led (i.e. search for alkaloids or flavonoids) to being biological activity-led.[18]

In the 1990s, the ability to readily produce purified human enzymes and receptors tipped the balance again towards drug discovery using artificial assays (such as enzyme inhibition assays and receptor-binding assays), which replaced the time-honoured functional assays (which measured biological activity) and this again marginalized the process of drug development from plants.[26]

Nonetheless, plants still retain an important role in drug development: 65% of drugs approved for marketing from 1983 to 1994 were based on natural products. Of these, 30 were pure natural products, 127 were derived from natural product sources and 46 were synthetic drugs modelled on natural products.[29] Nine of the 20 best-selling non-protein pharmaceuticals in 1999 (enalapril, four statins, three antibiotics and cyclosporin) are either natural products, or are derived from lead compounds of natural origin and their combined annual sales exceeded $US16 billion.[30] In 2000, over 50% of the best-selling pharmaceuticals were derived from natural products, with the diversity of natural products being the main draw card of a natural product drug development programme.[31]

A renewed interest in drug discovery using natural products was spearheaded by new technologies, such as combinatorial synthesis and high-throughput screening,[3] as natural products have a distinct advantage when searching for lead molecules against newly discovered targets if there are no known small molecule leads, and because they remain more cost-effective than the synthetic pathway.[30]

The greatest impact on the use of natural remedies in the West in recent years is due to an increased exchange of information with China, where this tradition goes back for thousands of years and continues even in the current era of Western pharmaceutical industry domination.[2]

USING PLANTS AS SOURCES OF THERAPEUTIC AGENTS

Over the years, the process of discovery has embraced different forms, with some of the more commonly employed ones being discussed below.

Plants as Drug Prototypes

Examples of plant-derived drugs include digoxin (derived from *Digitalis* species), morphine and codeine (obtained from *Papaver somniferum*) and atropine and hyoscine (obtained from *Atropa belladonna*).[1,6,21]

The discovery of these small molecules, which are effective treatments for a wide range of diseases, launched the pharmaceutical industry and in time served as a pharmacological tool for understanding the mechanisms of disease processes and the biochemical pathways that can influence them.[26] For example, the identification of digitalis from foxglove in the 18th century led to the discovery of digoxin, which provided a dose-controlled medicinal preparation for the treatment of heart failure and arrhythmias and over time contributed to the elucidation of the biochemical pathways involved in heart failure and led to the discovery of the sodium–potassium pump.[26]

Plants as a Source of Lead Compounds

The pharmaceutical industry views lead compounds with great interest, as synthetic products modelled on plant compounds can provide product claim protection, the strongest form of patent protection.[21,32]

Natural compounds with an identified chemical structure provided templates for the synthesis of pharmaceutical products, such as taxol (originally isolated from *Taxus brevifolia*), which was converted to active analogues such as taxotere and podophyllotoxin (isolated from *Podophyllum peltatum* or *Podophyllum emodii*), which was converted semi-synthetically to etoposide and teniposide.[1,33] It is critical that lead compounds are specific for the intended targets and are available in sufficient quantities to support the drug development process (for biological characterization and toxicity studies), but their potency may be lower than that of the final drug preparation.[28]

Plants as Complementary and Alternative Medicines

The use of plants as herbal remedies is very popular in the Western world, with plants such as *Echinacea*, *Gingko biloba*, St. John's wort and saw palmetto generating annual over-the-counter sales of tens of millions of $US in the US alone (see Table 1).[21] In the European Community, the sale of herbal medicinal products is worth approximately $US7 billion annually, whereas in the US this increased 25-fold from 1988 to 1997, from 200 million to $US5.1 billion.[34]

A public preference for natural products is driving the "green consumerism" movement, which is leading to a substantial increase in the use of herbal remedies in the Western world.[31] In 1997 Americans' out-of-pocket expenditures on alternative therapies were conservatively estimated at $US27 billion,[35] with herbal medicine the most commonly used complementary therapy (with 38 million users).[36] The over-the-counter sale of botanical supplements is on the increase and from 13 to 63% of cancer

Table 1. Top 10 selling herbal supplements in the US in 2002 and their clinical indications.

Rank	Herb	Clinical indication	US retail sales in 2002 ($US)
1	Garlic	Hypercholesterolemia	34,509,288
2	Ginkgo	Dementia, intermittent claudication	32,998,528
3	Echinacea	Prevention of common cold	32,448,966
4	Soy	Menopausal symptoms	28,252,518
5	Saw palmetto	Benign prostate hyperplasia	23,053,036
6	Ginseng	Physical and mental fatigue	21,686,192
7	St. John's wort	Mild depression	14,969,575
8	Black cohosh	Menopausal symptoms	12,333,188
9	Cranberry	Urinary tract infection	11,857,782
10	Valerian	Insomnia, stress	8,120,329

Modified from Sparreboom *et al.*[37]

patients are estimated to be using botanical preparations, often combining them with prescription medications.[37,38] It has been estimated that in 2000, Australians spent $AU2.3 billion on complementary and alternative medicine, or four times the public contribution to the Pharmaceutical Benefits Scheme[39] and the annual retail turnover of complementary medicine in 2003 was estimated at $AU800 million, with a further 20% of the national output being exported.[40]

Cassileth identifies the acceptance of unconventional therapies by mainstream care in the US as a defining moment for health-care in the 1990s.[41] Some of the reasons behind this trend include: the increased prevalence of chronic diseases (where conventional medicine is perceived as less effective) in ageing populations, the fact that orthodox medicine lost some of its legitimacy in representing the public interest in matters of health-care[42] and the public belief that botanicals have fewer side-effects than conventional drugs.[43] Furthermore, the perception that orthodox medicines are more likely to have adverse effects, to create dependency or cause microbial resistance and the increasing cost of Western medicine has also led many to choose self-medication with herbal products.[1] The increase in travel also brought opportunities to learn more about what used to be viewed as "exotic" cultures, many of which still have strong traditional medicine roots.[1]

APPROACHES TO DRUG DISCOVERY AND DEVELOPMENT

Drug development largely follows two different pathways, with many medications being derived as a result of a basic pharmacology/cell biology/biochemistry approach.[32] However, natural products remain significant contributors to drug discovery,[16] as the chemical structures found in nature greatly exceed the synthetic capabilities of medicinal chemistry.[44]

Fabricant & Farnsworth[21] outlined several approaches to drug development from plants, which include the following.

Random Selection Followed by Phytochemical Screening

Random selection followed by phytochemical screening (looking for specific active compounds such as alkaloids, triterpenes, flavonoids or isothiocyanates) is a time-honoured approach, still in use in many developing countries.[33] Botanicals that demonstrated promising activities are fractionated further and active compounds are isolated, their mechanism of action identified and toxicity studies, bioavailability and gene expression studies carried out, and ultimately the purified compounds are tested in clinical trials.[9]

Random Selection Using Biological Assays

These assays use animal models of human disease (many relying on murine leukaemias),[44] which by current standards is a slow, expensive and not very selective or easy to interpret process.[28] Although this is further compounded by significant difficulties in procurement of sufficient material for *in-vivo* testing,[44] this pathway was used by the National Cancer Institute from 1960 to 1981 and led to the discovery and understanding of the pharmacological action of paclitaxel, and played an important role in the discovery of vinblastine, vincristine and podophyllotoxin. Other drawbacks of *in-vivo* models include the limited number of parameters that can be observed during each experiment, high cost, time and a shift in public opinion against the use of animals in early drug research.[6] From 1960 to 1982, over 114,000 extracts were screened, with collection being mostly at random, across a broad taxonomic range.[6] As the programme developed, emphasis was placed on the collection of certain families of plants that provided larger numbers of useful extracts. In 1986 new screening algorithms were introduced, to fast-track the process of drug discovery from plants.[18]

Traditionally, two plant selection programmes have been employed: a random plant selection programme (popular in the 1960s), where plants were collected and screened irrespective of taxonomic or ethnobotanical context, with collectors dispatched around the world and asked to collect as many species of plants as possible (which had an overall low yield of useful products), and "targeted" surveys. The latter include phylogenetic surveys (where relatives of plants deemed useful are collected and analysed), ecological surveys (where plant selection is guided by plant habitat) and ethnopharmacological surveys (where plants used by indigenous people are the subject of research).[45]

As may be expected, indigenous cultures used medicinal plants useful for the treatment of health problems specific to developing countries, which are dominated by the treatment of infections, fever, jaundice, diarrhoea and reproductive health.[6] Of Western diseases, some are more likely to be recognized by indigenous healers (e.g. gastrointestinal diseases, inflammations, skin infections and some viral diseases) than others (such as cancer or cardiovascular diseases).[24]

Indigenous cultures that are most likely to have discovered natural products of import to pharmacology share certain features: an ethnomedical tradition able to record the information, residence in an area with a diverse flora and a continuity of residence in the same area over many generations.[45] The ethnobotanical approach is informed by the reported medicinal use of plants by certain cultures, so it may contribute less to drug discovery in cancer,[45] as the cancers with a significant burden of disease in the developed world (cancers of the lung, colon and prostate) occur later in life and are less likely to be encountered in cultures reliant on herbal medicines.[33]

Random Selection Followed by Screening Using Human Cancer Cell Lines

In 1985, the National Cancer Institute (NCI) decided to use human tumour cell lines representing major cancers, such as leukaemia, melanoma, colorectal cancer, brain cancers, ovarian and renal cancers, as assays for a primary cancer screen.[33,44] *In-vitro* tests (or bioassays), widely used in both drug discovery and ethnopharmacological research, are based upon the inhibition or stimulation of receptor binding, assaying the activity of an enzyme, or determining the effect on gene transcription.[6,28] The assays are faster, easier to perform and less expensive than animal experimentation, opening the way for the testing of a much larger number of substances in a relatively short time.[28] Furthermore, *in-vitro* screens have reduced the requirement for large quantities of material for testing, facilitating the throughput of compounds through the screening programme.[44]

The use of *in-vitro* tests brings some new challenges and pitfalls. At times the fractionation of an active extract may lead to a reduction of the activity of the original compound (due to the possibility of decomposition, or on account of synergy), the most active compound may not be the one responsible for most of the effect, *in-vitro* activity does not always correlate with *in-vivo* activity and *in-vitro* tests alone are not sufficient to test an extract against a particular disease.[46]

Advances in chemical methods, such as high-performance liquid chromatography, high-resolution mass spectroscopy and X-ray crystallography, made it possible to speed up the process of identification of chemical structures and to fully characterize these compounds. The miniaturization and automation of some of these processes rekindled interest in searching for new lead compounds, as thousands of samples can now be assayed in one day in automated laboratories.[6,28] It is estimated that only approximately 4% of screened agents have been referred for further testing, which involves secondary *in-vitro* testing and subsequently *in-vivo* testing, with novel approaches integrating computer science, molecular biology and medicinal chemistry playing a role in drug development.[44]

Chemotaxonomic Approach

A chemotaxonomic approach uses the plants that have yielded products of interest as "chemical templates" to identify other naturally occurring compounds that may be equally or more effective as drug lead compounds.

A chemotaxonomic approach is better suited when seeking to identify new leads for a narrow range of diseases, where using ethnobotanical or ethnomedical information data is more likely to be successful than aiming to develop a broad-based screening programme.[28] Using natural templates for the discovery of lead compounds is a lengthy and arduous process, as safety testing and clinical development take an average of 7–10 years and estimated costs exceed $US250 million.[32] It was estimated that the cost to bring a new drug to market ranges from $US100 to 360 million and involves a minimum of 10 years of work and the testing of some 10,000 compounds.[8]

In the field of oncology, some drug companies choose to focus their research on developing specific cytotoxic drugs from plants, with little chemical modification, whereas others focus their work on identifying active principles with more specific inhibitory activities. This marks the beginning of a lengthy medicinal chemistry process, aiming to produce a simpler molecule than the original natural compound, which ideally is more potent, selective and bioavailable and can be produced in a cost–effective manner; however, all of this requires considerable time, effort and financial investment.[32] Some examples where natural products act as industrial intermediates include hecogenin (a steroid obtained from the juice of *Agave sisalana*, which is a synthetic intermediate for cortisone and cortisol) and cephalosporin C (obtained from *Cephalosporium acremonium*, which is the synthetic intermediate for the production of cephalosporin antibiotics).[32]

Databases

Databases that are used include the NAPRALERT (acronym for Natural Products ALERT), which is the largest relational database on the ethnobotanical uses of medicinal plants.[34] By the year 2000, this database had detailed information on over 58,000 species of organisms and 155,000 distinct chemical constituents.[47] NAPRALERT is also the repository of over 200,000 scientific papers and reviews of natural products and includes ethnomedical, pharmacological and biochemical information on their effects *in-vitro* and *in-vivo*, including their human use and the results of clinical studies.[48]

The Follow-Up of Ethnomedical (Traditional Medicine) Uses of Plants

The study of how different cultures use plants can provide useful information about their intended medicinal use.[9] The information collected is derived through several sources.

1. The use of plants by sophisticated traditional medical systems, including ayurvedha, unani medicine, kampo and TCM, with a history going back in some cases for millennia and transmitted through regularly updated and written systems of documenting knowledge and theory.

2. The information derived from herbalism, folklore or shamanism, which centres on an apprenticeship system, with the information often passed on secretly from one generation to the next, with little information being recorded or available for examination. Plants are administered according to spiritual beliefs, which complicates the identification of their medicinal properties, as no standard method of identifying these plants is generally available.[9]
3. Reviewing information on plant use from published books on medical botany, review articles (including surveys of medicinal plants by geographic regions or by different ethnic groups) and field reports of botanists.[21]

A well-conducted ethnomedical research programme is likely to yield high success rates in terms of drug discovery and drug development, but requires input from a multi-disciplinary team and involves complex field research and the collection of information from multiple sources: interviews with traditional healers including case discussions, detailed collection of ethnomedical data and information about the use of traditional medicines in the region, disease epidemiology and plant and medical data searches.[31] The process is complex, slow and better suited to the study of natural products used to treat diseases familiar to traditional healers (such as malaria, intestinal worms or leishmaniasis) rather than diseases such as cancer,[6,31] where the healers' experience is likely to be limited, due to a generally shorter life expectancy and different disease patterns likely to be observable in these settings (see above).[6]

Direct "Adoption" of Medicinal Mushrooms by Western Medicine

In the Far East (especially in Japan and China), mushrooms and mushroom extracts have been key ingredients in TCM. Three polysaccharides extracted from mushrooms (krestin, lentinan and scizophyllum) are being used in Japan in cancer therapy, alongside conventional medicine.[16] The *Ganoderma* species have a history of use in TCM dating back four millennia (*Ganoderma lucidum* is known as *reishi* or *manetake* in Japan and *ling zhi* in China) and are now gradually gaining recognition in the West as "medicinal mushrooms".[49] The active compounds of these mushrooms have demonstrated anti-cancer and immunomodulating activities, as well as other medicinal properties relevant to cardiovascular disease, although research into their effectiveness according to Western standards of evidence remains limited.[49,50] One of these compounds, polysaccharide K (PSK), was isolated in 1960 and by 1987 accounted for >25% of the total national expenditure on anticancer drugs in Japan (where it is used in combination with conventional chemotherapy, mostly for gastrointestinal cancers), so it seems that, in Eastern countries at least, medicinal mushrooms have crossed the divide between traditional herbal medicine use and a pharmaceutical grade product.[49]

FACTORS INFLUENCING THE CONTRIBUTION OF ETHNOMEDICINE TO DRUG DEVELOPMENT

Accuracy of Recorded Observations

Ethnomedical information is commonly documented by botanists, but the records generally provide limited useful information that may assist in determining the potential role of a plant in drug development; details about the medical conditions being treated, what parts of the plant are being used and the type of preparation used (concoction, infusion, paste, etc.) are uncommonly documented.[6] Other challenges include the difficulties inherent in accurately recording scientific information originating in another language and in translating different concepts of medicine into Western medical concepts.[6]

Promising ethnomedical leads, suggesting the existence of active compounds include the use of a plant for the same purpose by different cultures separated geographically and/or the sharing of information between adjacent cultures.[51]

Low Toxicity, Ability to Demonstrate a Biological Effect and Reproducibility of the Effect Under Laboratory Conditions

In the 1940s a Chinese doctor named Zhang Changshao reported that patients with malaria caused by *Plasmodium vivax* recovered following treatment with a traditional concoction of Chinese hydrangea, called *changsan* (or *Dichroa febrifuga*).[22] However, the subsequent purification process exacerbated the product's toxicity (causing severe emesis) and reduced its effectiveness, which ultimately led to it having to be abandoned as an antimalarial agent.[22]

As many as 25% of plants with early evidence of biological activity may not have this property confirmed in subsequent batches,[21] or in other laboratory settings. Possible contributing factors include the following:

1. The poor nutritional status of the experimental animals in laboratories in developing countries can lead to a different response to the testing of drugs:
2. Variations in the chemical constituents and potency among different crops, related to the age of the plants, the time of harvesting, the season or the geographical area where they were collected.[5] For example, the concentration of active ingredients in ginseng preparations can vary from 0 to 300%.[52]
3. Possibility of contamination (by fungi, bacteria or pesticides).[53]
4. Use of incorrect plant species, or of extracts that may not be prepared according to traditional medicine methods.[1,9,54]

Ability to Access Biodiversity

Developing countries and their indigenous people are the custodians of much of the world's genetic resources, but until recently the prevailing attitude in the developed world has been that these resources should be freely available for the use of humankind, irrespective of their origins.[19] The United Nations Convention on Biological Diversity recognizes the sovereign right of countries over their biological resources and provides a legislative framework, allowing the preservation and rational use of biological resources,[19,20,30] although these provisions have not always led to the sharing of commercial rewards with the source country.[30] Bioprospecting projects are complex processes, where the scientific expertise from many fields comes together with expertise in the area of diplomacy, international law, social sciences and anthropology, the willingness to work collaboratively and, in the case of drug-targeted bioprospecting, the need to collaborate with the pharmaceutical industry to progress the potential discoveries along the drug development pipeline.[20] The issue of how to best ensure reciprocal benefits is a taxing one and new solutions and reciprocity strategies have been suggested to address these challenges.[55]

These challenges have provided opportunities to find new ways to investigate biodiversity, by identifying new plant species in different habitats and seeking to systematically explore the microbial diversity and the available bounty of marine plants and animals.[30] This led to appropriate genetic material from species of interest being removed and incorporated into more convenient organisms through genetic transfer (such as *Streptomyces* species), the genes coding for specific biosynthetic enzymes being used to create synthetic homologous products through genetically engineering biosynthesis in living organisms (in combinatorial genetics), or by using enzymes and other catalysts *ex vivo* to build "chemical libraries" from scaffolds such as nucleosides, flavonoids or taxanes (in combinatorial biocatalysis).[30]

Translating a Traditional Practice into Western Medicine

The widespread use of medicinal mushroom extracts in the Far East raises some interesting questions as to whether purified or crude extracts should be used as drugs. As the pharmacological effect of these preparations is assumed to be due to a synergistic effect of their different constituents,[50] converting them into single-agent, pharmaceutical-grade preparations may lead to a loss of effectiveness.[49] However, using crude extracts complicates the identification of possible pharmacokinetic–pharmacodynamic interactions with conventional cancer treatments, as they may affect the absorption, distribution or metabolism of conventional chemotherapeutic agents, or affect the effectiveness of targeted therapies.[49]

Challenges in Designing Botanical Studies

As mentioned earlier, traditional medicine tends to use multiple herbs and treatment modalities, which makes the application of modern research methodology challenging, although ingenious research designs have been devised to allow the treatment of patients in a clinical trial setting.[9]

Some challenged the suitability of RCTs to address the specific needs of complementary therapies as whole systems of care and suggested that a mixed-method approach is better suited to evaluate whole systems, provided it is matched by a different range of appropriate outcome measures to assess their effectiveness.[56]

Additional challenges in setting up trials using botanicals relate to the safety of using the botanicals in conjunction with chemotherapeutic agents, so even though many of these preparations have a long track record of use in traditional medicines, early-phase clinical studies remain important to test for safety and optimal dose.[9]

Role of the Placebo Effect

Carrying out RCTs with botanicals is complicated by the fact that many herbs have distinctive smells and tastes, which makes devising a suitable placebo a special challenge.[6,15] Mok *et al.* recently published the results of a rigorous double-blind RCT, where patients with early-stage breast or colon cancer receiving post-operative adjuvant chemotherapy were randomly assigned to also receive a combination of a packaged herbal extract prescribed by a Chinese herbalist, or a placebo package containing non-therapeutic herbs, which had the smell and taste of a typical herbal tea.[15]

SOME PROS AND CONS OF USING PLANTS AS STARTING POINTS FOR A DRUG DEVELOPMENT PROGRAMME

Using ethnomedical information can provide reassurance that plants that have already withstood the test of time are more likely to provide active compounds, be safer to use and provide a richer source of new compounds than what is expected from a *de-novo* synthetic programme.[21] Examples of successes using this approach include the discovery of vinblastine, vincristine, taxol, *d*-tubocurarine and digoxin.[21]

Using this approach to drug discovery may provide a range of "leads" that will become the basis for further drug testing and chemical modifications, leading to safer, more effective and easier to produce drugs — the key ingredients of what is being termed "rational drug design".[44]

Some barriers that need to be overcome include: time to lead (the time taken to when the crude extract can become a lead compound), issues of supply and considerations on how to compensate countries and communities providing the natural products for their biodiversity that forms the basis for new drug discoveries.[31] Some logistical challenges include the following:

1. The ability to procure appropriate material for the study in sufficient quantities to allow to study to proceed.[9,57] Ways to address this challenge include using the prototype natural product as a lead compound and developing simpler, semi-synthetic or synthetic analogues, using improved recovery techniques (successfully achieved for artemisin and paclitaxel) and potentially using tissue culture to generate the active compound.[57]
2. The sustainability of plant collections cannot always be guaranteed, due to restrictions imposed by countries that are repositories of such biological diversity, intellectual property rights and compensation sought by countries for the use of their genetic resources.[21]
3. The fact that many herbal preparations consist of a mixture of different compounds raises the possibility that the overall effect is a sum total of the interaction of different ingredients, so that the administration of purified single extracts may not achieve the same effect; this is in keeping with the overall philosophy of herbalism, which suggests that part of the activity of the herbal preparation may be directed at the effects that plant constituents have on other bodily functions, not directly related to the disease process.[1]
4. The collection of plants based upon ethnomedical claims requires a more detailed and systematic approach and documentation, which limits the number of successful collections.[21]
5. Difficulties in achieving product standardization.[52]
6. Although the safety of herbal preparations can be inferred by the widespread use of a plant by different cultures over a long period of time, the use of the same plant material in a different culture, by people of a different genetic makeup, using a different type of diet, and/or self-administering the herbal medicines (rather than using them as part of a prescription by a skilled traditional medicine practitioner) leaves open the

possibility of adverse effects, which may not be manifest in the original setting.[1]

STEPS IN MOVING FROM TRADITIONAL MEDICINE TO CANDIDATE DRUG AND BEYOND

Driscoll describes the drug development process as consisting of two pre-clinical phases: drug discovery (with a lead discovery and a lead improvement stage) and a drug development phase (where the biological testing commenced in the previous phase is continued, toxicology studies are performed and the drug goes into production and formulation).[58] Approaches to lead discovery include screening (the major tool in lead discovery) and rational drug design (used in lead improvement).[58] It is noteworthy that the drug development process based on TCM uses similar steps, as the two systems share common goals of improved pharmacological profile of the candidate drugs.[13]

Corson *et al.* describe the pipeline leading from traditional medicine to Western pharmaceutical as an obstacle course, where the various challenges encountered during this process pertain to the initial discovery process, drug synthesis, determination of mechanism of action and the steps required to bring the new drug to market.[23]

Western "Discovery" of Traditional Medicine

Although in the West the use of quinine to treat malarial fevers is credited to Pelletier and Caventou in 1820, Peruvian Indians had been using the *Cinchona* bark to treat malarial fevers since the 17th century, so it took some two centuries for Western medicine to "discover" quinine.[23] Similarly, the bark of the willow tree had been used for millennia to treat fever and inflammation in many traditional medical systems long before the active principle (aspirin) was discovered by Western medicine.[23]

Isolation/Synthesis of Active Compound(s)

The use of artemisin, derived from *Artemisin annua* (sweet wormwood or *quinghao*) was first documented in TCM in 168 BC as a treatment for haemorrhoids and since the 4th century AC as an antimalarial,[59] but its structure was not elucidated until the mid-1970s; its widespread adoption was further hampered by production challenges, as agricultural production alone was insufficient to provide the required quantities, and the fact that the concentration of the drug in plant extracts is highly variable.[23]

Elucidation of the Mechanism of Action

Although the basis for use, active ingredients and their mechanism of action have been validated for many medicinal plants, this is not the case for many others and, even when carried out, the methodology used was not always appropriate for the intended purpose.[1]

Development of a Pharmaceutical

Corson *et al.* use the example of curcurmin to highlight the difficulties encountered in the clinical testing of a natural compound, which is both a spice (turmeric or *Curcurma longa*) and a drug with a long history of use in ayurvedha and TCM for the treatment of conditions ranging from rheumatism, trauma, amenorrhoea and various intestinal disorders. This versatility makes the design of rigorous clinical testing challenging, as the relative ease of demonstrating effectiveness in pre-clinical and/or pilot studies can work against the formal validation of effectiveness in rigorous randomized, placebo-controlled double-blind studies, particularly as pharmaceutical companies have limited interest in a non-patentable agent and due to the perception that curcurmin is more of a nutraceutical than a "real" drug.[23]

Furthermore, after scaling all of these obstacles, these compounds may need to be transformed through semi-synthesis or total synthesis into agents with an optimized ADMET (the most favourable Absorption, Distribution, Metabolism, Excretion and Toxicity) profile.[23]

NATURAL COMPOUNDS CURRENTLY USED IN CANCER THERAPY

Nobili *et al.* recently published a comprehensive review of natural compounds used in cancer treatment and prevention, providing a detailed review of tubulin-binding agents of plant origin (vinca alkaloids and taxanes) and topoisomerase inhibitors (including camptothecins, epidophyllotoxins and anthracyclines) as well as other natural compounds.[3]

Vinca Alkaloids

Vinca alkaloids were originally isolated from *Vinca rosea* (also known as *Catharrantus roseus* or periwinkle), with vincristine, vinblastine and vindesine being the first-generation antitumour agents identified in this class.[3]

The discovery of these agents illustrates the role played by a combination of serendipity and sharp clinical acumen in drug discovery. During the 1940s and 1950s a group of investigators at the University of Western Ontario were studying the effect of periwinkle extracts on carbohydrate metabolism, prompted by ethnobotanical information from Jamaica suggesting that tea made from the white-flowered periwinkle (*Vinca rosea*) was effective in controlling diabetes mellitus. Although no effects were observed on diabetes, the researchers observed that rats treated with this extract had a reduced resistance to infection, associated by a reversible rapid fall in their white cell count (particularly of myeloid elements), accompanied by bone marrow suppression, which they correctly attributed to the antiproliferative properties of these extracts.[25]

Using vinblastine as a lead compound, structural modification subsequently led to the development of second-generation *Vinca* alkaloids, such as vinorelbine and more recently vinflunine, which is currently being evaluated in clinical trials.[3]

Taxanes

Taxanes, with the flagship drug taxol (paclitaxel), were discovered through plant collections conducted by botanists searching for steroids that could become cortisone precursors. Originally taxol was extracted from the bark of *Taxus brevifolia*, but it is now obtained through semi-synthesis[27] from 10-deacetylbaccatin III, extracted from the needles of the European yew tree, *Taxus baccata*.[3] Recently the pharmaceutical industry has been focusing on developing new more potent taxane formulations with increased tolerability and less drug resistance and finding new formulations. Some of the new, more potent taxanes include abraxane and docosahexenoic acid-paclitaxel.[3]

Plant-Derived Campthotecins

Plant-derived campthotecins were discovered through the NCI screening programme in the 1950s, which found that the leaves of *Campthoteca acuminata* (a tree native to China) were effective against leukaemias and some solid tumours; subsequently the active compound was identified as campthotecin.[3] Its antitumour activity was also identified in clinical trials in China, in patients with a variety of cancers.[60] As the effectiveness of the original campthotecin formulation was marred by unpredictable toxicity, many years of research went into producing two semi-synthetic derivatives, irinotecan and topotecan, which were released in the mid-1990s; a number of synthetic derivatives (e.g. lurtotecan, exatecan mesylate and gimatecan) are currently under evaluation.[3]

Podophyllotoxins

Podophyllotoxins derived from *Podophyllum peltatum* have been used by American Indians for their emetic and antihelminthic purposes and their antitumour activity has led to the chemical synthesis of etoposide and teniposide, which target DNA topoisomerase II.[3]

Anthracyclines

Anthracyclines of plant origin include daunorubicin and doxorubicin, with new formulations having come on the market (e.g. liposomal formulations) and synthetic analogues being evaluated in clinical studies.[3]

WHAT IS THE FUTURE OF NATURAL MEDICINES IN DRUG DISCOVERY?

Some compounds under active investigation today have a long record of use in traditional medicine and may provide new drug remedies for a variety of conditions. They include green tea (mentioned in ancient Japanese texts), saffron (stigmata of *Crocus sativum*), and turmeric and myrrh (the dried resin of *Commiphora myrrha*, mentioned in the Bible).[3] Green tea contains epigallocatechin-3-gallate, shown to reduce the growth of some cancers in experimental animals, whereas myrrh, traditionally used for its anti-inflammatory effects is also being investigated for its ability to kill cancer cells resistant to other anti-cancer drugs.[3]

It may be possible that treating cancer in the future will involve a combined approach, in which Western medicine (including surgery, chemotherapy and radiotherapy) will be used to destroy the tumour, whereas other treatments, such as TCM, will address the entire "unhealthy" condition, so that a change in the body environment could facilitate cure, by addressing disease determinants more broadly and from an alternative perspective.[11]

In order to fulfill the promise of natural medicines, it is critical to adopt commonly agreed criteria for assessing their safety and effectiveness, and to ensure the sustainability of these products. This will remain of particular relevance for developing economies, where plant materials, used as traditional medicines, could help to meet the needs of primary care medicine and lead to improvements in the quality of health-care for a large proportion of the world's population.[61]

In technologically advanced countries, a multi-disciplinary approach to drug discovery, encompassing both the rational exploitation of natural resources and synthetic methodologies, could enhance the productivity of the drug-discovery process.[62] The process could be streamlined by using new technologies to select the appropriate targets, improve the extraction and separation of the active compounds and by using high-throughput screening and microfractionation techniques, which use up only small amounts of samples for characterization of the compounds.[62] At the dawn of the new millennium, it was estimated that approximately 170 companies and about 40 research institutions were engaged in the process of discovery, evaluation and development of natural medicinal products.[63] Meanwhile, international patent applications for natural medicinal substances are increasing, drug development costs are rising and the yields from synthetic pathways in drug discovery are falling. All of these factors, coupled with an ever-increasing public preference for natural products, suggest that the future of natural medicinal products remains bright indeed.

REFERENCES

1. Houghton PJ. The role of plants in traditional medicine and current therapy. *J Altern Complement Med* **1**(2):131–143 (1995).
2. Phillipson JD, Anderson LA. Ethnopharmacology and Western medicine. *J Ethnopharmacol* **25**(1):61–729 (1989).
3. Nobili S, Lippi D, Witort E, *et al*. Natural compounds for cancer treatment and prevention. *Pharmacol Res* **59**(6):365–378 (2009).
4. Wang MW, Hao X, Chen K. Biological screening of natural products and drug innovation in China. *Philos Trans Roy Soc Lond* **362**(1482):1093–1105 (2007).
5. Farnsworth NR, Akerele O, Bingel AS, *et al*. Medicinal plants in therapy. *Bull World Health Org* **63**(6):965–981 (1985).
6. Farnsworth NR. The role of ethnopharmacology in drug development. *Ciba Found Symp* **154**:2–11; discussion 11–21 (1990).
7. Phillipson JD. Natural products as drugs. *Trans R Soc Trop Med Hyg* **88**(suppl 1):S17–S19 (1994).
8. Rates SM. Plants as source of drugs. *Toxicon* **39**(5):603–613 (2001).
9. Yeung KS, Gubili J, Cassileth B. Evidence-based botanical research: applications and challenges. *Hematol/Oncol Clin North Am* **22**(4):661–670, viii (2008).
10. Zhu YP, Woerdenbag HJ. Traditional Chinese herbal medicine. *Pharm World Sci* **17**(4):103–112 (1995).
11. Ruan WJ, Lai MD, Zhou JG. Anticancer effects of Chinese herbal medicine, science or myth? *J Zhejiang Univ Sci* **7**(12):1006–1014 (2006).
12. Moyad MA, Hathaway S, Ni HS. Traditional Chinese medicine, acupuncture, and other alternative medicines for prostate cancer: an introduction and the need for more research. *Semin Urol Oncol* **17**(2):103–110 (1999).
13. Lee KH. Research and future trends in the pharmaceutical development of medicinal herbs from Chinese medicine. *Pub Health Nutri* **3**(4A):515–522 (2000).
14. Molassiotis A, Potrata B, Cheng KK. A systematic review of the effectiveness of Chinese herbal medication in symptom management and improvement of quality of life in adult cancer patients. *Complement Ther Med* **17**(2):92–120 (2009).

15. Mok TS, Yeo W, Johnson PJ, *et al.* A double-blind placebo-controlled randomized study of Chinese herbal medicine as complementary therapy for reduction of chemotherapy-induced toxicity. *Ann Oncol* **18**(4):768–774 (2007).
16. Patwardhan B, Gautam M. Botanical immunodrugs: scope and opportunities. *Drug Discov Today* **10**(7):495–502 (2005).
17. Mishra LC, Singh BB, Dagenais S. Scientific basis for the therapeutic use of Withania somnifera (ashwagandha): a review. *Altern Med Rev* **5**(4):334–346 (2000).
18. Phillipson JD. 50 years of medicinal plant research — every progress in methodology is a progress in science. *Planta Med* **69**(6):491–495 (2003).
19. Baker JT, Borris RP, Carte B, *et al.* Natural product drug discovery and development: new perspectives on international collaboration. *J Nat Prod* **58**(9):1325–1357 (1995).
20. Soejarto DD, Fong HH, Tan GT, *et al.* Ethnobotany/ethnopharmacology and mass bioprospecting: issues on intellectual property and benefit-sharing. *J Ethnopharmacol* **100**(1–2):15–22 (2005).
21. Fabricant DS, Farnsworth NR. The value of plants used in traditional medicine for drug discovery. *Environ Health Perspect* **109**(suppl 1): 69–75 (2001).
22. Burns WR. East meets West: how China almost cured malaria. *Endeavour* **32**(3):101–106 (2008).
23. Corson TW, Crews CM. Molecular understanding and modern application of traditional medicines: triumphs and trials. *Cell* **130**(5):769–774 (2007).
24. Cox PA. The ethnobotanical approach to drug discovery: strengths and limitations. *Ciba Found Symp* **185**:25–36; discussion 36–41 (1994).
25. Noble RL, Beer CT, Cutts JH. Role of chance observations in chemotherapy: Vinca rosea. *Ann N Y Acad Sci* **76**(3):882–894 (1985).
26. Rishton GM. Natural products as a robust source of new drugs and drug leads: past successes and present day issues. *Am J Cardiol* **101**(10A):43D–49D (2008).
27. Kinghorn A. Pharmacognosy in the 21st century. *J Pharm Pharmacol* **53**(2):135–148 (2001).
28. Borris RP. Natural products research: perspectives from a major pharmaceutical company. *J Ethnopharmacol* **51**(1–3):29–38 (1996).
29. Cragg GM, Newman DJ, Snader KM. Natural products in drug discovery and development. *J Nat Prod* **60**(1):52–60 (1997).

30. Harvey A. Strategies for discovering drugs from previously unexplored natural products. *Drug Discov Today* **5**(7):294–300 (2000).
31. Schuster BG. A new integrated program for natural product development and the value of an ethnomedical approach. *J Altern Complement Med* **7**(suppl 1):S61–S72 (2001).
32. Turner DM. Natural product source material use in the pharmaceutical industry: the Glaxo experience. *J Ethnopharmacol* **51**(1–3):39–43; discussion 44 (1996).
33. Cragg GM, Boyd MR, Cardellina JH, 2nd, *et al.* Ethnobotany and drug discovery: the experience of the US National Cancer Institute. *Ciba Found Symp* **185**:178–190; discussion 90–96 (1994).
34. Mahady G. World health and international collaboration in traditional medicine and medicinal plant research. In Eskinazi D (ed), *What Will Influence the Future of Alternative Medicine? A World Perspective,* World Scientific Publishing Co Pte Ltd., Singapore, pp. 89–104 (2001).
35. Eisenberg DM, Davis RB, Ettner SL, *et al.* Trends in alternative medicine use in the United States, 1990–1997: results of a follow-up national survey. *JAMA* **280**(18):1569–1575 (1998).
36. Tindle HA, Davis RB, Phillips RS, *et al.* Trends in use of complementary and alternative medicine by US adults: 1997–2002. *Altern Ther Health Med* **11**(1):42–49 (2005).
37. Sparreboom A, Cox MC, Acharya MR, *et al.* Herbal remedies in the United States: potential adverse interactions with anticancer agents. *J Clin Oncol* **22**(12):2489–2503 (2004).
38. Kaufman DW, Kelly JP, Rosenberg L, *et al.* Recent patterns of medication use in the ambulatory adult population of the United States: the Slone survey. *JAMA* **287**(3):337–344 (2002).
39. MacLennan AH, Wilson DH, Taylor AW. The escalating cost and prevalence of alternative medicine. *Prevent Med* **35**(2):166–173 (2002).
40. Expert Committee on Complementary Medicines in the Health System. *Complementary Medicines in the Australian Health System.* Report to the Parliamentary Secretary to the Minister for Health and Ageing. Commonwealth of Australia, Canberra (2003).
41. Cassileth B, Vickers A. Complementary and alternative cancer therapies. In Holland JF, Frei E (eds), *Cancer Medicine,* 6th edn, B.C. Decker Inc., Hamilton, pp. 1101–1111 (2003).

42. Coulter ID, Willis EM. The rise and rise of complementary and alternative medicine: a sociological perspective. *Med J Aust* **180**(11):587–589 (2004).
43. Cassileth B, Deng G, Vickers A, *et al. PDQ Integrative Oncology. Complementary Therapies in Cancer Care*, B.C. Decker Inc., Hamilton (2005).
44. Grever MR, Schepartz SA, Chabner BA. The National Cancer Institute: cancer drug discovery and development program. *Semin Oncol* **19**(6):622–638 (1992).
45. Cox PA. Ethnopharmacology and the search for new drugs. *Ciba Found Symp* **154**:40–47; discussion 47–55 (1990).
46. Houghton PJ, Howes MJ, Lee CC, *et al.* Uses and abuses of *in vitro* tests in ethnopharmacology: visualizing an elephant. *J Ethnopharmacol* **110**(3):391–400 (2007).
47. Graham JG, Quinn ML, Fabricant DS, *et al.* Plants used against cancer — an extension of the work of Jonathan Hartwell. *J Ethnopharmacol* **73**(3):347–377 (2000).
48. Farnsworth N. NAPRALERT^{sm}.
49. Sullivan R, Smith JE, Rowan NJ. Medicinal mushrooms and cancer therapy: translating a traditional practice into Western medicine. *Perspect Biol Med* **49**(2):159–170 (2006).
50. Normile D. Asian medicine. The new face of traditional Chinese medicine. *Science* **299**(5604):188–190 (2003).
51. Farnsworth NR. Ethnopharmacology and drug development. *Ciba Found Symp* **185**:42–51; discussion 51–59 (1994).
52. Glickman-Simon R. Highlights of evidence based medicine from the American College of Physicians 2005 Annual Session. Complementary and alternative medicine: an evidence-based approach. *Medscape Medicine* (2005).
53. Ko RJ. Adulterants in Asian patent medicines. *N Engl J Med* **339**(12):847 (1998).
54. Murch S, KrishnaRaj S, Saxena P. Phytopharmaceuticals: problems, limitations and solutions. *Sci Rev Altern Med* **4**:33–37 (2000).
55. King SR, Carlson TJ, Moran K. Biological diversity, indigenous knowledge, drug discovery and intellectual property rights: creating reciprocity and maintaining relationships. *J Ethnopharmacol* **51**(1–3): 45–57 (1996).
56. Verhoef MJ, Lewith G, Ritenbaugh C, *et al.* Complementary and alternative medicine whole systems research: beyond identification

of inadequacies of the RCT. *Complement Ther Med* **13**(3):206–212 (2005).
57. Clark AM. Natural products as a resource for new drugs. *Pharm Res* **13**(8):1133–1144 (1996).
58. Driscoll JS. The preclinical new drug research program of the National Cancer Institute. *Cancer Treat Rep* **68**(1):63–76 (1984).
59. Liu C, Zhao Y, Wang Y. Artemisinin: current state and perspectives for biotechnological production of an antimalarial drug. *Appl Microbiol Biotechnol* **72**(1):11–20 (2006).
60. Wall ME, Wani MC. Camptothecin and taxol: from discovery to clinic. *J Ethnopharmacol* **51**(1–3):239–253; discussion 53–54 (1996).
61. Cordell GA, Colvard MD. Some thoughts on the future of ethnopharmacology. *J Ethnopharmacol* **100**(1–2):5–14 (2005).
62. Vuorelaa P, Leinonenb M, Saikkuc P, *et al*. Natural products in the process of finding new drug candidates. *Curr Med Chem* **11**(11):1375–1389 (2004).
63. Meng C. On the development of traditional Chinese medicine in 21st century China. In Eskinazi D (ed), *What Will Influence the Future of Alternative Medicine? A World Perspective*. World Scientific Publishing Co Pte Ltd, Singapore, pp. 23–30 (2001).

9

Creating an Integrative Oncology Centre: The SolarisCare Experience

David Joske

ABSTRACT

Cancer constitutes a large burden of disease upon developed countries in terms of cost, loss of workforce productivity, mortality, suffering and distress. Although cancer survival is improving, ways are needed to improve the cancer treatment experience. In September 2001, an innovative and unique cancer support facility, the SolarisCare Centre, opened in Sir Charles Gairdner Hospital, a major teaching hospital in Perth, Western Australia with over 600 beds and a strong cancer treatment focus. Facilities at the Centre include a quiet area, access to information and supportive care organisations, counselling and complementary therapy sessions. Nearly nine years later, many thousands of cancer patients have been helped and treated in various ways. Our evidence shows that patients who participate in complementary therapy sessions have reduced symptom distress, and improved quality of life. The Centre also provides a sense of community for some, that is otherwise lacking, and focuses community support. Two more centres now operate, using a similar novel model of care. This chatper outlines the processes by which this novel integrative oncology Centre was established, including selection of therapies and therapists, models of governance and funding, credentialling of therapists, training of volunteers, minimisation of medico-legal risk, prevention of harm to a vulnerable patient population, and development of research methods to measure efficacy. Five barriers to this approach in cancer care are identified: health system resistance, funding, identifying and keeping therapists, credentialling of therapists, and spirituality clashes. Recommendations are made towards sustainable models of integrative cancer care and future research. A new model of cancer care is proposed with one-stop treatment and support facilities and a national collaboration of like-minded cancer support centres to investigate further the benefits of this approach.

Keywords: Cancer; Cancer Treatment; Complementary and Alternative Medicine (CAM); Complementary Integrative Therapy (CIT); Psycho-Oncology.

INTRODUCTION

Cancer is a large burden upon developed countries, in terms of cost, lost workplace productivity, and human mortality, suffering and anguish. In Australia in 2001, some \$2.9 billion[1] was spent on mainstream cancer treatments, and \$215 million on cancer research.[1] In recent years, there have been undoubted improvements in survival for many cancer subtypes, including breast cancer,[2] myeloma,[3,4] chronic myeloid leukaemia[5] and lymphomas.[6] Although much improvement is still needed in other types of cancer, there is now an increased focus upon improving the cancer journey.[7] In Australia, interventions have mostly been based upon counselling, behavioural or psychosupportive approaches.[8]

Cancer patients consistently turn to complementary and alternative medicine (CAM). Surveys in developed countries show that some 30–75% of cancer patients use complementary therapies,[9,10] often without informing the mainstream health team. Reasons include a desire to feel hopeful, a belief that the treatments are non-toxic, wanting more control, or seeking a cure.[11] Another reason may be frustration with poor communication, or the sense of being production-line fodder. Health inflation continues to outstrip fiscal inflation, but cancer patients and Federal and State Governments all expect access to effective or expensive new treatments. For example, Glivec for chronic myeloid leukaemia costs around $50,000 pa,[12] whereas iodine seed therapy for low-risk prostate cancer costs around $20,000 (personal communication, Dr David Joseph, Radiation Oncologist, Sir Charles Gairdner Hospital, June 2010). Costs have been reined in by making staff "more efficient", meaning that more patients are treated by the same or fewer staff. This leaves health professionals with less time to give a human face to cancer care.

As a practising physician in haematology, my awareness of the pressures on our health system grew in the late 1990s. I felt that my patients needed more support than I was able to offer them in 15-minute appointments. A chance comment led to a reappraisal of the possible role that CAM could play in cancer care. What follows here is an exposition of the unique circumstances and initiatives that allowed a personal response to this situation as a physician — to lead a charitable cancer support foundation, providing services for over 200 cancer patients each week in three centres. This chapter outlines simultaneously the development of the SolarisCare model of integrative cancer care using complementary therapies and my own personal journey from a doctor who felt he had to show an open mind on CAM to one **with** an open mind — far from being the same thing!

HISTORY AND FIRST STEPS

In 2000, a gentleman with lymphoma said to me in consultation that it took him three months to learn how to be a patient. When quizzed, he replied that by this he meant that he had to learn the geography of the hospital, the biology of his tumour, the language of medicine, and "who I could talk to about what I was doing to help myself". This chance comment led to some deep self-reflection and a realisation that I must learn something about complementary therapies, or forever have a barrier between me and my patients. I started researching, found more data than I expected and learnt of some cancer support centres in the UK. A few months later, I was approached by a then-local dairy product manufacturer, Peters & Brownes Dairy, seeking ideas for a community campaign they wanted to conduct. They were immediately keen to be involved in the concept of a cancer support centre. Following a special meeting of their Board, I was filmed as the talking head for an 8-week advertising campaign that went to air on free-to-air television stations before Christmas, 2000. The company donated 5c for each litre of milk sold and $208,000 was raised. With the closure of a bank branch within the hospital, an area was refurbished to become the Department of Haematology and the Peters & Brownes Cancer Support Centre. Organisations including the Wylie Corporation and Kailis Foods also donated a further $150,000 to the project and their generosity is gratefully acknowledged.

The Cancer Council of Western Australia funded a visit to Western Australia by radiation oncologist, Dr Jane Maher. Her visit gave me the opportunity to gain insight into her experiences, challenges and successes in her establishment of a similar centre at the Mount Vernon Hospital in Middlesex, UK. Her advice can be distilled to three key points: (1) don't ignore the "squeaky wheels", as they are often saying the same thing as the silent majority, if more stridently; (2) focus on alleviating symptoms; and (3) choose therapists with whom you feel you can share a dialogue on clinical endpoints.

In designing the Centre we took inspiration from the traditional Australian country homestead. The centre is 150 m^2 in size and focuses around a kitchenette, with a quiet area and sofas, large and small treatment rooms, one small office and a library area. It is located directly next door to the Haematology Department and only a short walk from the entrances to the Radiation Oncology and Medical Oncology Departments.

The Centre opened its doors on 15 September 2001 and, from week one, has seen on average 150 visitors per week. About half of these patients access the complementary therapy sessions. Others just sit and have a cup of tea, or browse the extensive collection of brochures and information from a variety of organisations, including the Cancer Council and the Leukaemia Foundation. For those who chose complementary therapies, initially we provided six sessions, free of charge and asked for donations thereafter. The selection of therapy modality by patients was and is *ad hoc*, depending upon availability and, to a lesser extent, on patient preference. The philosophy was and is to be as inclusive as possible, involving other cancer-related organisations and treating patients and their carers from any hospital or practice.

SELECTION OF THERAPIES

Our literature review, since published, guided us to the selection of complementary therapies.[13] Treatment modalities can be broken down into five domains, as described by Goldrosen and Straus:[14] manipulative and body-based techniques (massage in various forms), biologically-based approaches (diets, herbs), energy therapies (Reiki, magnets), mind–body interventions (yoga, relaxation techniques) and alternative belief systems (ayurvedic and Chinese traditional medicine). In summary, we found level II evidence (single-centre randomised controlled trials) in support of touch- and massage-based therapies to reduce anxiety, acupuncture to reduce chemotherapy-related nausea,[15] music therapy to improve mood and some benefit with counselling. There is no evidence that massage promotes the spread of cancer.[16] After deliberation, we selected mostly massage- and touch-based therapies, limited counselling interventions, acupuncture, some meditative or mindfulness therapies, and activities such as Chi breathing and beauty therapy. Oral or herbal interventions were not considered, due to the absence of clear benefit[14] and lack of infrastructure to adequately research them. Table 1 contains a list of therapies offered by SolarisCare Centres.

SELECTION OF THERAPISTS

The initial advertisement for therapists drew many responses and gave a deep insight into the world of complementary therapists. Although some were clearly seeking the cachet of teaching hospital "accreditation", many were motivated by a deep sense of altruism. Public sector guidelines for volunteer selection were followed, including police clearance. We sought practitioners with the highest possible training we could discern for their therapy and at least 12 months of clinical experience. All selected therapists completed 4 weeks as a meet-and-greet volunteer to assess their motivation and interaction with cancer patients; this practice continues. Many CAM practitioners use several therapy modalities, but all were asked to restrict their practice with SolarisCare to the selected therapy, with which they have the most experience. Some therapists with powerfully-held belief systems that clashed too strongly with the planned *modus operandi* were deemed unsuitable.

Table 1. Complementary therapies administered and collated by SolarisCare therapists during the period February 2002–November 2008.

Therapy type	Number of sessions	% of all sessions
Energy-based		
Reiki	675	24.93
Pranic healing	298	11.00
Kinesiology	89	3.29
Massage/touch		
Reflexology	385	14.22
Aromatherapy	320	11.82
Bowen therapy	210	7.75
Acupuncture*	105	3.88
Healing touch	98	3.62
Cranio-sacral therapy	92	3.39
Relaxation massage	81	2.99
Beauty therapy	80	2.95
Mind–body-based		
Chi breathing and Chi meditation	120	4.43
Creative art therapy	15	0.55
Breathe for health	14	0.52
Creative visualisation	13	0.48
Tai Chi	11	0.40
Qi Gong	5	0.18
Sound and music therapy	2	0.07
Other		
Counselling	95	3.51
Total	2708	100

*Note that acupuncture is normally used as part of Chinese traditional medicine, and not classified as a massage/touch therapy, but was included here for the analysis provided in Fig. 1.

TRAINING OF VOLUNTEERS

The role of meet-and-greet volunteers in the Centre is to greet patients and visitors, provide a listening ear and manage the therapists' appointments. Formal counselling skills are not needed. However, as a back-up, permission was obtained to refer patients *in extremis* to the Hospital's Department of Psychiatry. This has never been required. A Centre Manager was appointed, with a background in Technical and Further Education (TAFE) and an understanding of many complementary therapies. His role was to help to select therapists, coordinate the volunteer programme and to monitor meet-and-greet and therapist volunteer interactions with patients.

GOVERNANCE AND NEXT STEPS

The immediate popularity of the Centre indicated a previously unmet need. It also created problems of space, governance, relationship to the hospital and therapist numbers. The space issue proved insoluble within the Centre and eventually we were ceded an additional room adjacent to the cancer ward of the hospital. This later served as a base for treating inpatients, with the episode of care documented in the inpatient notes.

The hospital gave its support through a peppercorn rental, use of accounting and financial systems, payroll functions for the small number of employees and third-party insurance and indemnity. Although the Hospital Executive was strongly supportive throughout, it appeared not to know how to manage this new entity. The governance was essentially provided by the Centre Manager and myself, for 5 years. I opted to create a Steering Committee, including an experienced cancer nurse, the administrative assistant to the Cancer Clinical Service Unit and the Head of Physiotherapy, all of whom had an interest and were prepared to become involved. The Steering Committee was responsible for providing reports to the Hospital Executive every 6 months, to provide feedback on activity, patient numbers, misadventure (see below) and, later, results.

Within 2 years, it was decided to form a Board of interested persons, with the goal of becoming a stand-alone charitable Foundation and to drive a research programme. The SolarisCare Foundation, a non-Governmental charitable Foundation, with donor gift recipient status, was launched by Dr Neale Fong, then Director-General of the Health Department of Western Australia, in November 2006.

RESEARCH AND MEASURING EFFICACY

In 2002, a research committee was formed involving clinicians and researchers from the hospital and external agencies. An initial patient assessment survey was developed for patients to provide therapists with the information needed for their practice, such as their cancer type, known sites of disease or spread, other health problems, recent operations and basic details about their mainstream cancer care (chemotherapy, radiotherapy and surgery).

The McCorkle and Young Symptom Distress Scale (SDS)[17,18] was adapted for use in the Centre. Patients were asked to complete seven-point Quality of Life (QoL) Scale SDS and before the first, and before and immediately after the third and sixth complementary therapy session. The SDS includes scores for pain, fatigue, nausea, bowel problems, breathing difficulty, poor appetite and impaired sleep. The seven-point QoL Scale includes scores for disempowerment, depression, anxiety, frustration, confusion, impaired coping and worry. The data were collected between February 2002 and November 2008, collated and subjected to independent statistical analysis.

Results

Data on over 1400 cancer patients and 400 carers completing complementary therapy sessions have now been collated. Full results are in preparation for publication. In summary, of 1240 cancer patients treated, 952 were female (77%) and 288 male (23%). The mean age was 55 years (54 for women, 59 for men). There were 970 outpatients (81.7%) and 218 inpatients (18.4%). Breast cancer was the predominant cancer type; 596 (45%) were women with breast cancer. Some 358 (27%) reported known metastases (41.6% lymph, 24.3% bone, 17% liver). In terms of ongoing mainstream treatments, 12.3% were undergoing concurrent chemotherapy, 17% radiotherapy, 28% surgery and 52.3% were not undergoing active cancer treatment. Patients' medical treatment was based at several different hospitals, both public and private, but the majority were being treated at Sir Charles Gairdner Hospital (68%).

Some 2724 complementary treatment sessions were recorded in the database. Details of the treatments are given in Table 1 and Fig. 1. In total, data on 1303 first sessions, 977 third sessions and 444 sixth sessions were collected There were some variations in

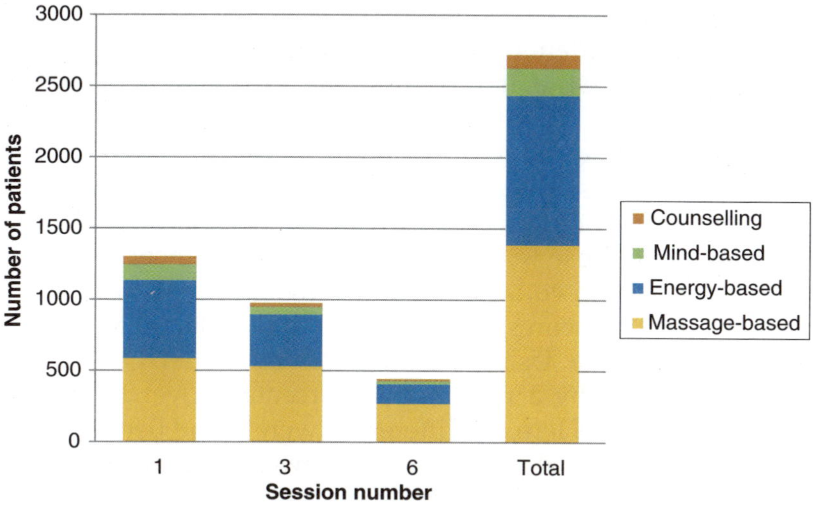

Therapy choice	Session number			
	1	3	6	**Total**
Massage-based	585	530	270	**1385**
Energy-based	548	365	137	**1050**
Mind-based	114	55	23	**192**
Counselling	56	27	14	**97**
Total	**1303**	**977**	**444**	**2724**

Fig. 1. Patient enrolment and choice of complementary therapy type at sessions 1, 3 and 6.

types of treatments between the cumulative data for the first, third and sixth sessions, with relatively more massage-based therapies delivered in the sixth session (Fig. 1).

Both the SDS and QoL Scale showed large effects in the before and after assessments at treatment sessions 3 and 6, which would suggest a strong very short-term beneficial effect. However, for the results given above the data points before sessions 1, 3 and 6 only were analysed, on the assumption that the pre-session scores are indicative of longer term effect or lack thereof of the prior treatment or treatments.

The mean symptom distress score for the SDS is an average of the scores for all patients, across all symptoms. It was found to fall linearly from before the first to before the sixth session ($P < 0.0001$). Using a statistical technique referred to as summary measure analysis, this was found to correspond to a measurable reduction in symptom distress over the six treatments. Patients with lung cancer and metastatic disease had higher baseline scores (more symptoms) than those with breast and prostate cancer, but all cancer types showed an equal reduction in symptom distress.

The mean QoL scores, using an inverted scale, improved from session 1 to session 6. Using a random effects model, QoL was estimated to improve by a measurable percentage over baseline per session ($P < 0.0001$). Here, no differences were found between cancer types at baseline and all cancer types showed equal improvement.

There was a correlation found between symptom distress and QoL. Improvements in QoL for some 400 carers were also found; however these data are not shown here.

Discussion

These results are not randomised controlled data, and involve essentially self-selected patients. Consequently they should be interpreted with caution. Possible explanations for a clearly positive result include: placebo effect, benefit from concurrent mainstream treatment, an effect of missingness (i.e. that the drop-out in numbers between sessions 1, 3 and 6 biases the results as these are the patients who are not responding or worsening during the treatments) or a true beneficial effect of the treatment intervention. The placebo effect is likely to be strong here, as the volunteers are highly motivated to listen and/or provide their therapy. Some 53% of patients reported no concurrent mainstream treatment and this alone is therefore unlikely to be the explanation. Four different techniques were used to allow for missingness. Essentially unchanged results were found after repeated analyses using predictors of attrition, the Heckman method, a clustered linear regression model, multiple imputation methods and maximum likelihood estimation.

I believe that the data unambiguously show a benefit of the Centre in reducing symptom distress and improving QoL with statistical and clinical significance. Whether this is due to placebo effect, empowerment of individuals or a biologically-mediated psycho-physiological effect is of less importance than the results themselves.

This is gratifying and extraordinary. Using what many would consider an inadequately trained, uncredentialled volunteer work-force, employing treatment modalities discarded for hundreds of years by mainstream Western medicine, cancer symptoms and treatment side-effects can be alleviated and QoL powerfully improved in selected cancer patients. Put another way, a community-based complementary cancer care model is effective and provides health benefits in oncological medicine that cannot be achieved otherwise. The model addresses many of the concerns and recommendations made by the Cooke Enquiry.[19] Moreover, we find that for some cancer patients who are alone or isolated (those with no partner or a cancer-phobic partner), the Centre provides a caring community, which is not otherwise available.

MINIMISING MEDICO-LEGAL RISK AND MEDICAL MISADVENTURE

With a recurring nightmare vision of a senior colleague bursting into my office and accusing a therapist of turning someone against chemotherapy, a number of steps were taken to minimise the risk of harm to patients, and the medico-legal risk to the organisation and the hospital. These steps are detailed in Table 2. Our policies of limiting therapists to their selected modality, following public sector volunteer guidelines, recognising optimal training and insisting upon 12 months' prior experience and the four-week meet-and-greet trial period (now two weeks) have been effective in workforce recruitment and selection. There have been no significant episodes of medical misadventure. One hospital staff member reported pain after an overly vigorous neck massage; the therapy was discontinued. During an acupuncture teaching session, a needlestick injury occurred and hospital protocols were followed.

SOLARISCARE CURRENT STRUCTURE AND ACTIVITIES

A second centre opened at a large private hospital campus with a dedicated cancer centre in 2008, at the St. John of God Health Campus including the Jack Bendat Family Comprehensive

Table 2. Early steps to minimise medico-legal and harm risk.

Volunteer selection	Ability to share clinical endpoints with mainstream model
	Adherence to public sector volunteer guidelines (police check, references)
	At least 12 months' experience in the selected modality
	Initial 4 weeks as "meet-and-greet" volunteer
	Modalities selected after literature review
Volunteer "do's"	Do refer to other support organisations where appropriate
	Do encourage further treatments outside SolarisCare
Volunteer "don'ts"	Don't massage near known sites of disease
	Never dissuade patients from mainstream care
	Don't practice any therapy except that for which you were selected
	Don't claim accreditation with the hospital

Cancer Centre in Subiaco, Perth, Western Australia. This is funded by a Service Agreement between St. John of God Healthcare and SolarisCare.

SolarisCare has recently acquired and refurbished a property in Bunbury, Western Australia, 250 km south of Perth. It is a regional centre, where cancer services are being increased (e.g. two radiation therapy bunkers) to service the State's southwest. Thus, a third centre has started operations using complementary therapies for cancer patients in 2010. Finally, in response to the growing evidence of the efficacy of exercise during and after cancer treatment,[20,21] the SolarisCare "Chemo Club" has provided supervised exercise and resistance training for cancer patients twice a week, free of charge, at a Perth gymnasium (Aspire Fitness, in Claremont). This is staffed by volunteer exercise physiologists and others.

Thus, the current SolarisCare structure is of two metropolitan, hospital-based centres, one at a public teaching hospital and one in a private hospitals, a third rural/regional centre located off-campus and the Chemo Club at a private gymnasium. Current paid staff include a general manager, three centre coordinators, a postdoctoral research fellow plus part-time information technology, public relations and marketing staff. There are over 120 volunteers, about half meet-and-greet and half therapists.

FIVE BARRIERS TO COMPLEMENTARY THERAPY USE IN CANCER CARE

Health System Resistance

There is a long history of enmity and discord between the mainstream medical world and the world of complementary therapies. The former can be characterised as reductionist, hypothesis-testing, quantitative, population-based and founded upon disease-based models of health. The latter is more qualitative, open-ended and retains a focus upon the individual in whom the disease has occurred. Put more simply, some would see this as a clash of rigorous science versus anecdotalism or, at worst, snake-oil charlatanism. Mainstream health practitioners are rightly concerned that vulnerable patients will be lured into expensive and futile health practices on the promise of cure. However, to be dismissive of cancer patients who report CAM use to their health-care professional is to humiliate people who are, after all, attempting to be pro-active about their health.[22] Such a derisory attitude may well have prevented some from accessing SolarisCare, for example. However, having an open door and an inclusive policy has meant that the main "referral" source has been nursing staff in various institutions. At a macro level, it manifests as an absence of funding or planning for cancer support facilities in infrastructure projects.

Funding

In our experience, the cost of running one centre, treating around 150 patients per week, is around $250,000 p.a., using volunteers for meet-and-greet duties and therapy sessions. For the first seven years, funding came from private donations and the fundraising activities of SolarisCare staff and volunteers. An early donation from the Leukaemia Foundation of Western Australia was also very helpful. It was a precarious existence. Twice, we were almost unable to pay staff, with a private benefactor stepping in with donations. In 2007, a group of highly motivated business people, the RedSkyRide (www.redskyride.com.au) resolved to ride for cancer charities and to make SolarisCare the beneficiary. Their donations enabled SolarisCare to continue for the next two years. In 2008, the incoming Liberal-National Party Government of Western Australia provided an unencumbered grant of $1.5 m to SolarisCare, which has enabled the organisation to be revamped more professionally, to treat more cancer patients in a satellite project in the department of Medical Oncology at Sir Charles Gairdner Hospital and for the Bunbury centre to become a reality.

Funding for research into CAM is also an issue. Until 2007, funding was best described as "homeopathic" (thanks to Professor Marc Cohen for the pun). After the Cooke Senate Enquiry, the National Health and Medical Research Council (NHMRC) called for grant applications for CAM research. However, much of the focus of this research funding has been on oral and herbal CAM, rather than complementary therapies. The term complementary integrative therapies (CIT) is now preferred, when such practices are used alongside and ideally integrated into mainstream care. Published, high-quality evidence that CIT improves QoL, efficacy and possibly promotes secondary cancer prevention (e.g. exercise may reduce bowel cancer relapse rates) is needed as the first step to change.

Finding and Keeping Therapists

In recent years, maintaining adequate numbers of therapist staff has been a key issue for SolarisCare and clinical activity has at times been constrained by available therapist numbers. Many of our staff have been active in SolarisCare for five years and remain with us from a strong sense of altruism and professional satisfaction. Any further expansion would require careful consideration of the likelihood of successfully finding more therapists. Financial reward, if this were feasible, might attract some.

Credentialling of Therapists

This issue is very much "the elephant in the room" when planning CIT. It has been our good fortune to devise a successful model for attracting, identifying and often retaining good therapists, with the ability to work alongside mainstream beliefs and practices. In recent years, we have strived organisationally to define and document our standards for each therapy modality. We have embarked upon professional development of therapists with training days and are moving towards a training programme that provides CIT therapists with an understanding of mainstream cancer care, psychological awareness and listening competency, and communication skills. Our therapists appreciate that they are respected for their skills and donation, and have the opportunity to work in a professionally appropriate, private, quiet and unhurried manner.

Spiritual or Religious Belief System Clashes

Many complementary therapies have a more Eastern religious framework that can put them at odds with Western religious beliefs. A recent call from a senior Roman Catholic bishop in the US[23] to distance the church from Reiki in particular highlights the potential for tension that can exist between formal religious practitioners and complementary therapists. SolarisCare is careful to refrain from claiming any formal spiritual role although, anecdotally, some patients have had profound life experiences during treatment sessions (personal communication with Associate Professor Anne Williams, Edith Cowan University, June 2010). Any such conflict was beautifully defused by Reverend Edward Hewitt at the opening of the Centre at St. John of God Health Campus in 2008, as he dedicated and blessed the new centre for the relieving of suffering according to each individual's belief.

RECOMMENDATIONS FOR SUSTAINABILITY AND FUTURE RESEARCH

Sustainability

There are two looming issues for SolarisCare. Firstly, the model is effective, but is it sustainable? How can funding be shifted from what has been a hand-to-mouth, stressful, time-consuming, fund-raising existence, to a more certain and ensured future? The constraints upon health funding are here to stay. If the evidence is amassed of improved QoL using CITs, governments can and should have a role. Beyond individual grants and seed funding, one way forward would be the introduction of Medicare rebates for complementary therapies that show health and possibly health-economic benefit.[24] The current onco-political recognition of the need for better supportive care for cancer patients and carers[19,25] makes this increasingly likely. A number of private health insurance funds are already moving in this direction. Such recognition could create a sustainable model for developing integrative oncology for our patients' benefit.

Future Research and a Proposal

Secondly, how do we move from the broad research approach and results described above, to a more specific programme addressing the next research questions of how best to integrate complementary therapies in cancer care? Do specific complementary therapies work best for particular clinical indications, such as cancer type (for example our blunt data suggest a benefit from Reiki in women with breast cancer), mainstream treatment type (chemotherapy or radiotherapy), symptoms (such as pain[26] or fatigue[27]) or even certain personality types.[28] Methodological problems around this area[29,30] make randomised controlled trials extremely difficult, but the long-term future of this approach can only be achieved with high-quality research that will convince the sceptics and fund-holders of its value. If other hospitals and institutions followed the SolarisCare example, it should be possible to develop a national collaboration between like-minded centres and start to work more effectively and rapidly towards gathering the evidence required to determine the most effective interventions.

CONCLUSIONS

In retrospect, the SolarisCare model has been effective for at least six reasons. First, the close link with the teaching hospital and the location centrally within the hospital gave patients easy access to and indicated institutional acceptance of the Centre. Second, it required a clinical champion with an acceptable mainstream reputation to take the necessary professional risks in establishing the

Centre and developing a process for selection of therapists and therapies, which accords closely enough with mainstream medical practices. This process provides safety and quality in the absence of regulation. Third, patients' expectations of the Centre were never allowed to become unrealistic; the focus was and is upon addressing symptoms. Fourth, the readiness of our practitioners to donate their time and expertise, and to modify or limit their approach to accommodate the guidelines. Fifth, our processes and measures to prevent harm or risk proved effective. Sixth, the institutional support of the Sir Charles Gairdner Hospital for a then-radical approach was imperative.

SolarisCare and I have received many requests for information and advice from individuals and institutions contemplating embracing new cancer support methods. My core advice to them is distilled in this chapter: find a clinical (medical) champion (usually the most difficult step it seems); gain institutional support at a high and broad level; find a location, ideally on campus; define a governance model that either involves or feeds back to the parent institution; and select therapies and therapists with care and be careful to provide them with a professionally fulfilling work experience. At the time of writing, cancer support centres with a similar focus upon individual healing and wellness are in gestation at the Austin Hospital in Melbourne, which has received high-profile celebrity support from Olivia Newton-John and State Government fundings, and at various campuses in Sydney, including St. Vincent's Hospital.

The SolarisCare experience indicates that the door can be safely opened to a new, wider model of health-care delivery. Our data, pending publication, suggests that, at least in some patients, marked improvements in the cancer journey can be achieved. I propose a new model for cancer care, based around major and tertiary centres, comprising one-stop diagnostic, treatment and wellness facilities, ideally with a national collaboration of the latter to study the role of CIT in cancer care. This would enlarge patient numbers in clinical trials involving multi-centre studies and thus improve access to research funding.

For me as a doctor and person, the SolarisCare experience has been a fascinating and formative journey. As a physician, it is fulfilling to prescribe non-pharmacological therapies for cancer symptoms and treatment side-effects, and to see my immediate colleagues on ward rounds prescribe acupuncture for intractable chemotherapy-induced nausea with patients benefiting from this. I have come to see that healing is not the sole province of health "professionals", and to know the importance of healing, especially when cure is impossible. As Hippocrates said "Cure sometimes, treat often, comfort always".

ACKNOWLEDGEMENTS

I acknowledge here the generous gifts of SolarisCare volunteers; research ideas and inspiration from Professor Linda Kristjanson and Dr Elizabeth Lobb; statistical analysis from Dr Mike Philips; and editorial assistance with this manuscript from Dr Anna Petterson and Dr Kate Poland.

REFERENCES

1. Australian Institute of Health and Welfare. *Health System Expenditures on Cancer and Other Neoplasms in Australia*, 2000–2001, AIHW, Canberra (2005).
2. Tracey E, Roder D, Zorbas H, *et al.* Survival and degree of spread for female breast cancers in New South Wales from 1980 to 2003: implications for cancer control. *Cancer Causes Control* **19**:1121–1130 (2008).
3. Barlogie B, Attal M, Crowley J, *et al.* Long-term follow-up of autotransplantation trials for multiple myeloma: update of protocols conducted by the Intergroupe Francophone du Myelome, Southwest Oncology Group, and University of Arkansas for Medical Sciences. *J Clin Oncol* **28**:1209–1214 (2010).
4. Turesson I, Velez R, Kristinsson SY, *et al.* Patterns of improved survival in patients with multiple myeloma in the twenty-first century: a population-based study. *J Clin Oncol* **28**:830–834 (2010).
5. Druker BJ, Guilhot F, O'Brien SG, *et al.* Five-year follow-up of patients receiving imatinib for chronic myeloid leukemia. *N Engl J Med* **355**:2408–2417 (2006).
6. Yu XQ, Chen WH, O'Connell DL. Improved survival for non-Hodgkin lymphoma patients in New South Wales, Australia. *BMC Cancer* **10**:231 (2010).

7. National Breast Cancer Centre and National Cancer Control Initiative. *Clinical Practice Guidelines for Psychosocial Care of Adults with Cancer,* National Breast Cancer Centre, Camperdown, NSW (2003).
8. Hutchison SD, Steginga SK, Dunn J. The tiered model of psychosocial intervention in cancer: a community based approach. *Psycho-Oncology* **15**:541–546 (2006).
9. Sewitch M, Rajput Y. A literature review of complementary and alternative medicine use by colorectal cancer patients. *Complement Ther Clin Pract* **16**:52–56 (2010).
10. Corner J, Yardley J, Maher E, *et al.* Patterns of complementary and alternative medicine use among patients undergoing cancer treatment. *Eur J Cancer Care* **18**:271–279 (2009).
11. Richardson MA, Sanders T, Palmer JL, *et al.* Complementary/alternative medicine use in a comprehensive cancer center and the implications for oncology. *J Clin Oncol* **18**:2505–2514 (2000).
12. Joske DJ. Chronic myeloid leukaemia: the evolution of gene-targeted therapy. *Med J Aust* **189**:277–282 (2008).
13. Joske DJ, Rao A, Kristjanson L. Critical review of complementary therapies in haemato-oncology. *Intern Med J* **36**:579–586 (2006).
14. Goldrosen MH, Straus SE. Complementary and alternative medicine: assessing the evidence for immunological benefits. *Nat Rev Immunol* **4**:912–921 (2004).
15. Vickers AJ. Can acupuncture have specific effects on health? A systematic review of acupuncture antiemesis trials. *J R Soc Med* **89**: 303–311 (1996).
16. Corbin L. Safety and efficacy of massage therapy for patients with cancer. *Cancer Control* **12**:158–164 (2005).
17. McCorkle R, Young K. Development of a symptom distress scale. *Cancer Nurs* **1**:373–378 (1978).
18. Lobchuk MM, Kristjanson L, Degner L, *et al.* Perceptions of symptom distress in lung cancer patients: I. Congruence between patients and primary family caregivers. *J Pain Symptom Manage* **14**:136–146 (1997).
19. Senate Community Affairs References Committee Secretariat. *The Cancer Journey: Informing Choice,* Commonwealth of Australia, Canberra (2005).
20. Adamsen L, Quist M, Andersen C, *et al.* Effect of a multimodal high intensity exercise intervention in cancer patients undergoing chemotherapy: randomised controlled trial. *BMJ* **339**:b3410 (2009).

21. Schmitz KH, Courneya KS, Matthews C, *et al.* American College of Sports Medicine roundtable on exercise guidelines for cancer survivors. *Med Sci Sports Exerc* **42**:1409–1426 (2010).
22. Frenkel M, Ben-Arye E, Cohen L. Communication in cancer care: discussing complementary and alternative medicine. *Integr Cancer Ther* **9**(2):177–185 (2010).
23. Committee on Doctrine United States Conference of Catholic Archbishops. *Guidelines for Evaluating Reiki as an Alternative Therapy*, United States Conference of Catholic Archbishops (2009).
24. Herman PM, Craig BM, Caspi O. Is complementary and alternative medicine (CAM) cost-effective? A systematic review? *BMC Complement Altern Med* **5**:11 (2005).
25. National Health Priority Action Council. *National Service Improvement Framework for Cancer*, Australian Government Department of Health and Ageing, Canberra (2006).
26. Deng G, Cassileth BR. Integrative oncology: complementary therapies for pain, anxiety and mood disturbance. *Cancer J Clin* **55**:109–116 (2005).
27. Sood A, Barton DL, Bauer BA, *et al.* A critical review of complementary therapies for cancer related fatigue. *Integr Cancer Ther* **6**:8–13 (2007).
28. Segerstrom SC. Individual differences, immunity, and cancer: lessons from personality psychology. *Brain Behav Immun* **17**(suppl 1):S92–S97 (2003).
29. Sikorskii A, Wyatt G, Victorson D, *et al.* Methodological issues in trials of complementary and alternative medicine interventions. *Nurs Res* **58**(6):444–451 (2009).
30. Broom A, Adams J. Current issues and future directions in complementary and alternative medicine (CAM) research. *Complement Ther Med* **15**:217–220 (2007).

10

The Emergence of New Consumerism in Health-Care: The Empowered Health Consumer and the Role of Complementary and Alternative Medicine

Liz Paslawsky

ABSTRACT

Where traditionally health professionals, policy-makers and health-funders considered the drivers of change in health service delivery to be the ageing of the population, rising costs, advances in medical technology and skills shortage, to name but a few, the "attitude of consumers" and their behavioural change have not received due consideration. Consumer attitude is changing, as the current societal trends are moving towards self-management in all sectors of the economy. This is also evident in the health sector in Australia, being fuelled by government policy initiatives to move to self-management and home-based care to address the burden of chronic disease. With increased access to information, better informed patients are able to establish choices in the types of health-care they are seeking. Patients are becoming "empowered consumers". The move towards self-management brings about a change in attitude and behaviour, demonstrated by a changing set of needs and expectations. Rather than reacting to ill-health as passive recipients, empowered consumers will increasingly decide what treatment they want, how they want to receive it, when they want to receive it and who should be its providers.

Keywords: Complementary and Alternative Medicines; Empowered Consumers.

BACKGROUND

The rapid growth of complementary and alternative medicine (CAM) suggests that empowered consumers are seeking something different to standard, disease-specific medical care. The empowered consumer's definition of health broadens from disease-specific to that which fulfils consumer's individual needs, including their quality of life, symptom relief and sense of expediency.

How empowered consumers define what health-care means to them as individuals and shape the choices they make will have a diverse range of repercussions throughout the health system. From insights gained from the CAM literature, this chapter will identify the required changes in the role of the health professional and the implications for health policy-makers and health facility designers.

CHANGES IN THE HEALTH-CARE LANDSCAPE

The Trends Towards Self-Management and Home-Based Care in the Health Sector

In every aspect of life consumers are being educated towards doing more for themselves. The trend is towards self-care. A good example in Australia is observed in the airline industry. The purchase of tickets moved from a travel agent to telephone to purchasing over the Internet. The boarding pass is also now printed off at home or via the electronic check-ins. Electronic processing of passports is also speeding up the process.

Health is also moving towards an increased emphasis on self-management. In the health sector there are five key factors that are driving self-management and home-based care. These drivers have a subsequent impact on the behaviour and attitudes of the patient. They are:

1. government policy and initiatives towards self-management and home-based services, particularly the need to address the burden of chronic disease;
2. the increase use of CAM, particularly in managing chronic disease;
3. the private health insurance funding provider's initiatives towards self-management;
4. the availability of self-management and home-based health services with supporting research as to their success; and
5. personalised medicine and more transparency in the provision of health-care information.

The emerging forms of out-of-hospital care are building patient confidence and providing consumers with greater self-management skills in actively participating in their own health. They are empowering the patient to be able to make informed choices. Each of these issues will be considered below.

Changes in Government Policy

The Australian (Federal and State) public health policy has been following global health policy trends in establishing strategies to reduce expenditure on acute or hospital care. A recent key policy shift is towards home-care and self-care.

This shift has occurred for two reasons. Firstly, to reduce the growth in expenditure in hospital-based care by targeting prevention, early interventions can reduce admissions, particularly of "frequent flyers", or those who have several hospital admissions per year. Secondly, it is increasingly being realised that the bulk of the hospital expenditure is used for patients with chronic illness, much of it preventable and amenable to self-management.

The report by the Australian Institute of Health and Welfare entitled *Australia's Health 2010* indicated that health in Australia is a $100-billion-a-year industry, with governments footing 70% of that bill. Health is an industry that is growing at a faster rate than inflation, and faster than the growth of the population.[1]

The health system is struggling to keep up with demand. Hospital admissions in Australia rose by 37% in the 10 years to 2007–08, and health expenditure per person rose by around 45% in real terms. Employment in health occupations grew by 23% between 2003 and 2008, almost double the rate across all occupations. In the 5 years from 2003–04 to 2007–08, the median waiting time for elective surgery in public hospitals rose from 28 to 34 days.[1]

Health-care in Australia is predominantly built around an acute, episodic model of care. The Australian Government Health Reform Commission (NHHRC) report published in 2009 identified that Australians are 20–30% more likely to be admitted to hospital overnight than people in Britain or the US. This is not only very expensive as a health delivery system, but the current system is also not well-equipped to meet the requirements mandated by the delivery of effective care for chronic illness.[2]

A major area of concern is the growth of chronic disease in Australia, now consuming 70% of the health sector's spending. The nine chronic diseases with the greatest impact on the Australian health-care system are: coronary heart disease, stroke, lung cancer, colorectal cancer, depression, diabetes, asthma, chronic obstructive pulmonary disease and chronic kidney disease. Strategies to combat chronic disease are increasingly preventative and home- or community-based. A third of the chronic disease burden is due to preventable factors, such as smoking, obesity, physical inactivity, harmful drinking and stress.[2]

The concerns in resolving the health-care system in Australia are far reaching and not limited to the financial burden alone. The 2009 NHHRC report identified that for each person older than 65 years in 2007, there were five working-age people. In 2050 there will be fewer than three working-age people. This has implications for constraining the supply of informal carers, imposing new pressures on the recruitment and retention of the health workforce and leading to reductions in the taxation base required to fund governmental expenditure on health-care.[2]

In response to the ageing of the population, the subsequent cost of health-care and the need to manage the growth in the burden of chronic disease, the Federal Government's (2009) Health Reform Commission (NHHRC) report was based on two key principles.

1. Shared responsibility: *"The health system has a particularly important role in helping people of all ages become more self-reliant and better able to manage their own health care needs"*.[2]
2. Strengthening prevention and wellness: *"Our health system also needs greater emphasis on helping people stay healthy through stronger investment in wellness, prevention and early detection and appropriate intervention to maintain people in as optimal health as possible"*.[2]

A similar approach has been taken in other primary care Federal reviews, including the National Primary Health Care Strategy[3] and the National Preventative Health Task Force report completed in 2009.[4]

The Growth in CAM is Also Evidence that the Health System is Moving Towards Self-Care

The usage of complementary medicine is difficult to ascertain, due to varying definitions of what constitutes complementary or alternative medicine (CAM). However, the numbers of users are high and increasing rapidly. A 2007 survey indicated that in Australia out-of-pocket expenditure for CAM was estimated to be AU $4.13 billion per year.[5]

The Australian Federal Government established an expert committee into complementary medicine to examine the use of complementary therapies.[6] The report indicated that between 50 and 75% of the Australian adult population use at least one complementary medicine product and one in four Australians use complementary medicine services every year.

The prevalence of chronic disease will continue to drive the growth of CAM. CAM has a high prevalence in usage for chronic conditions such as diabetes and cardiovascular disease, for which strong evidence already exists that it is used to complement Western medicine.[7] The prevalence of diabetes continues to increase markedly, having trebled over the last two decades, with over 800,000 Australians diagnosed with the disease in 2009. Type 2 diabetes is projected to become the leading cause of disease burden by 2023. Costs from diabetes alone are projected to increase 436% from $1.6 billion to $8.6 billion from 2002–03 to 2032–33.[7]

An increasing proportion of the Australian population are using CAMs and a South Australian survey indicated that in 2004 over 50% of the South Australian population surveyed had used at least one CAM.[8]

The use of CAM is self-funded by consumers; this issue is considered further below in the section on Increase of User Pay.

Private Health Insurance Funds

In Australia, the private health funds are taking deliberate steps in moving care away from hospitals, towards a self-management model. The funds have a population-based approach to the management of their members. They also have more incentives to control outlays, because of government pressure on keeping premiums low.

The larger private health funds (Medibank Private, HCF, Bupa) are encouraging self-awareness in wellness, health prevention and promotion programmes by linking the consumer into a health portal. This is an online tool that elicits and assesses information provided by a member through a health risk assessment and, in response, provides targeted health and wellness information and tools to assist members achieve and maintain optimum health and wellness. As currently deployed, health portals are used as 'platforms' for offering a diversity of information, programmes and links to service providers.

The Availability of Self-Management and Home-Based Health Services

The move towards self-management is resulting in the introduction of new terminology, for example the "chronic care continuum", which commences with wellness, moving towards increased acuity and ultimately hospitalisation. The general aim of programmes along the chronic care continuum is to keep people out of hospital and in their home, by empowering them to more effectively manage their own illnesses. Instead of being passive recipients of care, patients participating in these programmes become active participants in their own health and care plans. Most programmes involve cooperation with the patient's general practitioner and other relevant community-based programmes.

Examples of health services along the chronic care continuum include the following.

1. Health portals — including health risk assessments (described above), introduced by the private health insurance industry.
2. Telephone-based disease management programmes and home-care programmes.

   Many programmes in the public sector are attempting to increase the coordination of patient care. This is evident particularly in the delivery of cancer services, where the public sector is providing more care coordinators whose tasks include: improving patients' understanding of complicated medical information and technical terminology, assisting patients to navigate the system, assisting them with web-enabled decision support tools, and motivating patients to follow through on their care plan set by their medical practitioner. This includes ensuring that patients keep medical appointments, have good medication compliance and are informed about available preventative or early intervention services.

   The trend in Australia is for these services to be provided through high technology-backed telephonic disease management services. The patient is allocated a personalised coach, and is able to call at any time. The telephonic coaching programmes are backed by web-enabled health portals, decision support tools and videos. These systems are designed to support the role of the general practitioner or the patient's primary carer. Examples of overseas companies now offering these services in Australia include Bupa Health Dialog and Healthways.
3. Hospital substitution programmes, including Hospital in the Home (HITH) programmes. These include patients who need admission to hospital, but can be supported to recover at home at a much earlier point in their recovery, provided that home-based services are available to assist them. In Australia in 2009 there were 40 private hospitals with HITH services paid by health funds associated with the Australian Health Services Management Association. Common programmes include: chronic wound care, administration of intravenous drugs, orthopaedic rehabilitation, cardiac rehabilitation, transitional care from hospital to nursing home and palliative care.

4. Trends in home-care are being supported by an increasing array of diagnostic tools, allowing the remote monitoring of blood pressure, heart rate and skin temperature. Patients with diabetes have moved from requiring urine tests as an indirect measure to know whether they have abnormal levels of glucose in their blood to having miniature blood glucose metres with them wherever they go. Diabetic patients themselves can manage most aspects of their disease that previously had required much more professional involvement. Leading technology includes the provision of diagnostic toilets (manufactured by Toto in Japan) and advances in using the cell phone in diagnostic monitoring, including microscopy added to cell phones.

There is increasing research evidence supporting the positive impact of engaging individuals in self-management. The key element for success in programmes such as telephonic coaching is active involvement of members in managing their own health — a term referred to as 'active member engagement'.[9] Further, multi-component health promotion programmes that engage participants in self-care activities and increase their involvement in health-care decision-making can achieve long-term behaviour change and health risk reductions in large populations.[10]

A 2010 Cochrane systematic review of home-based versus centre-based cardiac rehabilitation found equivalence between these two rehabilitation modalities in improving clinical and health-related quality-of-life outcomes in patients diagnosed with acute Myocardial Infarction (MI) and /or having revascularisation procedures. There is a substantive evidence base for home-based, cardiac rehabilitation models. Hence, there is potential benefit to be realised for a greater number of patients by combining telephone coaching and home-based rehabilitation, compared with clinic-based programmes.[11]

Personalised Medicine and Individualised Information is Allowing Motivated Consumers to Increasingly Make an Informed Decision

There are three trends observed in this area:

1. The advent of personalised medicine. The promise of individualised medicine is that it can tailor treatment to an individual's

genetic make-up. Individuals who know their genetic sequence can seek information to predict their own risk of many diseases.
2. Increased access to individualised information. There is an increasing ability of consumers to find out information on individuals with similar conditions on the Internet and by using blogs or Twitter. Self-help groups, networks and support groups are becoming global. With the introduction of the electronic medical record, consumers will increasingly endeavour to access their own information.
3. Improvements in information transparency. Information transparency in health-care is increasingly an ethical obligation and is giving consumer access to an array of information. The Federal Government and the States are increasingly transparent on access, costs, waiting lists, patient satisfaction measures and patient safety measures — including hospital error rates and infection rates.

In conclusion, consumers are taking greater control of decision-making and will be demanding the ability to make an informed choice and actively participate in the management of their own care.

SOCIETAL FACTORS INFLUENCING CONSUMER ATTITUDES AND BEHAVIOUR

Introduction

In addition to the changes in the health-care landscape driving change towards self-management in health-care, societal factors will also influence behaviour and attitude change of consumers making choices about their own health-care. They include an increase in user pay health-care systems and generational changes in expectations.

Increase of User Pay

A factor that will influence attitude and behaviour is the trend in Australia for consumers to pay more for health-care. The consumers' "value equation" will expand and expectations will increase. In all aspects of health service delivery consumers are now paying a gap payment. The gap payment is increasing for visits to general practitioners, diagnostics and specialists. Pressure continues for health insurance premiums to increase.

Furthermore, many of the services currently demanded by those with chronic conditions and quality of life have no funding mechanism. These services are user pay. Federal funding of pharmaceuticals is through the Pharmaceutical Benefits Schedule and that of general practitioner medical services is through the Medicare Benefits Schedule. There is no equivalent when it comes to funding CAM, or in fact services for chronic care generally involving community-based activities, allied health-care and preventative activities.

Disproportionately only 2% of government-funded total health expenditure in Australia is for preventative services or health promotion.[1] The Federally-funded Medicare Benefits Schedule for general practitioners principally subsidises one-off visits to manage and diagnose health problems, rather than looking after a patient over a time period, or keeping the patient well.

This will lead consumers to change their "value equation" resulting in rising consumer expectations.

Generation X and Generation Y

Choices also become easier with generational change. Product marketing and company human resources departments are identifying Generation X and Generation Y as the new generations thinking differently about their health. Generation X includes those born between 1965 and 1979. They are considered resourceful, self-reliant and individualistic. Lifestyle is important and they have increased expectations. They are more likely to be more computer/information literate than the baby boomers.

Generation Y includes those born since 1980. This generation has a sense of civic duty, buys locally and is confident and comfortable with new concepts. They communicate informally, electronically and access the most up-to-date technology and continue to be kept updated.

Generation X and Y will be concerned with their health and want to simply feel their best. The new generations bring new terminology such as "new age" in the search for a more holistic approach to healing and health-care.

PATIENTS CURRENTLY USING CAM ARE SEEKING SOMETHING DIFFERENT TO STANDARD MEDICAL CARE

Patients using CAM are Empowered Consumers

Patients currently using CAM are clearly seeking something different to standard medical care. They are empowered consumers.

Australian studies reveal that 65% of cancer patients use some form of complementary therapies.[12,13] The first survey of cancer patient satisfaction in NSW (2008) identified: "*the need for greater emotional support, help with fear and anxiety, information and education and the need to feel comfortable when talking with staff about Complementary, Alternative or Non-traditional therapies*".

The factors often quoted as influencing the choice to use CAM[14–18] are outlined below. CAM takes for granted the necessity of quality of life and placing patient values and lifestyle habits at the core of any design and delivery of care.[19] These factors are often outside the scope of Western medicine but represent the embodiment of characteristics sought by empowered consumers. The main reasons that patients choose CAM include the following.

1. Consumerism — the fact that CAM information is readily available. The trend is towards a higher level of patient sophistication in accessing medical knowledge, coupled with information from friends and family and the media.
2. Sense of empowerment and the ethos of "actively doing something for themselves". Patients are taking greater control, demanding to make an informed choice and actively participate in the management of their care.
3. The individualised approach of CAM practitioners.
4. Expedience assists with patients' need for immediacy — "what will help me right now".
5. Quality of life/symptom relief. Patients and their carers who are coping with radical treatments such as surgery, radiation and chemotherapy often seek additional means of maintaining

their health and of coping with the difficult emotional and physical side-effects associated with treatment.

6. A pragmatic pursuit of better outcomes for chronic health problems. This is particularly relevant for conditions where Western medical treatment is not very effective, as is the case with many chronic diseases. Preference could also be for holistic, natural therapies, as a gentler alternative to Western medicine, with fewer side-effects.
7. Trust of and familiarity with CAM in the family since childhood (particularly for Chinese people towards Chinese medicine). Often this is also associated with the belief that disease causation differs from the Western medical paradigm and CAM that are congruent with their values and beliefs.

CAM AND THE CONCERN OF LACK OF DISCLOSURE

As health moves more towards self-care, more consumers will choose CAM as it addresses many of their needs and expectations.

The fact that the Australian health system is not keeping up with the changing attitudes and behaviours of patients is made evident by the increasing problem of the lack of disclosure by patients of their use of CAM to their Western-trained medical practitioners. An Australian study identified that 50% of patients did not discuss their use of complementary or alternative medicine with their oncologist[20] and general practitioners generally underestimate the extent to which their patients access complementary medicine.[21]

There are a variety of reasons why open communication about complementary treatments is not taking place in some Western medical clinics. The most common reason that patients give is that it just never came up in the discussion, meaning that no one asked them about CAM use, and that patients did not think it was important to bring it up. Patients may fear that the topic will be received with indifference, or will be dismissed without discussion, and health-care professionals may fear not knowing how to respond to questions, or wanting to avoid initiating a time-consuming discussion.[22]

A key question raised by this issue of non-disclosure relates to a doctor's duty of care for his or her patients when patients 'treat' their health problems outside the medical setting.

The widespread use of CAM identifies the need for all medical practitioners (particularly Western-trained) to have a level of competence in advising patients accurately about CAM application to their clinical care in order to optimise health outcomes.[23]

To address this issue the Royal Australian College of General Practitioners (RACGP) and the Australian Integrative Medicine Association (AIMA) endorsed in July 2005 a joint position paper on CAM, emphasising the need for increased education of the medical workforce and increased research.[24] The RACGP/AIMA joint position paper reported a growing interest in complementary medicine among medical specialties such as oncology, paediatrics, obstetrics and gynaecology, and rheumatology.

> "There are many reasons for the medical profession to be fully informed about complementary medicines and/or therapies..... General practitioners also need to be aware of what medicines and therapies their patients are using, as well as their potential benefits, and adverse effects. GPs also need to be aware of possible interactions between western pharmaceuticals, complementary medicines and foods.
>
> It is important that the medical profession sets standards for medical practices and practitioners who wish to augment their practice with the use of complementary medicines and/or therapies. It is also important that patients have improved access to information and are aware of the different roles of general practitioners and complementary therapists. It is essential that patients understand the importance of consulting their GP in relation to medical symptoms and health concerns and the need to obtain a medical diagnosis for any underlying condition."[24]

IMPLICATIONS FOR THE MEDICAL PROFESSION, HEALTH POLICY-MAKERS, FUNDERS AND HEALTH DESIGNERS

The New Consumerism: Lessons Gained from Empowered Consumers Seeking CAM

Based upon the knowledge of why consumers are choosing to use CAM, the medical profession, health policy-makers, funders and health designers can prepare for the implications of attitudinal changes as the health system moves towards self-management.

How consumers define what health means to them as individuals, and the choices they make, will have a diverse range of influences throughout the health system. Without doubt the outcome of health moving to consumer empowerment is that one size will not fit all.

The Western-trained medical professionals will need to develop an ability to embrace change, extending outside their professional discipline and Western medical training paradigms.

One way in which health professionals can consider the changes required in their decision-making is by considering the three contexts that influence individual decision-making.

1. Individual preferences — or how the consumers' attitude, preparedness and knowledge are influencing decision-making.
2. Defining the health-care team that is the locus of the health consumer decision-making for the provision of health-care.
3. The societal context that influences the health consumer choices. In turn the collective view of consumers will change the way that health-care is defined by policy-makers.

The required changes in health professional decision-making are discussed in three contexts.

Individual Preference

Increased patient sophistication in their medical knowledge, ethos of self-care, having choices and actively doing something for themselves will challenge traditional medical convention and force behaviour change in health providers.

Traditionally the medical profession had autonomy in patient decision-making. Empowered consumers with informed knowledge and a range of choices will consider the options available in different modalities of health-care on offer from a range of practitioners from both Eastern and Western medicine.

Previously the medical professional had professional control surrounding decision-making about the patient's care. The control was based on years of training and experience and evidence-based medicine. Empowered consumers will embrace the most reliable health information and have an ability to access the knowledge when required. Their criteria will be evidence-based on what has worked.

Traditional Western medicine identifies best practice care plans for common treatments. This includes what should happen every day during a hospital stay and what drugs and treatments the patient requires. The empowered consumer will have an expectation of the medical practitioner being able to personalise the treatment for the individual.

High in expectation, the empowered consumer will demand to be treated with respect and dignity, as they now have an increasing array of choices in health-care. Personal and cultural differences will be more pronounced and individual needs, preferences and expectations will be paramount. Rather than reacting to ill-health as passive recipients, consumers will increasingly decide what treatment they want, how they want to receive it and who provides the treatment.

The extent of the Western-trained medical practitioners' involvement in the treatment of self-managed and community-based chronic care will be dictated by the patient and not by the medical provider's choice.

At the very least, the consumers will be equal partners in decision-making and demand to be respected as equal partners in the choices that they make, along with their medical provider. The empowered consumer will be seeking a doctor who will consider all aspects of a person's well-being and all factors that can have an impact on health outcomes. At the extreme, the doctors will be viewed as just one of the consultants.

It is likely that the role of the medical provider will evolve from a purely diagnostic and management one into interpreting information and acting as information navigator, being the source of reliable recommendations for therapeutic options. The medical profession will not be expected to know all of the answers, but to expeditiously find answers to patients' queries. Patients will expect timely, accurate and complete information to allow informed decision-making. Patients will also be a source of information to practitioners.

Defining the Health-Care Team That is the Locus of Health Consumer Decision-Making

As health moves towards self-management, the focus is shifting away from the health-care specialist and the medical-imposed structures to multiple networks that may include family, friends and an international network of blogs and twitters.

With the increased role of family and friends as a source of information, the extended family may anticipate an increasing role in care and decision-making. The medical profession will need to be able to communicate more effectively with the patient's family, as well as the patient.

A paradigm shift for Western-trained medical professionals is the definition of the multi-disciplinary team that they will be working with to improve patient outcomes. There will be a need for the medical professional to work cooperatively as part of a non-traditional multi-disciplinary team, which can incorporate multiple modalities of health-care.

These professional networks will work across organisational boundaries and health-care delivery will be defined by a networked group of services.

The Societal Context that Influences Choices

Societal contexts including who pays for health-care, legislative changes in health policy and, more widely, social and economic contexts will continue to influence people's attitudes. This will include climate change and social responsibility.

As consumers will be increasingly paying for health services from their own pocket, they will be looking for value for money. Being Generation X and Y, they will be concerned with their health and will want to simply feel their best. Searching for answers to many questions, they will realise that disease-focused Western medicine cannot provide absolutely everything that they require.

> The collective view of consumers will change the way health care is defined by policy makers and health care professionals.

An example of how the collective view of empowered consumers will change is the way that health-care is delivered and the design of hospitals. Western thinking of evidence-based and quantitative analysis as the foundation of decision-making may need re-evaluation, as quantitative decision-making is often to the exclusion of individual differences. Qualitative research methods will become more relevant, as individual experiences will need to be more fully explored and understood. Consumer 'stories', reflecting the complexity of inter-relationships in health-care settings will be paramount in the future design of health service delivery. Focus groups, surveys and recorded observations of care practices in use will become more important. These practices today are less often acknowledged as credible evidence.

Moving to home-based care leads to a redefinition of a hospital, from being defined by the number of its beds to being defined by its value-added services. Consumer attitude will lead to hospital design requiring increased patient education services and facilities in a welcoming, engaging environment, as they will be expecting more convenience and personal comfort.

The question will be raised of what is the relevance of many of the hospital-defined systems. Where previously guidelines, accreditation systems and patient safety clinical audits had their boundaries clearly defined by the hospital, these quality systems will now only be a subset of consumer health-care. At the very least, there will be an increasing need for hospital departments and pharmacies to produce policies in response to patients requesting continued access to their complementary medicines and/or therapies during hospitalisation.

Improved coordination will occur along the continuum of chronic care. However, the locus of coordination of care will be increasingly from the community, not the hospital, and the consumer, not the consumer's medical professional.

The question arises whether more Australian hospital designs should embrace integrative medicine. Australia's first Centre of Excellence in Integrative Medicine is currently being built in Sydney, in collaboration with the government of the Peoples' Republic of China. The centre will deliver traditional Chinese medicine (TCM) and Western general practitioner medical services. The clinical services will be supported by education and research. The focus of the centre will be on wellness, health prevention and early intervention in chronic diseases. The intention is to expand the centre to accommodate inpatient beds.

The centre will be established as a dedicated training and academic general practice facility and will provide opportunities for clinical placement of undergraduate and post-graduate students training in TCM. It is proposed that teaching facilities and information technology will be optimised to facilitate teaching and linking with other teaching facilities in Australia and China.

At the very least, the features of integrative medicine design concepts should be embraced in future hospital design.

CONCLUSION

In every aspect of life consumers are being educated towards doing more for themselves and this is also evident in the evolution of the health sector in Australia. Patient sophistication in accessing medical knowledge, the ethos of self-care, and having choices will increasingly lead to an empowered consumer.

CAM is anticipated to grow exponentially. Further empowered consumers have a set of needs, expectations and characteristics that Western medicine only partly fulfils. The characteristics of an empowered consumer reflect the characteristics of people choosing CAM.

The empowered consumer will challenge traditional medical convention and force behaviour change in health providers, as they move from passive recipients of medical treatment plans to active participants in their own health. The required changes in the role of health professionals and the implications for health policy-makers have been outlined. Integrative medicine will need to become an established discipline and there is clear evidence in NSW of services being developed to respond to the changing consumer demand.

REFERENCES

1. Australian Institute of Health and Welfare (AIHW). *Australia's Health 2010*, in AIHW (ed), AIHW, Canberra (2010).
2. National Health and Hospital Reform Commission. *A Healthier Future for all Australians*, Final Report of the National Health and Hospitals Reform Commission, Department of Health and Ageing (ed), AIHW, Canberra (2009).
3. Commonwealth of Australia. *Building a 21st Century Primary Health Care System*, Australia's First National Primary Health Care Strategy, Commonwealth of Australia, Canberra (2010).

4. Commonwealth of Australia. *Australia: The Healthiest Country by 2020 — National Preventative Health Strategy – Overview*, Commonwealth of Australia, Canberra (2009).
5. Arcury TA, Bell RA, Snively BM, *et al.* Complementary and alternative medicine use as health self-management: rural older adults with diabetes. *J Gerontol B Psychol Sci Soc Sci* **61**(2):S62–70 (2006).
6. Moolasarn S, Sripa S, Kuessirikiet V, *et al.* Usage of and cost of complementary/alternative medicine in diabetic patients. *J Med Assoc Thai* **88**(11):1630–1637 (2005).
7. Dixon T. Costs of diabetes in Australia, 2000–01. In AIHW (ed), *Bulletin*, AIHW, Canberra (2005).
8. Maclennan AH, Myers SP, *et al.* The continuing use of complementary and alternative medicine in South Australia: costs and beliefs in 2004. *Med J Aust* **184**(1):27–31 (2006).
9. RAND Health. *Evidence Report and Evidence-Based Recommendations: Health Risk Assessments and Medicare*, RAND Corporation (ed) (2004). http://www.rand.org/content/dam/rand/pubs/reprints/2007/RAND_RP1225.sum.pdf [Accessed 15 December 2010].
10. Institute for Clinical Systems Improvement (ICSI). *Primary Prevention of Chronic Disease*, in *ICSI* (ed. ICSI) (2010).
11. Dalal HM, Zawada A, Jolly K, *et al.* Home based versus centre based cardiac rehabilitation: cochrane systematic review and meta-analysis. *BMJ* **340**:b5631 (2010).
12. Xue C, Zhang A, Lin V, *et al.* Complementary and alternative medicine use in Australia: a national population-based survey. *J Altern Complement Med* **13**(6):643–650 (2007).
13. Expert Committee on Complementary Medicines in the Health System. *Complementary Medicines in the Australian Health System*, Report to the Parliamentary Secretary to the Minister for Health and Ageing, Commonwealth of Australia, Canberra (2003).
14. Sirois F, Gick M. An investigation of the health beliefs and motivations of complementary medicine clients. *Soc Sci Med* **55**:1025–1037 (2002).
15. Robotin MC, Penman GP. Integrating complementary therapy into mainstream cancer care: which way forward. *Med J Aust* **185**:377–379 (2006).
16. Astin JA. Why patients use alternative medicine: results of a national study. *JAMA* **279**(19):1548–1553 (1998).

17. Hyodo I, Amano N, Eguchi K, *et al.* Nationwide survey on complementary and alternative medicine in cancer patients in Japan. *J Clin Oncol* **23**:2645–2654 (2005).
18. Molassiotis A, Fernadez-Ortega P, Pud D, *et al.* Use of complementary and alternative medicine in cancer patients: a European survey. *Ann Oncol* **16**:655–663 (2005).
19. Ernst E. Complementary therapies in palliative cancer care. *Cancer* **91**:2181–2185 (2001).
20. Coulter I, Willis E. The rise and rise of complementary and alternative medicine: a sociological perspective. *Med J Aust* **180**:587–589 (2004).
21. Pirotta M, Cohen M, Kotsirilos V, *et al.* Complementary therapies: have they become accepted in general practice? *Med J Aust* **172**(3):105–109 (2000).
22. Cohen MM, Braun LA. Towards the evidence-based integration of complementary medicines into hospital settings. *Evid Based Integr Med* **1**(4):241–244 (2004).
23. Cassileth B, Deng G, Vickers A, *et al. PDQ Integrative Oncology. Complementary Therapies in Cancer Care,* BC Decker Inc, Hamilton (2005).
24. RACGP AIMA. *Joint Position Statement on Complementary Medicine* (2005).

11

Interaction Between Complementary and Alternative Medicines and Conventional Medicines

Stephen J. Clarke and
Andrew J. McLachlan

ABSTRACT

An increasing proportion of the population use complementary and alternative medicines (CAM) including herbal medicines. This use is frequently undertaken in addition to their prescribed treatments, often without their physician's knowledge. For many types of CAM, this concomitant use of treatments is without risk. However, for systemically administered CAM such as herbal medicines, there are significant risks of adverse drug interactions between herbal medicines and conventional treatments, which may result in either increased drug toxicity or therapeutic failure. This review highlights the mechanisms through which CAM may interact with conventional medicines and emphasises the paucity of high-quality randomised controlled data that are available to guide clinicians in regard to potential adverse interactions between standard treatments and commonly used herbal medicines. It is clear that certain combinations of herbal medicines and conventional medicines carry significant risks of reduced efficacy or adverse effects and the combinations are contraindicated. For instance, *in-vivo* studies have shown that concomitant use of St. John's wort with therapeutic agents that are CYP3A4 substrates has the potential to cause therapeutic failure. *In-vitro* and *in-vivo* studies show that caution is warranted when considering concomitant Asian ginseng or fenugreek with CYP3A4 substrates and guarana with CYP1A2 substrates. In cancer treatments there is also potential for pharmacodynamic interactions between herbal medicines and anticancer agents. For example, patients with oestrogen receptor-positive breast cancers should be advised to avoid administration of phyto-oestrogen-containing herbal preparations. Physicians should be proactive in obtaining a complete medication history including herbal medicine use in all of their patients receiving cancer chemotherapy in order to advise them appropriately.

Keywords: Chinese Herbs; Drug–Herb Interactions.

INTRODUCTION

Complementary and alternative medicine (CAM) includes a diverse group of treatments ranging from music therapy, exercise and massage to systemically administered treatments including nutritional therapies and herbal medicines. The last 15 years have seen a significant increase in the use of CAM. In 1990, a survey performed in the US estimated that 34% of the respondents had used at least one form of complementary therapy in the previous 12 months.[1] This figure had increased to 42% by 1997.[2] The popularity of CAM use has been mirrored in Australia.[3] In 2004, a South Australian survey reported that 52% of respondents had used at least one non-medically-prescribed CAM in the previous year. More than 57% of respondents reported using CAM without their health practitioner's knowledge and 50% took conventional medicines on the same day, creating the potential for interactions between conventional medicines and CAM.[3]

In certain diseases such as cancer there has been an even greater increase in the use of CAM. In 1998, a systematic review of the literature revealed a mean CAM use of 31% among cancer patients.[4] A number of recent studies have suggested that this figure may now exceed 80%, although there is variability in use depending on tumour type and ethnic group studied, CAM use being more common in breast cancer patients and individuals from Asian backgrounds.[5,6] The increased use of CAM in people with cancer is relevant as even in optimal circumstances there is a low therapeutic index for anti-cancer drugs, which may be further lowered by adverse interactions between CAM and the conventional cancer drugs.

The possibility that herbal and complementary medicines may lead to significant pharmacological interactions with conventional therapies is not surprising given the long list of medicines that have been derived from plants (see Table 1). There is a growing emphasis on evaluating potential herb–drug interaction in drug development,[7] but systematic evidence is lacking to aid consumers and clinicians in assessing the risk.

A recent systematic review attempted to identify the principal reasons for CAM use in cancer patients. Although there was a wide range of responses, the most frequent were a perceived beneficial response (38%), wanting "control" (17%), CAM as a "last resort" (10%) and "finding hope" (10%).[8]

Not surprisingly therefore CAM is big business. In the US alone, it has been estimated that cancer patients spend over $30 billion in out-of-pocket expenses on CAM, even though there are few data to indicate the cost-effectiveness of CAM.[9] This increased use by patients and expense of CAM have highlighted issues in regard to the safety and efficacy of these treatments. This is particularly the case for systemically administered CAM including herbal medicines, where there is the potential for clinically significant interactions with conventional treatments. Consequently, in this chapter we have focused our discussions on CAM principally to systemically administered vitamins and medicines in order to highlight the potential for CAM interactions with conventional agents, to educate clinicians about these commonly used medicines and highlight the dearth of high-quality data that are available to guide practitioners.

MECHANISMS OF CAM–DRUG INTERACTIONS

Herb–Drug Interactions

The focus of much of the current discussion has been limited to the more commonly used herbal medicines[10] and those mentioned in

Table 1. Selected medicines derived from plants.

Medicine	Pharmacological actions	Plant source
Caffeine	CNS stimulant	*Camellia sinensis*
Camptothecin	Anticancerous	*Camptotheca acuminata*
Cocaine	Local anaesthetic	*Erythroxylum coca*
Codeine	Analgesic, antitussive	*Papaver somniferum*
Colchicine	Antitumour agent, antigout	*Colchicum autumnale*
l-Dopa	Antiparkinsonism	*Mucuna* sp.
Digitalin	Cardiotonic	*Digitalis purpurea*
Digitoxin	Cardiotonic	*Digitalis purpurea*
Digoxin	Cardiotonic	*Digitalis purpurea*
Emetine	Amoebicide, emetic	*Cephaelis ipecacuanha*
Ephedrine	Sympathomimetic, antihistamine	*Ephedra sinica*
Etoposide	Antitumour agent	*Podophyllum peltatum*
Galantamine	Cholinesterase inhibitor	*Lycoris squamigera*
Gossypol	Male contraceptive	*Gossypium* sp.
Hyoscyamine	Anticholinergic	*Hyoscyamus niger*
Irinotecan	Anticancer, antitumour agent	*Camptotheca acuminata*
Methyl salicylate	Rubefacient	*Gaultheria procumbens*
Morphine	Analgesic	*Papaver somniferum*
Nicotine	Insecticide, stimulant	*Nicotiana tabacum*
Papavarine	Smooth muscle relaxant	*Papaver somniferum*
Physostigmine	Cholinesterase inhibitor	*Physostigma venenosum*
Pilocarpine	Parasympathomimetic	*Pilocarpus jaborandi*
Podophyllotoxin	Antitumour, anticancer agent	*Podophyllum peltatum*
Pseudoephedrine	Sympathomimetic	*Ephedra sinica*
Quinidine	Antiarrhythmic	*Cinchona ledgeriana*
Quinine	Antimalarial, antipyretic	*Cinchona ledgeriana*
Reserpine	Antihypertensive, tranquillizer	*Rauvolfia serpentina*
Rutin	Capillary fragility	*Citrus* sp.
Salicin	Analgesic	*Salix alba*
Scopolamine	Sedative	*Datura* sp.
Sennosides A, B	Laxative	*Cassia* sp.

(*Continued*)

Table 1. *(Continued)*

Medicine	Pharmacological actions	Plant source
Silymarin	Antihepatotoxic	*Silybum marianum*
Strychnine	CNS stimulant	*Strychnos nux-vomica*
Taxol	Antitumour agent	*Taxus brevifolia*
Teniposide	Antitumour agent	*Podophyllum peltatum*
α-Tetrahydrocannabinol	Antiemetic, decrease occular tension	*Cannabis sativa*
Theophylline	Diuretic, bronchodilator	*Theobroma cacao* and others
Topotecan	Antitumour, anticancer agent	*Camptotheca acuminata*
Tubocurarine	Skeletal muscle relaxant	*Chondodendron tomentosum*
Vinblastine	Antitumour, antileukaemic agent	*Catharanthus roseus*
Vincristine	Antitumour, antileukaemic agent	*Catharanthus roseus*

Adapted from www.rain-tree.com/plantdrugs.htm [Accessed 25 May 2010].

recent literature as causing or having the potential to cause herb–drug interactions with conventional medicines.[11–13] With many conventional agents, herb–drug interactions may not lead to any serious sequelae; however, for some classes of conventional therapeutic agents that have a low therapeutic index (i.e. a fine line between a safe/effective dose and a toxic dose), such as anticancer drugs, even minor changes in drug clearance could produce dramatic effects on patient outcomes. Herb–drug interactions occur via several broad mechanisms, including pharmaceutical, pharmacokinetic and pharmacodynamic interactions (Table 2).

Pharmacokinetic interactions can result when common pathways of absorption, metabolism, distribution or elimination exist between the constituents of herbal medicines and conventional therapeutic agents. These interactions most commonly involve intestinal and hepatic metabolising enzymes (cytochrome P450 or "CYP" enzymes) and drug transporters such as the ABC transporters [including P-glycoprotein (P-gp)], breast cancer resistance protein and multi-drug

Table 2. Level of caution required for the concomitant use of selected anticancer agents with herbal medicines. The coloured classification system was derived by the authors based upon their critical, clinical evaluation of available literature. “Extreme” caution denotes high potential for adverse reactions confirmed from *in-vivo* studies, concomitant use should be avoided. “Moderate” caution denotes medium potential for adverse reactions (*in-vitro* studies indicate possible interaction), concomitant use should only be administered under strict, clinical supervision. “Low” caution denotes little potential for adverse reactions (*in-vivo* and *in-vitro* studies indicate little potential for interactions), concomitant use may be considered. “Unknown” caution denotes a lack of available clinical evidence to make an appropriate recommendation.

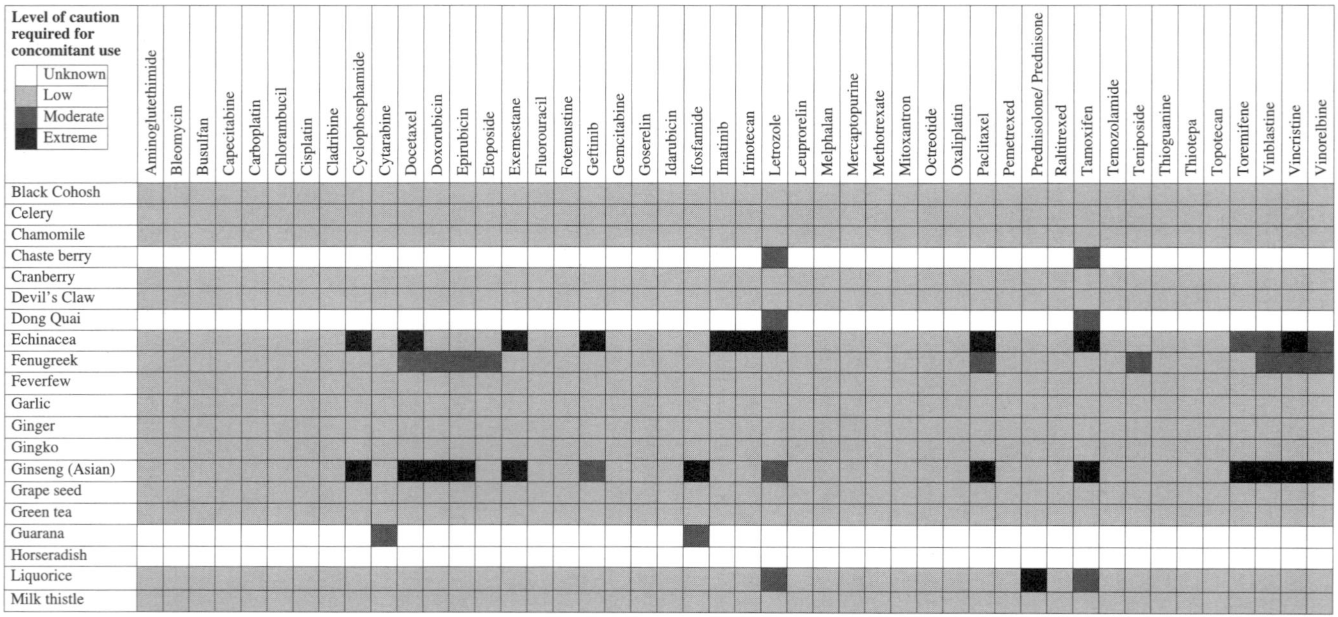

Table 2. (*Continued*).

Level of caution required for concomitant use: Unknown (white), Low (light grey), Moderate (dark grey), Extreme (black)

Level of caution required for concomitant use	Aminoglutethimide	Bleomycin	Busulfan	Capecitabine	Carboplatin	Chlorambucil	Cisplatin	Cladribine	Cyclophosphamide	Cytarabine	Docetaxel	Doxorubicin	Epirubicin	Etoposide	Exemestane	Fluorouracil	Fotemustine	Geftinib	Gemcitabine	Goserelin	Idarubicin	Ifosfamide	Imatinib
Passionflower																							
Pau'Darco																							
Red clover	Extreme	Low	Low	Low	Low	Low	Low	Low	Low	Low	Low	Low	Low	Low	Extreme	Low	Low	Low	Low	Extreme	Low	Low	Low
Saw palmetto	Low	Low	Low	Low	Low	Low	Low	Low	Low	Low	Low	Low	Low	Low	Low	Low	Low	Low	Low	Low	Low	Low	Low
Soy beans																							
St John's wort									Extreme		Extreme	Moderate	Moderate	Moderate	Extreme			Extreme				Extreme	Extreme
Valerian																							
Wild yam																							

Level of caution required for concomitant use	Irinotecan	Letrozole	Leuprorelin	Melphalan	Mercaptopurine	Methotrexate	Mitoxantron	Octreotide	Oxaliplatin	Paclitaxel	Pemetrexed	Prednisolone/ Prednisone	Raltitrexed	Tamoxifen	Temozolamide	Teniposide	Thioguanine	Thiotepa	Topotecan	Toremifene	Vinblastine	Vincristine	Vinorelbine
Passionflower																							
Pau'Darco																							
Red clover	Low	Extreme	Extreme	Low	Low	Low	Low	Low	Low	Low	Low	Low	Low	Extreme	Low	Low	Low	Low	Low	Extreme	Low	Low	Low
Saw palmetto	Low	Low	Low	Low	Low	Low	Low	Low	Low	Low	Low	Low	Low	Low	Low	Low	Low	Low	Low	Low	Low	Low	Low
Soy beans		Moderate												Moderate									
St John's wort	Extreme	Extreme								Extreme				Extreme		Moderate				Extreme	Extreme	Extreme	Extreme
Valerian																							
Wild yam		Moderate												Moderate									

resistance proteins, which are found in numerous healthy tissues including the gut epithelium, liver and central nervous system, as well as chemotherapy-resistant tumour cells.[14] Two of the most important CYP enzymes for metabolism of xenobiotics in humans are CYP3A4 and CYP2D6 (see Table 2). CYP3A4 is responsible for the metabolism of numerous therapeutic drugs. For instance, in cancer, CYP3A4 plays at least some role in the metabolism of agents such as the taxanes (docetaxel and paclitaxel), vinca alkaloids (vincristine, vinblastine, vindesine and vinorelbine), camptothecins (irinotecan), the hormones exemestane, tamoxifen, and letrozole, and the epidermal growth factor receptor inhibitors (gefitinib and erlotinib).[13] CYP3A4 is also involved in the metabolism of calcium channel blockers (e.g. amlodipine, diltiazem, felodipine, nifedipine and verapamil), HMG CoA reductase inhibitors (e.g. atorvastatin and simvastatin) and immunosuppressants (cyclosporine and tacrolimus).[15] Substrates for the drug transporter, P-gp, among cancer drugs include many of the naturally derived anticancer drugs including taxanes, vinca alkaloids, epipodophyllotoxins and anthracyclines.[16]

Drug interactions can result if herbal constituents induce or inhibit these drug-metabolising pathways, thereby altering the bioavailability of the conventional therapeutic agent. If bioavailability is increased, this might lead to increased drug toxicity, whereas a reduction in bioavailability might lead to compromised therapeutic efficacy. It has recently been proposed by a number of authors that some of the effects on these drug-metabolising pathways might be mediated through activation of the pregnane X receptor (PXR), a ligand-activated nuclear receptor that is part of the superfamily of nuclear receptors. PXR regulates induction of CYP3A gene expression by xenobiotics, but may also regulate the induction of other genes involved in drug-metabolising pathways, and drug transporters, including CYP2B, CYP2C, CYP24, glutathione S-transferases, sulfotransferases, glucuronosyltransferases, organic anion-transporting polypeptide 1A4, P-gp (MDR1) and multi-drug resistance-associated proteins 2 and 3.[17,18] It has been recently shown that PXR is activated by a number of herbal remedies including *Gingko biloba* (higher doses), St. John's wort (SJW), and traditional Chinese remedies including tian xian, wu wei zi and gan cao, demonstrating that herbal remedies have the potential to have a major impact on drug metabolism.[19–21]

Pharmacodynamic interactions may occur when the bioavailable constituents of an herbal compound act in an additive, synergistic or antagonistic fashion with a therapeutic agent.

It is worth noting that disease states themselves can change the Pharmacokinetics or Pharmacodynamics of a drug and extrapolating data from healthy volunteers to patients is not always possible.[22] For example, CYP3A-mediated drug metabolism may be impaired in patients with an acute phase response, as occurs in numerous illnesses including rheumatological conditions, acute infections and patients with advanced cancer and probably contributes to the marked variability in drug pharmacokinetics and toxicity that has been noted in these circumstances.[23]

Although the potential for herb–drug interactions remains theoretical for many therapeutic agents, the consequences are potentially significant in terms of disease outcome and morbidity, and any theoretical interaction should be regarded as clinically relevant.

The following section reviews some of the more commonly ingested herbal medicines and discusses the evidence to support the potential for significant herb–drug interactions. Although CAM covers a broad range of therapies, this review will only focus on herbal and complementary medicines.

Asian Ginseng (Panax ginseng)

Several different types of ginseng are used in herbal medicine products (Asian, Siberian, American and Japanese ginseng varieties) although Asian Ginseng is the most commonly used. Ginseng is widely used in an attempt to enhance the natural immune system, assist in recovery and reduce fatigue.[24] This herb is also purported to improve physical performance, strength and increase stamina, although rigorous data from controlled trials are lacking.

The main constituents of Asian ginseng include saponin glycosides, i.e. ginsenosides (also known as panaxosides), antioxidants, volatile oils, fatty acids, vitamins and polysaccharides. The ginsenosides are believed to be responsible for Asian ginseng's effects.[24]

The effects of Asian ginseng on drug efficacy/drug metabolism *in-vitro* and *in-vivo* have not yet been fully elucidated and available data have been contradictory. Several *in-vitro* studies have shown its constituents to have no significant effect on cytochrome P450 enzyme activity; however, one study performed using human liver microsomes suggested that a crude ginseng extract had moderate inhibitory effects on CYP1A1, 1A2, 1B1, 2D6, 2C19, 2C9, 2E1 and 3A4.[16] Further *in-vitro* studies have shown high concentrations of ginsenosides (>200 mg/L) to have a moderate inhibitory effect on P-gp activity.[25]

Several reports of drug interactions between ginseng products and conventional medicines, including monoamine oxidase inhibitors, warfarin, antidiabetic therapies, central nervous system (CNS) drugs (including tranylcypromine and isocarboxazid), nifedipine and digoxin, have been described in the literature.[26,27] There have been no reports of any interaction between Asian ginseng and anticancer agents. However, in view of the interaction with these other compounds, caution may still be warranted with the administration of Asian ginseng together with anticancer agents that are CYP3A4 substrates.

Black Cohosh (Cimicifuga racemosa)

Black cohosh is promoted for use in the treatment of menopausal symptoms and menstrual conditions, although its efficacy has yet to be conclusively substantiated in clinical trials. It may be misconceived as having oestrogenic properties due to its effect in menopausal herbal medicine products such as Remifemin®. However, black cohosh's effect may be due to more of a dopaminergic, rather than an oestrogenic profile,[28] or the result of constituents that have selective oestrogen receptor modulator activity.[29] Therefore, the theoretical caution in regard to administration of black cohosh in patients with oestrogen-dependent tumours may be unfounded.

Although there have been no direct *in-vivo* studies, an *in-vitro* study suggests that black cohosh may also influence the efficacy of selected chemotherapeutic agents used in the treatment of breast cancer.[30] Results showed that black cohosh enhanced the sensitivity of mouse mammary cancer cells to doxorubicin and docetaxel, but reduced sensitivity to cisplatin. Although the mechanisms of interaction and clinical relevance of this study are not yet clear, caution may be warranted in cancer patients receiving black cohosh in conjunction with chemotherapy. An *in-vivo* study in rats also investigated the use of black cohosh and tamoxifen on implanted endometrial adenocarcinoma cells and showed that black cohosh did not enhance or reduce the inductive effect of tamoxifen on tumour growth, but may have reduced the metastasising potential of the tumour potentiated by tamoxifen.[31]

A number of randomised studies have failed to show benefit for black cohosh compared with placebo in the treatment of hot flushes[32] or vasomotor symptoms of menopause, which are common problems for women undergoing chemotherapy.[33]

A clinical trial has shown that black cohosh may have an inhibitory effect on CYP2D6 activity, but no significant effect on the activities of CYP3A4, CYP1A2 and CYP2E1, in healthy volunteers.[34] Caution may be warranted therefore in patients receiving therapeutic agents metabolised by CYP2D6. A further study, again in healthy volunteers, has shown that black cohosh has no effect on the drug disposition of digoxin, which may be indicative of a lack of effect of the herb on the activity of P-gp.[35] There have also been reports of black cohosh inducing acute hepatotoxicity, leading in some instances to hepatic failure necessitating liver transplantation.[36]

In summary, evidence regarding the potential interaction between black cohosh and therapeutic agents is limited, and further clinical and pharmacokinetic studies are required.

Celery (Apium graveolens)

Celery has been traditionally used for the treatment of arthritic conditions and gout, as well as urinary tract infections. Celery extracts have also been shown to have a chemopreventive effect in pre-clinical models.[37,38] A pre-clinical study in mice pre-treated with celery and parsley juices also showed potentiation of the effects of pentobarbital; however, statistical significance was only observed in parsley-co-treated animals.[39] The likelihood of celery producing adverse interactions with other therapeutic agents is low; however, further investigation is warranted.

Chamomile (Matricaria recutita)

Chamomile is used topically for its anti-inflammatory effects and to treat skin disorders. It is also ingested orally for use as a mild sedative. Chamomile mouthwash may be of use in the prevention or treatment of mucositis induced by radiation and chemotherapy in patients, and a number of clinical trials have been carried out, albeit with conflicting results.[40,41] In terms of the potential for adverse drug interactions, a pre-clinical study found that the activity of CYP1A2 in rat liver microsomes treated with chamomile tea was significantly decreased by 24% ($P < 0.05$); however, no significant changes were observed in the activities of the CYP2D, CYP2E and CYP3A subfamilies.[42] This finding suggests that there is limited potential for interactions between chamomile and other therapeutic agents when ingested systemically; however, more data will be needed to produce a more conclusive finding.

Echinacea (Echinacea purpurea)

Echinacea is traditionally used as an immunostimulant, antibacterial and antiviral, and is commonly used in cough and cold preparations, in an attempt to alleviate symptoms.[43] Echinacea consists of a range of constituents including caffeic acid conjugates (caftaric acid, cichoric acid and echinacoside), alkylamides, glycoproteins and polysaccharides.[44,45]

In-vivo evidence regarding the effect of echinacea on the activity of CYP enzymes has been conflicting. One clinical study showed that echinacea inhibits CYP1A2 activity and induces CYP3A activity, but had no effect on the activities of CYP2C9 or CYP2D6;[46] however, another study observed no effect on CYP3A4, CYP2D6, CYP1A2 or CYP2E1 activity.[47] It is likely that the effects of echinacea on CYP enzyme activity may be dependent on the preparation and/or dosage of echinacea used, which could explain these apparently conflicting results. Thus, caution is still warranted with the use of agents that are metabolised by CYP3A4, as they may interact with co-administered echinacea products.

Fenugreek (Trigonella foenum graecum)

The German Commission E has approved the internal use of fenugreek as an appetite stimulant and topically as a poultice to treat local inflammation. Although no herb–drug interactions have been reported for fenugreek, it has several constituents that could theoretically cause interactions with some medicines. It has been suggested that the coumarin content could theoretically potentiate the anticoagulant effect of warfarin. However, a clinical study in patients with coronary artery disease receiving 5 g of fenugreek powder for 3 months found no significant effect on blood coagulation parameters, although *in-vitro* investigations showed inhibition of platelet aggregation.[48]

Fenugreek also contains several flavonoids, including quercetin, which has been implicated in CYP3A4 inhibition. One study demonstrated that quercetin increased the bioavailability of verapamil in rabbits *in-vivo*, suggesting CYP3A4 inhibition as a possible mechanism.[49] Another trial showed that the area under the curve (AUC) of cyclosporine (a CYP3A4 substrate) was increased when it was co-administered with quercetin to healthy volunteers ($n = 8$), the largest increase occurring when participants received quercetin for 3 days prior to commencement of cyclosporine.[50] An animal study also demonstrated that quercetin can increase the bioavailability of orally administered paclitaxel.[51] Increases in AUC and Cmax were observed when paclitaxel was administered with quercetin, possibly as a result of intestinal P-gp and CYP3A4 inhibition. Previous *in-vitro* studies also demonstrated an inhibitory effect of quercetin on P-gp.[52] However, information regarding plasma concentrations and bioavailability of quercetin following oral administration of recommended doses of fenugreek is largely unknown. Thus, there is the potential for interaction between fenugreek and conventional therapeutic agents as a result of the quercetin content and caution is warranted in co-administering fenugreek together with agents that are CYP3A4 substrates and/or substrates for P-gp.

Feverfew (*Tanacetum parthenium*)

Feverfew is commonly used for migraine prophylaxis or treatment, although supporting randomised trial data are lacking.[53] Parthenolide is thought to be the constituent responsible for feverfew's therapeutic effect.[54] There have been no reports of interactions with conventional medicines. Thus, it is probably safe to use feverfew with other therapeutic agents. Recent reports suggest an apoptotic effect from feverfew in cancer cell lines, which might provide possible therapeutic benefit in cancer treatment; however, further clinical studies are required.[55]

Garlic (Allium sativum)

Garlic has traditionally been reported to have expectorant, diaphoretic, disinfectant, diuretic, antimicrobial, antihypertensive, lipid-lowering, fibrinolytic, antiplatelet and cancer protective properties. A number of systematic reviews have provided evidence for its efficacy in the treatment of hypertension and hypercholesterolaemia.[56,57] A further systematic review has indicated a potential protective effect of high levels of raw or cooked garlic against colorectal and stomach cancers, although the evidence for this indication is of varying quality.[58]

An *in-vitro* study found that garlic extracts may have an inhibitory effect on CYP2C9*1, 2C9*2, 2C19, 2D6, 3A4, 3A5 and 3A7 and P-gp activity.[59] However, garlic extracts have been shown to not alter the disposition of co-administered medications primarily dependent on the CYP2D6 or CYP3A4 pathway of metabolism in healthy volunteers.[60]

A number of clinical studies investigating the potential interaction between garlic and the human immunodeficiency virus (HIV) protease inhibitor, saquinavir, have shown that garlic reduced drug bioavailability in healthy volunteers.[61,62] Although the mechanism of this interaction is not clear, the results indicate a possible inductive effect on CYP enzyme or P-gp activity, and suggest that caution may be warranted with concomitant use of garlic and drugs metabolised by these mechanisms.

These studies highlight the unreliability of *in-vitro–in-vivo* correlations, and in the absence of confirmatory clinical studies combined with the relative lack of involvement of the CYP2C class of isoenzymes in drug metabolism (except tamoxifen)[63] potentially significant herb–drug interactions appear unlikely.

Ginger (Zingiber officinale)

Ginger is used for its antiemetic and antispasmodic effects, often in pregnancy.[64] Its main constituents include starch, lipids, volatile oils, monoterpenes, amino acids and proteins. *In-vitro* studies have demonstrated its antiplatelet activity, its inhibitory effects on COX-2 and its glucose-lowering effects through enhanced insulin sensitivity.[65–67] Ginger may cause potential pharmacodynamic interactions with anti-inflammatory or antidiabetic medicines, although there is no *in-vivo* evidence to support this. Although the *in-vitro* evidence suggests that ginger may cause an increased risk of bleeding with antiplatelet agents or anticoagulants, a recent study reported no interactions with warfarin at recommended doses and suggested that ginger has no effect on CYP2C9 activity *in vivo*.[68]

From the available clinical evidence, it would appear that ginger is a relatively safe herbal medicine and should not produce adverse interactions with most classes of therapeutic agents.

Ginkgo (Ginkgo biloba)

Ginkgo extracts are used mainly as enhancers of peripheral circulation in the treatment of cerebrovascular disorders, memory loss, Alzheimer's disease, multi-infarct dementia and free radical damage.[69] The majority of these studies have been conducted using the standardised EGb 761 extract of *Ginkgo biloba*. Ginkgo consists of ginkgo flavonol glycosides: quercetin, kaempferol and isorhamnetin. Ginkgo extracts also contain biflavones including bilobetin, ginkgetin and isoginkgetin, as well as ginkgolides.[68,70]

As with garlic, clinical studies have shown that ginkgo extracts at recommended doses are unlikely to significantly alter the disposition of co-administered medications primarily dependent on the CYP2D6-, CYP3A4-,[70] CYP1A2- or CYP2E1-mediated pathways of elimination.[71]

Clinical studies have also shown that *Ginkgo biloba* does not affect the drug disposition of digoxin, indicating that there should be minimal potential for induction or inhibition of P-gp activity. Therefore, clinically significant interactions with agents that are substrates for P-gp are unlikely.[72]

Grape Seed (Vitis vinifera)

Grape seed extract is known for its potent antioxidant activity as well as purported antibacterial, anti-inflammatory and antiallergic properties. Grape seed extract at a concentration of 600 ng/mL has been shown to significantly increase the expression of CYP3A4 mRNA.[73] However, as suggested by Sparreboom *et al.*,[12] it is unlikely that these levels can be reached in humans following the intake of commercial grape seed preparations.[12]

Green Tea (Camellia sinensis)

The principal active constituents of green tea are catechins. Catechins have purported antioxidant, anticarcinogenic and antiatherogenic properties. In studies conducted in rodents, catechins have produced increases in the metabolism of substrates of CYP1A, 1A2, 2B and glutathione-S transferase, although decaffeinated extracts did not show these increases, implicating caffeine as the causative factor.[74] *In-vitro* studies of individual purified catechins have shown inhibition of numerous CYPs, including 1A1, 1A2, 2A6, 2C19, 2E1 and 3A4.[75] *In-vitro* cell line assays have also shown that catechins decrease P-gp activity and are able to decrease the efflux of doxorubicin, a theoretical interaction that may increase the efficacy of doxorubicin although no *in-vivo* studies have been performed to confirm this interaction.[76]

Few data for clinically significant *in-vivo* herb–drug interactions between catechins and therapeutic agents have been published. A pharmacokinetic study performed in healthy volunteers given green tea extracts showed no changes in the pharmacokinetics of dextromethorphan and alprazolam, indicating that decaffeinated green tea has no effect on the activity of CYP2D6 and CYP3A4, the major metabolising enzymes for these medicines, respectively.[77]

There has been a single case report of a possible interaction between green tea and Warfarin.[78]

Guarana (Paullinia cupana)

No *in-vivo* drug interaction studies examining the effect of guarana or its extracts have been reported. Caffeine,[79] the main constituent of guarana, is a CYP1A2 substrate and the potential exists for competitive inhibition with other CYP1A2 substrates including the chemotherapeutic agents cyclophosphamide and ifosfamide. Patients undergoing chemotherapy with these medicines should be advised to avoid ingesting extreme quantities of caffeine-containing beverages. Similar precautions should be undertaken in other disease states where CYP1A2 substrates are utilised.

Liquorice (Glycyrrhiza uralensis)

Liquorice root is used for its anti-inflammatory, antiulcer and antiarthritic actions. The active components are glycyrrhizin and its more potent metabolite glycyrrhetinic acid.[80] Glycyrrhizin and glycyrrhetinic acid are inhibitors of cortisol metabolism.[81] Fluid retention, hypokalemia, hypertension and aggravation of congestive heart disease are known adverse effects of long-term or high-dose use of liquorice root, due to accumulation of mineralocorticoids.[82] As glucocorticoids with significant mineralocorticoid effects (mainly dexamethasone and prednisone) are widely used in the treatment of inflammatory and malignant diseases, patients should be cautioned against the administration of liquorice root, to reduce the risk of excessive mineralocorticoid side-effects.

The major flavonoid component of liquorice, glabridin, has been shown *in-vitro* to irreversibly inhibit CYP3A4 and 2B6, possibly through the destruction of the heme moiety by a reactive metabolite of glabridin.[83] In studies conducted in rodents, significantly different effects are seen on total CYP protein and mRNA, depending on dosage regimens. Although single doses of liquorice extracts or purified glycyrrhizin had no effect, repeated dosing significantly induced CYP3A4 production in rats and mice, and CYP1A2 production in rats alone.[84] The clinical implications of these findings remain to be established in many disease settings.

Milk Thistle (Silybum marianum)

Milk thistle is commonly used for its hepatoprotective properties and silymarin, a mixture of closely related flavonoids, is the principal constituent believed to be responsible for this effect.[85] Although clinical evidence to support the efficacy of this herb remains elusive, milk thistle continues to be one of the most commonly promoted and used herbal medicines.[86,87]

A number of *in-vitro* studies have been carried out investigating the combination of milk thistle constituents and selected chemotherapeutic drugs. Results indicate that silybin may synergistically enhance the inhibition of ovarian cancer cell growth in combination with cisplatin and doxorubicin,[88] however, the clinical relevance of this observed positive effect is unclear and there is a lack of information regarding the potential toxic consequences of this combination *in-vivo*.

Evidence regarding the effect of milk thistle on CYP enzymes *in-vitro* is conflicting. One study investigated the effect of several silymarin flavonolignans, i.e. silybin, silydianin, silycristin, and dehydrosilybin (the oxidised product of silybin) on CYP3A4, 2D6 and 2E1 in human liver microsomes. The authors concluded that the activity of the human CYP enzymes was largely unaffected by flavonolignans in the silymarin complex at pharmacologically effective concentrations and, as a result, no drug interactions should be expected.[89] Other studies have demonstrated that milk thistle decreases CYP3A4 activity and inhibits P-gp cellular efflux *in-vitro*.[90,91]

In-vivo evidence from clinical studies has shown that recommended doses of a milk thistle preparation had no effect on the activity of CYP3A4, CYP2D6, CYP1A2 or CYP2E1 in healthy volunteers.[47] Furthermore, a recent randomised controlled clinical trial in 16 healthy volunteers investigated the combination of milk thistle with indinavir, a CYP3A4 substrate used in the treatment of HIV.[92] No significant difference was seen in the AUC for indinavir when milk thistle was added to the drug regimen, indicating that it does not inhibit CYP3A4 *in-vivo*. The findings of this latest study support results from earlier studies that indicated that milk thistle had no inhibitory or inductive effects on P-gp or CYP3A4.[93,94]

The lack of an effect of milk thistle on the activity of P-gp has been further supported by a recent study in which the combination of milk thistle and digoxin in healthy volunteers was investigated.[35] There was no apparent effect of milk thistle on the disposition of digoxin, indicating a lack of effect of the herb on P-gp activity.

The balance of available evidence suggests that milk thistle can be safely combined with agents that are CYP3A or P-gp substrates, but close monitoring of changes in drug effects is appropriate.

St. John's Wort (Hypericum perforatum)

SJW is commonly used for the treatment of mild to moderate depression, as well as other psychiatric disorders such as seasonal affective disorder and mild anxiety.[95] Although its overall mechanism of action is unclear, hyperforin is believed to be the constituent responsible for its antidepressant effect. Several *in-vitro* studies have indicated that hyperforin acts by inhibiting the reuptake of neurotransmitters such as serotonin, noradrenaline and possibly dopamine.[96] Despite these findings, SJW herbal medicine products with minimal concentrations of hyperforin have been demonstrated to have some efficacy as antidepressants, suggesting that other constituents may also have a role.

SJW has been shown to be a potent modulator of several cytochrome P450 enzymes. Its constituents have both inductive and inhibitory effects. *In-vitro* studies have shown that extracts of SJW significantly inhibit the activity of CYP1A2, 2D6, 2C9, 2C19 and 3A4. *In-vivo* studies have shown SJW derivatives produce significant induction of hepatic and intestinal CYP3A4 if administered for longer than a 2-week period, while having no inductive effect on cytochromes P450 2C9 or 2D6[97] and a possible inductive effect on CYP1A2.[98] In the clinical setting, the predominant effect of co-administration of SJW is induction of metabolism, with the associated risk of lack of efficacy due to subtherapeutic concentrations.

Hyperforin, a major constituent of SJW, is believed to be responsible for inducing intestinal expression of the MDR1 P-gp, enhancing its drug efflux function.[99,100] Two studies have directly investigated clinically significant interactions between SJW and anticancer agents. The first of these examined the effect of SJW on the metabolism of irinotecan, a pro-drug of SN-38 and a known CYP3A4 substrate.[101] A 42% decrease in the AUC was observed for the combination of irinotecan and SJW, compared with irinotecan alone. The second study investigated the effect of SJW on imatinib and found that the clearance of imatinib increased by 43% when co-administered with SJW.[102] CYP3A4 is the major enzyme responsible for the metabolism of imatinib, with CYP1A2, 2D6, 2C9 and 2C19 contributing to a lesser extent. These studies clearly indicate the potential for clinically significant interactions between SJW and anticancer agents.

Other trials have demonstrated clinically significant interactions between SJW and conventional medicines.[103] Several case reports suggest that SJW is responsible for interactions with cyclosporine, with one case resulting in acute heart transplant rejection.[104] Two possible mechanisms of interaction between SJW and cyclosporine include induction of intestinal and hepatic CYP3A4, as well as induced expression of intestinal P-gp drug transporters.

SJW has also been shown to interact with fexofenadine, which is not metabolised by CYP enzymes, but is a measure of MDR1 function, providing further evidence as to the involvement of SJW in multiple induction mechanisms.[105] Thus, concomitant treatment with SJW and other agents that are CYP3A4 substrates or substrates for the P-gp drug transport system may affect clinical outcomes.

Saw Palmetto (Serenoa repens)

Saw palmetto is primarily used for treating prostatic conditions, such as benign prostatic hypertrophy (BPH), because of its antiandrogenic properties and a systematic review supports the positive effects of saw palmetto on symptoms of BPH.[106] Although the exact mechanism of action is unknown, studies have shown that it acts as a mild inhibitor of 5-alpha-reductase, the enzyme responsible for the conversion of testosterone to the more active form, dihydrotestosterone.[107]

Its role in relieving symptoms of BPH also arises from its inhibition of cyclo-oxygenase and lipo-oxygenase pathways, thereby preventing the synthesis of prostaglandins and leukotrienes involved in inflammation.[108] This action has been implicated in a case report, in which a patient suffered intraoperative haemorrhaging following the use of a saw palmetto extract.[109] There have been no reported interactions between saw palmetto and conventional medicines.

An *in-vitro* study found a potent inhibitory effect of saw palmetto on CYP3A4, 2D6 and 2C9;[110] however, *in-vivo* pharmacokinetic studies have demonstrated that saw palmetto had no significant effect on cytochrome P450 isoenzymes including CYP1A2 and CYP2E1, CYP2D6 or CYP3A4 in healthy volunteers.[47,111]

In light of its antiandrogenic properties and until interaction studies prove otherwise, it would be advisable to avoid the use of saw palmetto in cancer patients who are receiving hormonal therapy, due to the risk of possible additive pharmacodynamic effects.

Valerian (Valeriana officinalis)

Valerian is purported to be useful as an antispasmodic, an anxiolytic and an antidepressant, but is most often used to treat insomnia. It has a complex composition and contains three major sesquiterpenes — valerianic acid, valeranone and kessyl glycol, and monterpenes (primarily borneol). *In-vitro* studies suggest that valerian inhibits CYP3A4 and P-gp.[112,113] However, *in-vivo* studies indicate that valerian does not interact with CYP1A2, 2E1, 2D6 or 3A4/5 metabolism pathways at recommended doses.[34,114] Although there may be some rationale against the concomitant use of barbiturates or other sedatives with valerian, there is no *in-vivo* evidence of any interactions between it and conventional medicines.

Other Frequently Used CAM

Evening primrose oil

Evening primrose oil contains high levels of gamma-linolenic acid (GLA), which exhibits anti-inflammatory, antiproliferative and antithrombotic properties.[115] Evening primrose oil or GLA has been shown to be useful in the treatment of atopic eczema,[116] diabetic neuropathy[117] and mastalgia.[118] There have also been a number of trials to investigate the use of evening primrose oil or GLA in improving survival rates and outcomes of patients with primary liver cancer,[119] but without demonstrable survival advantage.

A more recent clinical study investigated the combined treatment of a high-dose oral GLA supplement with tamoxifen in women with locally advanced or metastatic breast cancer, compared with tamoxifen alone.[120] Results indicate that GLA supplementation significantly enhanced the efficacy of tamoxifen, resulting in more rapid response to treatment, compared with patients receiving tamoxifen only. There were no adverse effects reported.

Overall, evening primrose oil and/or its constituent GLA have shown positive effects in a number of different settings. However, evidence is again limited, especially in terms of the assessment of potential negative interactions.

Phyto-oestrogen-containing herbal medicines

Many women self-medicate with complementary medicines to alleviate menopausal symptoms.[121] *In-vitro* studies have been performed investigating the proliferative effects of herbal substances and purified extracts that are marketed for menopausal symptom relief using MCF-7 cultured breast cancer cells. Products containing soy, red clover, dong quai and ginseng have all been shown to produce increases in MCF-7 cell proliferation in the absence of oestrogen.[122] A similar recently published *in-vitro* assay investigated purified genistein, daidzein and resveratrol, all phyto-oestrogens also showed increases in the proliferation of MCF-7 cells.[123] Research conducted in athymic mice with implanted MCF-7 cells showed that dietary genistein was able to negate the antioestrogenic effects of concurrent tamoxifen.[124] These proliferative effects have not been shown *in-vivo*; however, as it is unlikely that any such study would be attempted, it would be prudent to advise women with oestrogen receptor-positive breast cancers and who are undergoing treatment with antioestrogens to avoid self-medication with any herbs containing phyto-oestrogens.

Other Herbs

Devil's claw (Harpagophytum procumbens)

Devil's claw is used for the treatment of musculoskeletal conditions and has been shown to be effective in arthritic and chronic back pain.[125] It has been associated with an increased risk of bleeding in a patient receiving Warfarin;[126] however, this interaction has not been confirmed and no further studies on potential drug interactions with devil's claw have been carried out.

Cranberry (Vaccinium macrocarpon)

Cranberry is primarily used in the prevention of urinary tract infections, with some evidence of a beneficial effect.[127] Clinical studies have demonstrated that cranberry enhances the affect of Warfarin.[128] The exact mechanism of this interaction has yet to be characterised and it remains unclear whether cranberry will cause any significant interactions with other drugs; however, further investigations are required.

CONCLUSION

The increasing use of herbal medicines and complementary therapies has led to concerns about the appropriate concomitant use of pharmaceutical and herbal medicines. The data that we have examined highlight the validity of concerns about potential adverse interactions between CAM and conventional treatments. However, there are enormous gaps in our knowledge, because of the lack of well-conducted clinical and pharmacokinetic studies of CAM and conventional treatments in many therapeutic settings. It is imperative that these gaps be filled, to ensure that patients receive the safest and most effective therapies.

REFERENCES

1. Eisenberg DM, Kessler RC, Foster C, *et al*. Unconventional medicine in the United States. Prevalence, costs, and patterns of use. *N Engl J Med* **328**:246–252 (1993).
2. Eisenberg DM, Davis RB, Ettner SL, *et al*. Trends in alternative medicine use in the United States, 1990–1997: results of a follow-up national survey. *JAMA* **280**:1569–1575 (1998).
3. MacLennan AH, Myers SP, Taylor AW. The continuing use of complementary and alternative medicine in South Australia: costs and beliefs in 2004. *Med J Aust* **184**:27–31 (2006).
4. Ernst E, Cassileth BR. The prevalence of complementary/alternative medicine in cancer: a systematic review. *Cancer* **83**:777–782 (1998).
5. Richardson MA, Sanders T, Palmer JL, *et al*. Complementary/alternative medicine use in a comprehensive cancer center and the implications for oncology. *J Clin Oncol* **18**:2505–2514 (2000).

6. Boon HS, Olatunde F, Zick SM. Trends in complementary/alternative medicine use by breast cancer survivors: comparing survey data from 1998 and 2005. *BMC Womens Health* **7**:4 (2007).
7. Zhou SF, Zhou ZW, Li CG, *et al.* Identification of drugs that interact with herbs in drug development. *Drug Discov Today* **12**:664–673 (2007).
8. Verhoef MJ, Balneaves LG, Boon HS, *et al.* Reasons for and characteristics associated with complementary and alternative medicine use among adult cancer patients: a systematic review. *Integr Cancer Ther* **4**:274–286 (2005).
9. Herman PM, Craig BM, Caspi O. Is complementary and alternative medicine (CAM) cost-effective? A systematic review. *BMC Complement Altern* Med **5**:11 (2005).
10. Blumenthal M. Herbal sales down 7% in mainstream market. *Herbal Gram* **66**: (2005).
11. Pal D, Mitra AK. MDR- and CYP3A4-mediated drug-herbal interactions. *Life Sci* **78**:2131–2145 (2006).
12. Sparreboom A, Cox MC, Acharya MR, *et al.* Herbal remedies in the United States: potential adverse interactions with anticancer agents. *J Clin Oncol* **22**:2489–2503 (2004).
13. Meijerman I, Beijnen JH, Schellens JH. Herb-drug interactions in oncology: focus on mechanisms of induction. *Oncologist* **11**:742–752 (2006).
14. Beijnen JH, Schellens JH. Drug interactions in oncology. *Lancet Oncol* **5**(8):489–496 (2004).
15. Flockhart DA. *Drug Interactions: Cytochrome P450 Drug Interaction Table*, Indiana University School of Medicine (2007). *http://medicine.iupui.edu/clinpharm/ddis/table.asp* [Accessed 6 June 2010].
16. Takara K, Sakaeda T, Okumura K. An update on overcoming MDR1-mediated multidrug resistance in cancer chemotherapy. *Curr Pharm Des* **12**:273–286 (2006).
17. Ma X, Idle JR, Gonzalez FJ. The pregnane X receptor: from bench to bedside. *Expert Opin Drug Metab Toxicol* **4**:895–908 (2008).
18. Köhle C, Bock KW. Coordinate regulation of human drug-metabolizing enzymes, and conjugate transporters by the Ah receptor, pregnane X receptor and constitutive androstane receptor. *Biochem Pharmacol* **77**:689–699 (2009).
19. Moore LB, Goodwin B, Jones SA, *et al.* St. John's wort induces hepatic drug metabolism through activation of the pregnane X receptor. *Proc Natl Acad Sci USA* **97**:7500–7502 (2000).

20. Li L, Stanton JD, Tolson AH, *et al.* Bioactive terpenoids and flavonoids from Ginkgo biloba extract induce the expression of hepatic drug-metabolizing enzymes through pregnane X receptor, constitutive androstane receptor, and aryl hydrocarbon receptor-mediated pathways. *Pharm Res.* **26**:872–882 (2009).
21. Yeung EY, Sueyoshi T, Negishi M, *et al.* Identification of Ginkgo biloba as a novel activator of pregnane X receptor. *Drug Metab Dispos* **36**:2270–2276 (2008).
22. McLachlan AJ, Hilmer SN, Le Couteur DG. Variability in response to medicines in older people: phenotypic and genotypic factors. *Clin Pharmacol Ther* **85**:431–433 (2009).
23. Rivory LP, Slaviero KA, Clarke SJ. Hepatic cytochrome P450 3A drug metabolism is reduced in cancer patients who have an acute-phase response. *Br J Cancer* **87**:277–280 (2002).
24. Xiang YZ, Shang HC, Gao XM, *et al.* A comparison of the ancient use of ginseng in traditional Chinese medicine with modern pharmacological experiments and clinical trials. *Phytother Res* **22**:851–858 (2008).
25. Foster BC, Arnason JT, Briggs CJ. Natural health products and drug disposition. *Annu Rev Pharmacol Toxicol* **45**:203–226 (2005).
26. Bressler R. Herb-drug interactions: interactions between ginseng and prescription medications. *Geriatrics* **60**:16–17 (2005).
27. Janetzky K, Morreale AP. Probable interaction between warfarin and ginseng. *Am J Health Syst Pharm* **54**:692–693 (1997).
28. Mahady GB. Is black cohosh estrogenic? *Nutr Rev* **61**(5 Pt 1):183–186 (2003).
29. Seidlova-Wuttke D, Hesse O, Jarry H, *et al.* Evidence for selective estrogen receptor modulator activity in a black cohosh (Cimicifuga racemosa) extract: comparison with estradiol-17beta. *Eur J Endocrinol* **149**:351–362 (2003).
30. Rockwell S, Liu Y, Higgins SA. Alteration of the effects of cancer therapy agents on breast cancer cells by the herbal medicine black cohosh. *Breast Cancer Res Treat* **90**:233–239 (2005).
31. Nisslein T, Freudenstein J. Concomitant administration of an isopropanolic extract of black cohosh and tamoxifen in the *in vivo* tumor model of implanted RUCA-I rat endometrial adenocarcinoma cells. *Toxicol Lett* **150**:271–275 (2004).
32. Pockaj BA, Gallagher JG, Loprinzi CL, *et al.* Phase III double-blind, randomized, placebo-controlled crossover trial of black cohosh in

the management of hot flashes: NCCTG Trial N01CC1. *J Clin Oncol* **24**:2836–2841 (2006).
33. Newton KM, Reed SD, LaCroix AZ, *et al.* Treatment of vasomotor symptoms of menopause with black cohosh, multibotanicals, soy, hormone therapy, or placebo: a randomized trial. *Ann Intern Med* **145**:869–879 (2006).
34. Gurley BJ, Gardner SF, Hubbard MA, *et al. In vivo* effects of goldenseal, kava kava, black cohosh, and valerian on human cytochrome P450 1A2, 2D6, 2E1, and 3A4/5 phenotypes. *Clin Pharmacol Ther* **77**:415–426 (2005).
35. Gurley BJ, Barone GW, Williams DK, *et al.* Effect of milk thistle (Silybum marianum) and black cohosh (Cimicifuga racemosa) supplementation on digoxin pharmacokinetics in humans. *Drug Metab Dispos* **34**:69–74 (2006).
36. Chow EC, Teo M, Ring JA, *et al.* Liver failure associated with the use of black cohosh for menopausal symptoms. *Med J Aust* **188**:420–422 (2008).
37. Sultana S, Ahmed S, Jahangir T, *et al.* Inhibitory effect of celery seeds extract on chemically induced hepatocarcinogenesis: modulation of cell proliferation, metabolism and altered hepatic foci development. *Cancer Lett* **221**:11–20 (2005).
38. Zheng GQ, Kenney PM, Zhang J, *et al.* Chemoprevention of benzo[a]pyrene-induced forestomach cancer in mice by natural phthalides from celery seed oil. *Nutr Cancer* **19**:77–86 (1993).
39. Jakovljevic V, Raskovic A, Popovic M, *et al.* The effect of celery and parsley juices on pharmacodynamic activity of drugs involving cytochrome P450 in their metabolism. *Eur J Drug Metab Pharmacokinet* **27**:153–156 (2002).
40. Carl W, Emrich LS. Management of oral mucositis during local radiation and systemic chemotherapy: a study of 98 patients. *J Prosthet Dent* **66**:361–369 (1991).
41. Fidler P, Loprinzi CL, O'Fallon JR, *et al.* Prospective evaluation of a chamomile mouthwash for prevention of 5-FU-induced oral mucositis. *Cancer* **77**:522–525 (1996).
42. Maliakal PP, Wanwimolruk S. Effect of herbal teas on hepatic drug metabolizing enzymes in rats. *J Pharm Pharmacol* **53**:1323–1329 (2001).
43. Schoop R, Klein P, Suter A, *et al.* Echinacea in the prevention of induced rhinovirus colds: a meta-analysis. *Clin Ther* **28**:174–183 (2006).

44. Matthias A, Addison RS, Penman KG, *et al*. Echinacea alkamide disposition and pharmacokinetics in humans after tablet ingestion. *Life Sci* **77**:2018–2029 (2005).
45. Matthias A, Gillam EM, Penman KG, *et al*. Cytochrome P450 enzyme-mediated degradation of Echinacea alkylamides in human liver microsomes. *Chem Biol Interact* **155**:62–70 (2005).
46. Gorski JC, Huang SM, Pinto A, *et al*. The effect of echinacea (Echinacea purpurea root) on cytochrome P450 activity *in vivo*. *Clin Pharmacol Ther* **75**:89–100 (2004).
47. Gurley BJ, Gardner SF, Hubbard MA, *et al*. *In vivo* assessment of botanical supplementation on human cytochrome P450 phenotypes: Citrus aurantium, Echinacea purpurea, milk thistle, and saw palmetto. *Clin Pharmacol Ther* **76**(5):428–440 (2004).
48. Bordia A, Verma SK, Srivastava KC. Effect of ginger (*Zingiber officinale* Rosc.) and fenugreek (*Trigonella foenumgraecum* L.) on blood lipids, blood sugar and platelet aggregation in patients with coronary artery disease. *Prostaglandins Leukot Essent Fatty Acids* **56**:379–384 (1997).
49. Choi JS, Han HK. The effect of quercetin on the pharmacokinetics of verapamil and its major metabolite, norverapamil, in rabbits. *J Pharm Pharmacol* **56**:1537–1542 (2004).
50. Choi JS, Choi BC, Choi KE. Effect of quercetin on the pharmacokinetics of oral cyclosporine. *Am J Health Syst Pharm* **61**:2406–2409 (2004).
51. Choi JS, Jo BW, Kim YC. Enhanced paclitaxel bioavailability after oral administration of paclitaxel or prodrug to rats pretreated with quercetin. *Eur J Pharm Biopharm* **57**:313–318 (2004).
52. Scambia G, Ranelletti FO, Panici PB, *et al*. Quercetin potentiates the effect of adriamycin in a multidrug-resistant MCF-7 human breast-cancer cell line: P-glycoprotein as a possible target. *Cancer Chemother Pharmacol* **34**:459–464 (1994).
53. Pfaffenrath V, Diener HC, Fischer M, Friede M, *et al*. The efficacy and safety of Tanacetum parthenium (feverfew) in migraine prophylaxis — a double-blind, multicentre, randomized placebo-controlled dose-response study. *Cephalalgia* **22**:523–532 (2002).
54. Tassorelli C, Greco R, Morazzoni P, *et al*. Parthenolide is the component of tanacetum parthenium that inhibits nitroglycerin-induced Fos activation: studies in an animal model of migraine. *Cephalalgia* **25**:612–621 (2005).

55. Zhang S, Ong CN, Shen HM. Involvement of proapoptotic Bcl-2 family members in parthenolide-induced mitochondrial dysfunction and apoptosis. *Cancer Lett* **211**:175–188 (2004).
56. Silagy CA, Neil HA. A meta-analysis of the effect of garlic on blood pressure. *J Hypertens* **12**:463–468 (1994).
57. Stevinson C, Pittler MH, Ernst E. Garlic for treating hypercholesterolemia. A meta-analysis of randomized clinical trials. *Ann Intern Med* **133**:420–429 (2000).
58. Fleischauer AT, Arab A. Garlic and cancer: a critical review of the epidemiologic literature. *J Nutr* **131**(3s):1032S–1040S (2001).
59. Foster BC, Foster MS, Vandenhoek S, *et al*. An *in vitro* evaluation of human cytochrome P450 3A4 and P-glycoprotein inhibition by garlic. *J Pharm Pharm Sci* **4**:176–184 (2001).
60. Markowitz JS, Devane CL, Chavin KD, *et al*. Effects of garlic (Allium sativum L.) supplementation on cytochrome P450 2D6 and 3A4 activity in healthy volunteers. *Clin Pharmacol Ther* **74**:170–177 (2003).
61. Sussman E. Garlic supplements can impede HIV medication. *AIDS* **16**:N5 (2002).
62. Piscitelli SC, Burstein AH, Welden N, *et al*. The effect of garlic supplements on the pharmacokinetics of saquinavir. *Clin Infect Dis* **34**:234–238 (2002).
63. Desta Z, Ward BA, Soukhova NV, *et al*. Comprehensive evaluation of tamoxifen sequential biotransformation by the human cytochrome P450 system in vitro: prominent roles for CYP3A and CYP2D6. *J Pharmacol Exp Ther* **310**:1062–1075 (2004).
64. Borrelli F, Capasso R, Aviello G, *et al*. Effectiveness and safety of ginger in the treatment of pregnancy-induced nausea and vomiting. *Obstet Gynecol* **105**:849–856 (2005).
65. Tjendraputra E, Tran VH, Liu-Brennan D, *et al*. Effect of ginger constituents and synthetic analogues on cyclooxygenase-2 enzyme in intact cells. *Bioorg Chem* **29**:156–163 (2001).
66. Sekiya K, Ohtani A, Kusano S. Enhancement of insulin sensitivity in adipocytes by ginger. *Biofactors* **22**(1–4):153–156 (2004).
67. Nurtjahja-Tjendraputra E, Ammit AJ, Roufogalis BD, *et al*. Effective anti-platelet and COX-1 enzyme inhibitors from pungent constituents of ginger. *Thromb Res* **111**(4–5):259–265 (2003).
68. Jiang X, Williams KM, Liauw WS, *et al*. Effect of ginkgo and ginger on the pharmacokinetics and pharmacodynamics of warfarin in healthy subjects. *Br J Clin Pharmacol* **59**:425–432 (2005).

69. McKenna DJ, Jones K, Hughes K. Efficacy, safety, and use of ginkgo biloba in clinical and preclinical applications. *Altern Ther Health Med* **7**:70–86, 88–90 (2001).
70. Markowitz JS, Donovan JL, Lindsay DeVane C, *et al.* Multiple-dose administration of Ginkgo biloba did not affect cytochrome P-450 2D6 or 3A4 activity in normal volunteers. *J Clin Psychopharmacol* **23**: 576–581 (2003).
71. Gurley BJ, Gardner SF, Hubbard MA, *et al.* Cytochrome P450 phenotypic ratios for predicting herb-drug interactions in humans. *Clin Pharmacol Ther* **72**:276–287 (2002).
72. Mauro VF, Mauro LS, Kleshinski JF, *et al.* Impact of ginkgo biloba on the pharmacokinetics of digoxin. *Am J Ther* **10**:247–251 (2003).
73. Raucy JL. Regulation of CYP3A4 expression in human hepatocytes by pharmaceuticals and natural products. *Drug Metab Dispos* **31**: 533–539 (2003).
74. Maliakal PP, Coville PF, Wanwimolruk S. Tea consumption modulates hepatic drug metabolizing enzymes in Wistar rats. *J Pharm Pharmacol* **53**:569–577 (2001).
75. Muto S, Fujita K, Yamazaki Y, *et al.* Inhibition by green tea catechins of metabolic activation of procarcinogens by human cytochrome P450. *Mutat Res* **479**(1–2):197–206 (2001).
76. Sadzuka Y, Sugiyama T, Sonobe T. Efficacies of tea components on doxorubicin induced antitumor activity and reversal of multidrug resistance. *Toxicol Lett* **114**(1–3):155–162 (2000).
77. Donovan JL, Chavin KD, Devane CL, *et al.* Green tea (Camellia sinensis) extract does not alter cytochrome p450 3A4 or 2D6 activity in healthy volunteers. *Drug Metab Dispos* **32**:906–908 (2004).
78. Taylor JR, Wilt VM. Probable antagonism of warfarin by green tea. *Ann Pharmacother* **33**:426–428 (1999).
79. Bempong DK, Houghton PJ. Dissolution and absorption of caffeine from guarana. *J Pharm Pharmacol* **44**:769–771 (1992).
80. Fugh-Berman A, Ernst E. Herb-drug interactions: review and assessment of report reliability. *Br J Clin Pharmacol* **52**:587–595 (2001).
81. Ferrari P, Sansonnens A, Dick B, *et al.* *In vivo* 11beta-HSD-2 activity: variability, salt-sensitivity, and effect of licorice. *Hypertension* **38**:1330–1336 (2001).
82. Coxeter PD, McLachlan AJ, Duke CC, *et al.* Herb-drug interactions: an evidence based approach. *Curr Med Chem* **11**:1513–1525 (2004).

83. Kent UM, Aviram M, Rosenblat M, *et al.* The licorice root derived isoflavan glabridin inhibits the activities of human cytochrome P450S 3A4, 2B6, and 2C9. *Drug Metab Dispos* **30**:709–715 (2002).
84. Paolini M, Barillari J, Broccoli M, *et al.* Effect of liquorice and glycyrrhizin on rat liver carcinogen metabolizing enzymes. *Cancer Lett* **145**:35–42 (1999).
85. Jacobs BP, Dennehy C, Ramirez G, *et al.* Milk thistle for the treatment of liver disease: a systematic review and meta-analysis. *Am J Med* **113**:506–515 (2002).
86. Rambaldi A, Jacobs BP, Iaquinto G, *et al.* Milk thistle for alcoholic and/or hepatitis B or C virus liver diseases. *Cochrane Database Syst Rev* (2):CD003620 (2005).
87. Hoofnagle JH. Milk thistle and chronic liver disease. *Hepatology* **42**:4 (2005).
88. Scambia G, De Vincenzo R, Ranelletti FO, *et al.* Antiproliferative effect of silybin on gynaecological malignancies: synergism with cisplatin and doxorubicin. *Eur J Cancer* **32A**:877–882 (1996).
89. Zuber R, Modriansky M, Dvorak Z, *et al.* Effect of silybin and its congeners on human liver microsomal cytochrome P450 activities. *Phytother Res* **16**:632–638 (2002).
90. Venkataramanan R, Ramachandran V, Komoroski BJ, *et al.* Milk thistle, a herbal supplement, decreases the activity of CYP3A4 and uridine diphosphoglucuronosyl transferase in human hepatocyte cultures. *Drug Metab Dispos* **28**:1270–1273 (2000).
91. Zhang S, Morris ME. Effects of the flavonoids biochanin A, morin, phloretin, and silymarin on P-glycoprotein-mediated transport. *J Pharmacol Exp Ther* **304**:1258–1267 (2003).
92. Mills E, Wilson K, Clarke M, *et al.* Milk thistle and indinavir: a randomized controlled pharmacokinetics study and meta-analysis. *Eur J Clin Pharmacol* **61**:1–7 (2005).
93. DiCenzo R, Shelton M, Jordan K, *et al.* Coadministration of milk thistle and indinavir in healthy subjects. *Pharmacotherapy* **23**:866–870 (2003).
94. Piscitelli SC, Formentini E, Burstein AH, *et al.* Effect of milk thistle on the pharmacokinetics of indinavir in healthy volunteers. *Pharmacotherapy* **22**:551–556 (2002).
95. Barnes J, Anderson LA, Phillipson JD. St John's wort (Hypericum perforatum L.): a review of its chemistry, pharmacology and clinical properties. *J Pharm Pharmacol* **53**:583–600 (2001).

96. Singer A, Wonnemann M, Muller WE. Hyperforin, a major antidepressant constituent of St. John's Wort, inhibits serotonin uptake by elevating free intracellular Na+1. *J Pharmacol Exp Ther* **290**:1363–1368 (1999).
97. Chen Y, Ferguson SS, Negishi M, *et al.* Induction of human CYP2C9 by rifampicin, hyperforin, and phenobarbital is mediated by the pregnane X receptor. *J Pharmacol Exp Ther* **308**:495–501 (2004).
98. Wenk M, Todesco L, Krahenbuhl S. Effect of St John's wort on the activities of CYP1A2, CYP3A4, CYP2D6, N-acetyltransferase 2, and xanthine oxidase in healthy males and females. *Br J Clin Pharmacol* **57**:495–499 (2004).
99. Hennessy M, Kelleher D, Spiers JP, *et al.* St John's wort increases expression of P-glycoprotein: implications for drug interactions. *Br J Clin Pharmacol* **53**:75–82 (2002).
100. Durr D, Stieger B, Kullak-Ublick GA, *et al.* St John's Wort induces intestinal P-glycoprotein/MDR1 and intestinal and hepatic CYP3A4. *Clin Pharmacol Ther* **68**:598–604 (2000).
101. Mathijssen RH, Verweij J, de Bruijn P, *et al.* Effects of St. John's wort on irinotecan metabolism. *J Natl Cancer Inst* **94**:1247–1249 (2002).
102. Frye RF, Fitzgerald SM, Lagattuta TF, *et al.* Effect of St John's wort on imatinib mesylate pharmacokinetics. *Clin Pharmacol Ther* **76**:323–329 (2004).
103. Mills E, Montori VM, Wu P, *et al.* Interaction of St John's wort with conventional drugs: systematic review of clinical trials. *BMJ* **329**(7456):27–30 (2004).
104. Ruschitzka F, Meier PJ, Turina M, *et al.* Acute heart transplant rejection due to Saint John's wort. *Lancet* **355**(9203):548–549 (2000).
105. Dresser GK, Schwarz UI, Wilkinson GR, *et al.* Coordinate induction of both cytochrome P4503A and MDR1 by St John's wort in healthy subjects. *Clin Pharmacol Ther* **73**:41–50 (2003).
106. Wilt T, Ishani A, Mac Donald R. Serenoa repens for benign prostatic hyperplasia. *Cochrane Database Syst Rev* (3):CD001423 (2002).
107. Marks LS, Hess DL, Dorey FJ, *et al.* Tissue effects of saw palmetto and finasteride: use of biopsy cores for in situ quantification of prostatic androgens. *Urology* **57**:999–1005 (2001).
108. Goldmann WH, Sharma AL, Currier SJ, *et al.* Saw palmetto berry extract inhibits cell growth and Cox-2 expression in prostatic cancer cells. *Cell Biol Int* **25**:1117–1124 (2001).

109. Cheema P, El-Mefty O, Jazieh AR. Intraoperative haemorrhage associated with the use of extract of Saw Palmetto herb: a case report and review of literature. *J Intern Med* **250**:167–169 (2001).
110. Yale SH, Glurich I. Analysis of the inhibitory potential of Ginkgo biloba, Echinacea purpurea, and Serenoa repens on the metabolic activity of cytochrome P450 3A4, 2D6, and 2C9. *J Altern Complement Med* **11**:433–439 (2005).
111. Markowitz JS, Donovan JL, Devane CL, *et al*. Multiple doses of saw palmetto (Serenoa repens) did not alter cytochrome P450 2D6 and 3A4 activity in normal volunteers. *Clin Pharmacol Ther* **74**:536–542 (2003).
112. Strandell J, Neil A, Carlin G. An approach to the *in vitro* evaluation of potential for cytochrome P450 enzyme inhibition from herbals and other natural remedies. *Phytomedicine* **11**:98–104 (2004).
113. Lefebvre T, Foster BC, Drouin CE, *et al*. *In vitro* activity of commercial valerian root extracts against human cytochrome P450 3A4. *J Pharm Pharm Sci* **7**:265–273 (2004).
114. Donovan JL, DeVane CL, Chavin KD, *et al*. Multiple night-time doses of valerian (Valeriana officinalis) had minimal effects on CYP3A4 activity and no effect on CYP2D6 activity in healthy volunteers. *Drug Metab Dispos* **32**:1333–1336 (2004).
115. Das UN. Can essential fatty acids reduce the burden of disease(s)? *Lipids Health Dis* **7**:9 (2008).
116. Morse NL, Clough PM. A meta-analysis of randomized, placebo-controlled clinical trials of Efamol evening primrose oil in atopic eczema. Where do we go from here in light of more recent discoveries? *Curr Pharm Biotechnol* **7**:503–524 (2006).
117. Halat KM, Dennehy CE. Botanicals and dietary supplements in diabetic peripheral neuropathy. *J Am Board Fam Pract* **16**:47–57 (2003).
118. Blommers J, de Lange-De Klerk ES, Kuik DJ, *et al*. Evening primrose oil and fish oil for severe chronic mastalgia: a randomized, double-blind, controlled trial. *Am J Obstet Gynecol* **187**:1389–1394 (2002).
119. van der Merwe CF, Booyens J, Joubert HF, *et al*. The effect of gamma-linolenic acid, an in vitro cytostatic substance contained in evening primrose oil, on primary liver cancer. A double-blind placebo controlled trial. *Prostaglandins Leukot Essent Fatty Acids* **40**:199–202 (1990).

120. Kenny FS, Pinder SE, Ellis IO, *et al*. Gamma linolenic acid with tamoxifen as primary therapy in breast cancer. *Int J Cancer* **85**: 643–648 (2000).
121. Lethaby AE, Brown J, Marjoribanks J, *et al*. Phytoestrogens for vasomotor menopausal symptoms. *Cochrane Database Syst Rev* (4): CD001395 (2007).
122. Bodinet C, Freudenstein J. Influence of marketed herbal menopause preparations on MCF-7 cell proliferation. *Menopause* **11**:281–289 (2004).
123. Harris DM, Besselink E, Henning SM, *et al*. Phytoestrogens induce differential estrogen receptor alpha- or Beta-mediated responses in transfected breast cancer cells. *Exp Biol Med (Maywood)* **230**: 558–568 (2005).
124. Ju YH, Doerge DR, Allred KF, *et al*. Dietary genistein negates the inhibitory effect of tamoxifen on growth of estrogen-dependent human breast cancer (MCF-7) cells implanted in athymic mice. *Cancer Res* **62**:2474–2477 (2002).
125. Gagnier JJ, Chrubasik S, Manheimer E. Harpgophytum procumbens for osteoarthritis and low back pain: a systematic review. *BMC Complement Altern Med* **4**:13 (2004).
126. Fugh-Berman A. Herb-drug interactions. *Lancet* **355**(9198):134–138 (2000).
127. Jepson RG, Craig JC. Cranberries for preventing urinary tract infections. *Cochrane Database Syst Rev* (1):CD001321 (2008).
128. Mohammed Abdul MI, Jiang X, Williams KM, *et al*. Pharmacodynamic interaction of warfarin with cranberry but not with garlic in healthy subjects. *Br J Pharmacol* **154**:1691–1700 (2008).

12

Australian Doctors and Complementary Medicine — Don't Ask, Don't Tell and Don't Know

Lesley Braun

ABSTRACT

Complementary medicines are widely used by Australians in the community and hospital settings. They are often used as adjuncts to conventional medical health-care and not as true alternatives. Unfortunately, patients are not routinely asked about their possible use of complementary medicines by medical practitioners and surveys indicate that patients don't necessarily volunteer the information. If patients are identified as taking complementary medicines, physicians' poor knowledge about commonly used complementary medicines casts doubt on their ability to provide an informed opinion about safe and appropriate use. This gives rise to a 'don't ask, don't tell, don't know' situation that is potentially unsafe and does little to promote patient well-being. Patient expectations, the integration of some complementary therapies into conventional health-care and a growing evidence base compel medical practitioners to increase their knowledge about complementary medicines and have access to quality resources so that they can become providers of accurate, up-to-date information to improve patient outcomes, promote patient safety and encourage evidence-based policy.

Keywords: Australians; Complementary Medicines; Knowledge; Physicians; Safety.

Herbal medicines, nutritional and dietary supplements, also known as complementary medicines (CMs), have become increasingly popular in the US, UK, Canada and Australia, with self-medication making up the majority of use.[1–5]

Although exact usage figures are difficult to ascertain from the literature, it is obvious that a large proportion of Australians have used CM treatments and visited a CM practitioner in the community.[2,6–8] People using CMs in the community do not necessarily cease use before hospital admission and once in hospital; some continue using complementary treatments, but do not discuss their use with hospital staff.[9]

According to one survey, the estimated number of visits to CM practitioners by adult Australians in the 12-month study period (69.2 million) was almost identical to the estimated number of visits to medical practitioners (69.3 million).[2] Over a similar period, data from the Australian Bureau of Statistics show an 80% increase in people employed as CM practitioners in the 10 years to 2006 and the number of people visiting CM practitioners within a 2-week period rose from approximately 500,000 to 750,000.[10]

Taken together, these results indicate that CM makes up a sizeable component of the Australian health-care industry and that many people consulting medical practitioners in the community or in the hospital setting will also be using or considering CM treatments. This can present obvious safety issues, such as drug interactions and adverse reactions, which are unanticipated and potentially left unmanaged. It also presents an opportunity for medical practitioners to learn more about CM and its benefits and risks, and encourage the use of evidence-based CM therapies with proven efficacy and safety.

DEFINING CM — OUTSIDE THE SCOPE OF MEDICAL EDUCATION AND PRACTICE?

Defining the term 'complementary medicine' is a difficult task, as no one definition is globally accepted. In part, this is due to the multi-dimensionality of the concept. In some cases, CM has been defined by what it is not, rather than what it is, and definitions fail to acknowledge the relative nature of the concept. In most cases, the definition is also based on comparisons with orthodox medicine. It is interesting to observe the rapid shift in terminology that has occurred over the last decade in response to the changes in attitudes, perceptions and use of CM.

As early as 1993, an acceptable definition of CM was 'interventions neither taught widely in medical schools nor generally available in US hospitals'.[11] This definition by exclusion was published in the *New England Journal of Medicine* and implied that undergraduate medical education and hospital practice could be used as prime descriptors of what was accepted as medicine and that CM remained outside this domain.

In 1999, another definition surfaced, which described CM as 'a group of therapeutic and diagnostic disciplines that exist largely outside the institutions where conventional health-care is taught and provided'.[12] This definition reinforced the concept that CM remained outside medical education and institutional practice.

Both definitions are clearly outdated today, as the boundary between CM and mainstream medicine has blurred, largely as result of society's medical pluralism. Numerous surveys indicate that Australians use CM together with conventional medical services and pharmaceutical medicines.[7,13–15] It could be said that people have been managing their own health using an integrative medicine approach for years, although it has not always been discussed with their medical practitioner nor is it well informed or well coordinated.

In addition to community use, CM therapies are now available in some US hospitals. A national survey of 5,810 hospitals in the US identified that 15% offered CM services, with nearly half of these centres reporting that patient demand was the primary motivating factor.[16] The CM therapies offered include: acupuncture, massage, mind–body techniques (e.g. meditation), nutritional counselling and herbal medicine counselling. Most started as outpatient clinics either employing CM practitioners, or providing consultative and referral services, and nearly 80% have research ties.

Probably most challenging to practitioners who were supportive of these early definitions is the ongoing popularity of CM and the emergence of evidence to support the use of some complementary therapies. Today, medicine prides itself on using the best available evidence to inform practice. This means that medicine is in a constant state of flux and modifications to education, policy and practice are frequently required to respond to new information, so they remain relevant and help clinicians achieve best practice. So where does this leave CM?

In recent years the concept of 'integrative medicine' has been developed, which is more indicative of the changing usage patterns and attitudes to CM.

INTEGRATIVE MEDICINE — THE NEW CM

The National Centre for Complementary and Alternative Medicine, part of the National Institute of Health, has formulated a definition of integrative medicine: health-care that *'combines mainstream medical therapies and complementary medicine therapies for which there is some high-quality scientific evidence of safety and effectiveness'*.[17]

In 1999, the Consortium of Academic Health Centres for Integrative Medicine was established in the US and now boasts approximately 44 academic centres including: Stanford, Yale, Duke and John Hopkins Universities, Harvard Medical School and the Mayo Clinic and, in Canada, McMaster University.[17] These academic centres for integrative medicine conduct research and provide education about integrative approaches to health-care that are utilised alongside conventional medical care. Meditation, acupuncture, massage therapy and CM treatments are the main focus of interest.

In Australia, a slightly different definition is offered by the Royal Australian College of General Practitioners–Australasian Integrative Medicine Association position paper on CM. It defines integrative medicine as *'the blending of conventional and natural/complementary medicines and/or therapies with the aim of using the most appropriate of either or both modalities to care for the patient as a whole'*.[18]

According to a recent survey, approximately one-third of Australian general practitioners (GPs) consider that they practice integrative medicine/care, which was defined as 'a holistic approach to health care that integrates conventional medical care with complementary therapies'.[19] A national survey of pharmacists revealed that 47% describe their pharmacy practice as integrative, and a further 43% stated that they 'partly' practiced integrative medicines which was defined as recommending CM products together with conventional treatments in practice.[20]

A more meaningful exploration of integrative medicine reveals that it is actually much more than just incorporating CM treatments into a mainstream approach. True integrative medicine depends on its philosophical foundation and patient-centred approach, utilising systems that emphasise healing the person as a whole (bio-psycho-socio-spiritual dimensions) as a primary goal, drawing on both conventional and CM approaches, in the context of a supportive and effective physician–patient relationship. It is compatible with the World Health Organization definition of health that equates health with well-being 'Health is a state of complete physical, mental and social well-being, not merely the absence of disease or infirmity'.[21]

WHAT MEDICAL PRACTITIONERS KNOW AND THINK ABOUT CM

The widespread public use of CM means that medical practitioners are likely to be coming into increasingly frequent contact with people using CM, or asking for advice about CM treatments. As a reflection of this, an increasing number of studies have been conducted to investigate medical physicians' attitudes, perceptions, usage, training, referral and knowledge of CM.

A 1995 meta-analysis of 12 studies found that, in general, medical physicians viewed CM as moderately effective, with younger physicians more optimistic about these therapies than their older counterparts.[22] Zollman & Vickers reported that medical doctors also regard CM as scientifically unproven and are concerned about ensuring the best choice of treatment for their patients.[23] Common concerns include risk of delayed diagnosis, cessation of effective treatments, adverse effects and drug interactions, conflicting advice and treatments. Astin *et al*. analysed data from 19 surveys conducted between 1982 and 1995 of mainstream medical practitioners and identified similar and additional concerns amongst physicians who oppose its use: concerns that CM practitioners do not have sufficient knowledge to diagnose disease, CM lacks evidence of efficacy, and CM may be harmful either directly by inducing adverse events, or indirectly by delaying use of other treatments.[24]

Several studies have evaluated medical practitioners' self-perceived knowledge about CM, but few have determined actual knowledge about CM. Those that have that generally find medical practitioners are unfamiliar with the safety and efficacy evidence regarding popular herbal medicines.[25,26] One survey of emergency medicine and internal medicine physicians, which assessed their familiarity with the topic of herbal toxicities and adverse herb–drug interactions, found that the mean subject score on a knowledge quiz was only slightly higher than would have occurred from random guessing.[26] Neither the amount of the subjects' clinical experience nor their self-assessed familiarity with herbal toxicities and drug interactions correlated significantly with the score on the quiz.

Another survey distributed to physicians, residents and medical students and faculty of the State University of New York, Health Science Center at Brooklyn revealed that they had very little knowledge about popular herbal medicines and their side-effects.[25] The knowledge quiz that was employed asked people to match ten herbs and their side-effects. The highest score achieved was six out of ten correct answers and the average number of correct answers was 1.32, with a standard deviation of 1.39.

Not surprisingly, most GPs in the US have reported wanting more education about CM and many did not feel sufficiently knowledgeable about CM efficacy and safety.[27] Nearly half (46%) of academic physicians at a US institute thought that CM education should be included in the medical curriculum and 82% thought that it should be offered as an elective subject.[28] In the UK, 87% of physicians (excluding GPs) using CM themselves, or as part of their clinical team's commitment, had not had any CM training.[29]

AUSTRALIAN GPs' ATTITUDES AND KNOWLEDGE ABOUT CM

Australian surveys demonstrate that many GPs have an interest in complementary therapies, perceiving several as effective approaches, and that they would welcome further education. Some GPs have trained in various complementary therapies, specifically: meditation (34%), acupuncture (23%), vitamin and mineral therapy (23%), hypnosis (20%), herbal medicine (12%), chiropractic (8%), naturopathy (6%), homeopathy (5%), spiritual healing (5%), osteopathy (4%), aromatherapy (4%) and reflexology (2%).[30] A later survey found that 12% of GPs had a formal diploma or certificate in acupuncture and that more that 20% expressed interest in attending an introductory workshop on meditation, massage, hypnosis, yoga and herbal medicine.[31]

At least 80% of GPs have reported that they knew something about acupuncture, hypnosis, meditation and chiropractic; about half knew something about herbal medicine, naturopathy, and vitamin and mineral therapy, whereas 60%–70% had only heard of osteopathy, homeopathy,' spiritual healing, reflexology and aromatherapy.[30] A survey of oncologists found that they reported knowing most about acupuncture and meditation and least about cellular therapy, magnetotherapy and psychic surgery.[32] Most GPs (93%) agreed that there should be some education on complementary therapies in core medical undergraduate curricula.[30] Importantly, none of these studies evaluated practitioners' actual knowledge about complementary therapies, only their perceptions.

Clearly most GPs are convinced that several complementary therapies are effective, as several surveys indicate that they refer patients for CM services. One survey found that 93% had referred patients at least once in the previous year for CM services, with acupuncture and hypnosis being the most popular referrals.[30] The same year, another study demonstrated that GP referral for CM services in the previous year was far less, with only 66% and 55% having referred patients to non-medically-trained CM practitioners. Acupuncture, hypnotherapy and Feldenkreis were the most popular referral choices.[33] Five years later, the most frequent GP referrals for CM services were reported as massage, meditation, yoga and acupuncture.[31]

More recently, the National Prescribing Service conducted a study of GPs' information needs and knowledge about CM.[19] The sample of 1178 GPs across Australia found that almost all (92%) were of the opinion that they should be regularly asking patients about CMs use; however, only 38% of GPs indicated that they felt confident discussing CM therapy with their patients and only about half incorporated questions about CMs 'always' or 'often' when asking the medication history of a new patient. In terms of actual knowledge, less than half of the GPs surveyed were aware of some of the potential adverse effects and CM–drug interactions of three popular CMs.

HOSPITAL DOCTORS' ATTITUDES AND KNOWLEDGE ABOUT CM

It's not just community-based medical practitioners that have recognised the merits of some CM therapies; multi-centre surveys of medical physicians, surgeons and anaesthetists in hospitals in Victoria indicate that they too consider several complementary therapies as potentially useful.[9] Unfortunately, the surveys also reveal that few hospital doctors are familiar with commonly used CMs and scores on a simple tick-box knowledge quiz indicate that few would be able to provide patients with an evidence-based opinion about their usefulness or safety.

A survey of all hospital doctors and pharmacists at a metropolitan hospital in Melbourne found that, of the 105 doctors who responded (80% response rate), 39% rarely or never asked patients about their possible use of CMs.[9] For the surgeons, 54% stated they didn't have sufficient knowledge to ask patients. When compared with hospital pharmacists at the same site, fewer medical staff were found to be confident asking patients about possible use of CMs, compared will pharmacists.

With regards to knowledge, hospital pharmacists and doctors differed again, with pharmacists attaining significantly higher knowledge scores than medical staff (39% vs. 14%).

Approximately one-third of anaesthetists and 10% of medical physicians stated that their knowledge about CM was derived from post-graduate lectures and one-fifth of both groups undertook self-directed study. Only one surgeon reported attending seminars, receiving undergraduate training or undertaking self-directed learning. When taken as a complete group, 89% thought that it was important for CM information to be included in undergraduate medical education.

ANAESTHETISTS

One multi-centre study of 97 anaesthetists (61% response rate) found that only 26% always or occasionally asked patients about possible use of CM products.[9] If a patient was identified as using CMs only 15% felt confident that they had sufficient knowledge to identify when CM use could adversely affect patient care. As one might expect, those anaesthetists who felt confident discussing CM-related issues were more commonly those who asked patients about use of CMs.

If a complementary therapy can be viewed as 'accepted' if more than eight out of ten medical practitioners think that it's useful, then acupuncture, hypnosis, massage, meditation and yoga have become accepted by anaesthetists and are unlikely to be considered fringe therapies by this group.[9] In particular, acupuncture stood out as being well accepted in terms of effectiveness.

No formal training about CM had been received by 49% of the sample. Post-graduate lectures had been attended by 27%, undergraduate lectures by 9% and specific seminars by 8%, whereas 27% had undertaken self-directed learning. A total of 69% were interested in further training about CMs and therapies, and notably 25% stated that they were interested in practising acupuncture.[9] Despite the high interest in acupuncture, less than 5% have practiced this modality, in comparison with 18% of Australian GPs.[31]

In *Australasian Anaesthesia 2003*, published by the Australian New Zealand College of Anaesthetists, Grauer states that: "for the benefit of the patient and the physician, it is important for anaesthetists to inform themselves about the potential benefits, drug interactions and adverse effects of herbal medications and familiarity with the common 15–20 herbs .. is all that is really required".[34] Unfortunately, a knowledge quiz revealed that few anaesthetists were aware of the safety and efficacy evidence for 11 commonly used CMs, uncovering a significant unmet need for further education. This also confirmed the findings of a smaller survey that demonstrated that anaesthetists have limited knowledge about herbal medicines.[35]

Particularly disturbing were findings that anaesthetists lack confidence in dealing with CMs; lack of knowledge and the generally-held belief that CMs are potentially dangerous did not motivate them to seek information when patient use was identified, and many lacked awareness of common CMs that potentially increase bleeding risk.

Lack of enquiry from medical practitioners about patients' possible use of CMs is not unique to Australia as it has been documented in other parts of the world.[36,37]

POOR INFORMATION SOURCES USED

Australian GPs use a wide range of information resources when seeking answers to clinical questions about CM treatments. A national survey found that trade journals such as *Medical Observer* and *Australian Doctor* (75.5%), *MIMS* (67.8%), Internet searches (66.9%), peer-reviewed medical journals (62.3%) and colleagues (55.2%) were their most popular information sources. In contrast, the same group reported that CM textbooks (67%), specific websites (60%), Internet searches (55%), CM journals (50%) and drug information phone services (50%) were the most useful for this type of information.[19]

These discrepant results suggest that many GPs are not aware of or do not have access to useful CM resources. Further research indicates that most resources used by GPs do not provide quality information about CM.[19] As a result, it would not be surprising for GPs to be frustrated with the quality of information that they find for CM, or to perceive that there is a lack of good-quality CM information.

KNOWLEDGE AND COMMUNICATION ARE VITAL

Good communication between health-care professionals and patients is an essential part of providing safe and effective healthcare. Unfortunately, surveys consistently report that people using CM do not routinely tell their medical practitioner. A review of 12 North American studies indicated that the rate of non-disclosure may be as high as 77%. The main reasons that patients decided not to inform their doctor about CM use were concerns about eliciting a negative response from their doctor, a belief that the practitioner could not provide an informed opinion and they did not need to know, and because the practitioner did not ask.[38]

Consistent with findings from overseas studies,[39–41] patient disclosure about their use of CMs is inconsistent in Australian hospitals. Surveys of surgical inpatients attending two hospitals in Victoria revealed that the main reason that patients did not tell hospital staff about their use of CMs was because they were not asked and/or did not think it relevant, and not because they feared a negative response.[9]

The documented reluctance of patients to disclose their use of CM means that medical practitioners must take an active role in initiating this discussion. This requires them to be familiar with CM treatments and to have the confidence and knowledge to be able to conduct such a discussion in a meaningful manner.

EDUCATION IS URGENTLY REQUIRED

The rationale for developing effective education programmes about CM for medical practitioners includes: the prevalence and growth of CM in Australia, the need to enhance safety of CM use and to avoid or manage drug interactions, the need to enhance communication between health-care providers (medical and CM), the need to enhance communication between medical practitioners and their patients using or considering CM, and the potential for CM education to broaden core competencies, improve health-care coordination and patient outcomes by incorporating safe and effective CM approaches.[42]

Studies conducted with GPs in the US have found that over 80% want more CM education.[43,44] Similar results were obtained for Australian medical practitioners.[9,45] This indicates a general willingness to change the current situation and suggests that an opportunity for further education would be welcomed by many practitioners.

Ideally, education about CM should be incorporated into undergraduate and post-graduate training programmes for doctors. In the US, the integration of CM education into the medical school curriculum has increased substantially over the past decade, with two-thirds of US and Canadian medical schools including either core CM instruction in their curriculum, or CM electives.[46] In Australia, the teaching of CM in medical schools remains highly variable between sites and there are few dedicated CM familiarisation courses in Australian medical schools.[47]

FUTURE IMPLICATIONS FOR MEDICAL PRACTITIONERS

With the increasing use of CM, it is feasible that patients will expect their family physician to be more knowledgeable, skillful, have a balanced approach regarding CM use, and play a more central role in CM referral.[48] To a lesser extent, they may actually expect their family physician to provide CM treatments themselves. Already, some patients believe that the combination of CM and conventional medicine is better than either alone, and health is a combination of physical, emotional, and spiritual well-being, where nutrition and lifestyle play a role in wellness.[49]

Medical practitioners are aware of the need for greater knowledge and more education about CM. In fact, there is a feeling amongst some Australian GPs that a failure to engage adequately with this practice area may render general practice out of touch with a growing number of patients.[19]

Patient expectations, coupled with a growing evidence base, compel medical practitioners to increase their knowledge about CM and become providers of accurate, up-to-date information to improve patient outcomes and promote patient safety and evidence-based policy.

REFERENCES

1. Eisenberg DM, Davis RB, Ettner SL, *et al.* Trends in alternative medicine use in the United States, 1990–1997: results of a follow-up national survey. *JAMA* **280**:1569–1575 (1998).
2. Xue CC, Zhang AL, Lin V, *et al.* Complementary and alternative medicine use in Australia: a national population-based survey. *J Altern Complement Med* **13**:643–650 (2007).
3. Gavin JA, Boon H. CAM in Canada: places, practices, research. *Complement Ther Clin Pract* **11**:21–27 (2005).
4. McFarland B, Bigelow D, Zani B, *et al.* Complementary and alternative medicine use in Canada and the United States. *Am J Public Health* **92**:1616–1618 (2002).

5. Zollman C, Vickers A. ABC of complementary medicine. Users and practitioners of complementary medicine. *BMJ* **319**(7213):836–838 (1999).
6. Kristoffersen S, Atkin P, Shenfield G. Use of alternative medicines on Sydney's North Shore. *Aust J Hosp Pharm* **27**:367–372 Abstract (1997).
7. MacLennan AH, Myers SP, Taylor AW. The continuing use of complementary and alternative medicine in South Australia: costs and beliefs in 2004. *Med J Aust* **184**:27–31 (2004).
8. Wilkinson JM, Simpson MD. High use of complementary therapies in a New South Wales rural community. *Aust J Rural Health* **9**:166–171 (2001).
9. Braun L. *Complementary Medicines in Hospitals — A Focus on Surgical Patients*, RMIT University, Melbourne, Australia (2007).
10. Australian Bureau of Statistics. 4102.0 Australian Social Trends, Australian Bureau of Statistics, 13-7-0009 (2008).
11. Eisenberg DM, Kessler RC, Foster C, *et al.* Unconventional medicine in the United States. Prevalence, costs, and patterns of use. *N Engl J Med* **328**:246–252 (1993).
12. Zollman C, Vickers A. ABC of complementary medicine. Complementary medicine and the patient. *BMJ* **319**(7223):1486–1489 (1999).
13. Girgis A, Adams J, Sibbritt D. The use of complementary and alternative therapies by patients with cancer. *Oncol Res* **15**:281–289 (2005).
14. MacLennan AH, Wilson DH, Taylor AW. The escalating cost and prevalence of alternative medicine. *Prev Med* **35**(2):166–173 (2002).
15. Stankiewicz M, Smith C, Alvino H, *et al.* The use of complementary medicine and therapies by patients attending a reproductive medicine unit in South Australia: a prospective survey. *Aust NZ J Obstet Gynaecol* **47**:145–149 (2007).
16. Ruggie M, Cohen MH. Integrative medicine centers: moving health care in a new direction. *Sem Integr Med* **3**:9–16 (2005).
17. Ruggie M, Cohen MH. Integrative medicine centers: moving health care in a new direction. *Sem Integr Med* **3**:9–16 (2005).
18. Kotsirilos V. GPs' attitudes toward complementary medicine. *Aust Fam Physician* **36**:270–271 (2007).
19. McGuire T, Walters J, Dean A, *et al. Review of the Quality of Complementary Medicines Information Resources: Summary Report*, National Prescribing Service, Sydney (2009).

20. Braun L, Tiralongo E, Wilkinson JM, *et al.* The integration of CMs into pharmacy practice. 1, Australia (2009).
21. Bell IR, Caspi O, Schwartz GE, *et al.* Integrative medicine and systemic outcomes research: issues in the emergence of a new model for primary health care. *Arch Intern Med* **162**:133–140 (2002).
22. Ernst E, Resch KL, White AR. Complementary medicine. What physicians think of it: a meta-analysis. *Arch Intern Med* **155**:2405–2408 (1995).
23. Zollman C, Vickers A. ABC of complementary medicine: complementary medicine and the doctor. *BMJ* **319**(7224):1558–1561 (1999).
24. Astin JA, Marie A, Pelletier KR, *et al.* A review of the incorporation of complementary and alternative medicine by mainstream physicians. *Arch Intern Med* **158**:2303–2310 (1998).
25. Silverstein DD, Spiegel AD. Are physicians aware of the risks of alternative medicine? *J Community Health* **26**:159–174 (2001).
26. Suchard JR, Suchard MA, Steinfeldt JL. Physician knowledge of herbal toxicities and adverse herb-drug interactions. *Eur J Emerg Med* **11**:193–197 (2004).
27. Milden SP, Stokols D. Physicians' attitudes and practices regarding complementary and alternative medicine. *Behav Med* **30**:73–82 (2004).
28. Rosenbaum ME, Nisly NL, Ferguson KJ, *et al.* Academic physicians and complementary and alternative medicine: an institutional survey. *Am J Med Qual* **17**:3–9 (2002).
29. Lewith GT, Hyland M, Gray SF. Attitudes to and use of complementary medicine among physicians in the United Kingdom. *Complement Ther Med* **9**:167–172 (2001).
30. Pirotta MV, Cohen MM, Kotsirilos V, *et al.* Complementary therapies: have they become accepted in general practice? *Med J Aust* **172**:105–109 (2000).
31. Cohen MM, Penman S, Pirotta M, *et al.* The integration of complementary therapies in Australian general practice: results of a national survey. *J Altern Complement Med* **11**:995–1004 (2005).
32. Newell S, Sanson-Fisher RW. Australian oncologists' self-reported knowledge and attitudes about non-traditional therapies used by cancer patients. *Med J Aust* **172**:110–113 (2000).
33. Easthope G, Tranter B, Gill G. General practitioners' attitudes toward complementary therapies. *Soc Sci Med* **51**:1555–1561 (2000).

34. Grauer R. Herbal medicine and perioperative care — an Australian perspective. In Keneally J (ed), *Australasian Anaesthesia 2003*, ANZCAs Alexandria, pp. 105–115 (2003).
35. Lennox PH, Henderson CL. Herbal medicine use is frequent in ambulatory surgery patients in Vancouver Canada. *Can J Anaesth* **50**:21–25 (2003).
36. Kaczorowski J, Patterson C, Arthur H, *et al.* Complementary therapy involvement of physicians: implications for practice and learning. *Complement Ther Med* **10**:134–140 (2002).
37. Giveon SM, Liberman N, Klang S, *et al.* A survey of primary care physicians; perceptions of their patients use of complementary medicine. *Complement Ther Med* **11**:254–260 (2003).
38. Robinson A, McGrail MR. Disclosure of CAM use to medical practitioners: a review of qualitative and quantitative studies. *Complement Ther Med* **12**:90–98 (2004).
39. Adusumilli PS, Ben Porat L, Pereira M, *et al.* The prevalence and predictors of herbal medicine use in surgical patients. *J Am Coll Surg* **198**:583–590 (2004).
40. Kaye AD, Clarke RC, Sabar R, *et al.* Herbal medicines: current trends in anesthesiology practice — a hospital survey. *J Clin Anesth* **12**:468–4719 (2000).
41. Leung JM, Dzankic S, Manku K, *et al.* The prevalence and predictors of the use of alternative medicine in presurgical patients in five California hospitals. *Anesth Analg* **93**:1062–1068 (2001).
42. Gaylord SA, Mann JD. Rationales for CAM education in health professions training programs. *Acad Med* **82**:927–933 (2003).
43. Milden SP, Stokols D. Physicians' attitudes and practices regarding complementary and alternative medicine. *Behav Med* **30**:73–82 (2004).
44. Corbin WL, Shapiro H. Physicians want education about complementary and alternative medicine to enhance communication with their patients. *Arch Intern Med* **162**:1176–1181 (2002).
45. Cohen MM, Penman S, Pirotta M, *et al.* The integration of complementary therapies in Australian general practice: results of a national survey. *J Altern Complement Med* **11**:995–1004 (2005).
46. Torkelson C, Harris I, Kreitzer MJ. Evaluation of a complementary and alternative medicine rotation in medical school. *Altern Ther Health Med* **12**:30–34 (2006).
47. Brooks PM. Undergraduate teaching of complementary medicine. *Med J Aust* **181**:275 (2004).

48. Ben-Arye E, Frenkel M, Klein A, *et al.* Attitudes toward integration of complementary and alternative medicine in primary care: perspectives of patients, physicians and complementary practitioners. *Patient Educ Couns* **70**:395–402 (2008).
49. McCaffrey AM, Pugh GF, O'Connor BB. Understanding patient preference for integrative medical care: results from patient focus groups. *J Gen Intern Med* **22**:1500–1505 (2007).

13

Cancer, Primary Care and Complementary Therapies

Kerryn Phelps

ABSTRACT

General practitioners (GPs) are pivotal to all stages of cancer management. As up to 80% of cancer patients use complementary medicine (CAM), the GP should be well informed about these choices. The demographics of patients most likely to choose complementary therapies are known, they will want to discuss their use with their GP and education programmes are becoming available. Integrative medicine is based in conventional medicine but embraces non-conventional treatments and is practised by 30% of GPs. Interactions between complementary and conventional medicine must be understood. Integrative medicine can be practised by using actual or virtual teams that include a CAM practitioner who is appropriately credentialed. Self-prescribers risk unexpected toxicities or interactions. As they are without subsidies, complementary therapies can be unaffordable for many patients.

Keywords: Complementary; Conventional and Integrative Medicine; General Practitioner.

I have been a general practitioner (GP) for nearly 30 years. I have been a "health consumer" for a lot longer than that. So when I see a patient who has been diagnosed with a serious illness, the first question I ask myself is this: "What treatment(s) would I want and what choices would I make if I were in this patient's situation?" I have seen patients make all sorts of choices. Some of them I have agreed with. Some I have not. I believe the best thing I can do for my patients is to make sure I am as well-informed as I can be about the choices they face, so that I can provide them with the best possible advice about their range of options.

As GPs, we play crucial advocacy and advisory roles on behalf of our patients. The so-called "cancer journey" can be a very bumpy ride and the familiar face of the GP can provide a great sense of security for patients and their families, who are often trying to make sense of the diagnosis and its implications for their lives in the short and long term. The tertiary system can be a confusing maze for people and the GP ideally helps patients navigate their way through it.

General practice is the cornerstone of cancer management. That may seem like a sweeping statement, but consider this. The vast majority of cancer screening is arranged by GPs. This would include performing Pap smears, prostate checks or skin cancer checks, or referring for mammograms or colonoscopies, and so on.

The first presentation of any symptoms of cancer is likely to be to a GP. The initial investigations are ordered by the GP and results come back to the GP, who then needs to co-ordinate referrals for further investigation and treatment.

In an ideal world the specialists working in the tertiary sector will have kept us informed of any results, progress and setbacks experienced by patients. However, more often than not, from our perspective in general practice, once patients are diagnosed with a cancer, they are then seemingly swallowed up into the tertiary sector's cancer services for surgery and/or chemotherapy and/or radiotherapy, and then eventually turn up back in our offices somewhat the worse for wear.

Then it is our task to organise rehabilitation and monitoring of their (hopefully) recovery and remission. Sadly, it is sometimes only palliative and terminal care we are involved with.

Alongside their conventional cancer treatment, we estimate that at least 80% of cancer patients use some form of complementary therapies[1] during the course of their treatments and rehabilitation, almost always as an adjunct[2] to other treatments.

Some of the treatments work, some of them do not. Some are harmless, some have the potential to cause harm. Some interact with conventional treatments, others do not. Some complementary medicine (CAM) practitioners are highly qualified and extremely skilled, some are not. Some GPs have the necessary knowledge and skills to have an informed conversation with patients about the benefits and risks of adjunctive treatments, whereas others do not.

The delivery of so-called "complementary" or adjunctive treatments is almost exclusively in the primary community sector and often disjointed from general practice or oncology services. Yet it is so common that it should now be considered usual practice, if not yet mainstream.

MOTIVATIONS FOR PATIENTS SEEKING COMPLEMENTARY THERAPIES

The types of complementary treatment combinations that patients choose are as varied as are the options available. A significant number of patients who seek complementary therapies or are taking supplements are not disclosing this to their GP or oncologist and you can see that there is a major issue with communication and care co-ordination. This not only has the potential to cause problems for patients, with interactions between herbs or supplements and drug treatments, but patients might also be missing out on the health benefits they might get through detailed professional advice on the best possible combinations and doses.

In general terms, what all of this indicates is a significant level of unmet need within the system, and a disconnect between what patients feel they need and what the conventional system offers or is currently able to deliver.

An Israeli study[3] looked at the reasons patients had recently used complementary therapies. There were demographic characteristics associated with CAM use, which included:

- female sex;
- age 35–59 years;
- more education;

- coming to the hospital by private car;
- advanced disease status;
- having a close friend or a relative with cancer; and
- attending support groups or individual counselling.

After controlling for these factors, significant reasons included:

- needs unmet by conventional medicine;
- helplessness;
- incomplete trust in the doctor;
- changed outlook or beliefs since the diagnosis of cancer; and
- worse emotional and social function indicating considerable distress.

Patients who feel the need to explore CAM treatments in conjunction with their medical treatment will test their doctors for openness and their competence in discussing the options. They will encounter GPs and cancer specialists at various levels of enlightenment when it comes to "CAM" treatments, varying according to the doctor's training or education in aspects of complementary therapies and their general attitude to them. They may be:

- uninformed and openly hostile;
- interested but underinformed; or
- informed and encouraging of safe and effective treatments, while warning appropriately of unsafe or ineffective treatments.

The first group is represented by a blog entry in the Medical Observer[4] newspaper recently.

"Let's call it for what it is, what ever name, be it homeopathy or some other form of "intergrative (sic) *medicine" as the good Professor Phelps calls it, it is all witchcraft. Now I don't have a problem with witchcraft. I am sure it has a place. If the general support of a terminal or chronically ill patient for whom there is no real orthodox effective management then witchcraft is in order. But please let us not, however, pretend it is anything other than witchcraft".*

I doubt if this doctor would be capable of the sort of open, well-informed, evidence-based and non-judgemental conversation that a patient diagnosed with cancer and wanting to explore treatment options would need. Not yet anyway.

Fortunately, the second group is growing ... the doctors who are interested but under-informed. Most GPs are definitely interested in knowing more about CAMs.[5] This move is being supported by the Royal Australian College of General Practitioners which, in conjunction with the Australasian Integrative Medicine Association, is developing a Special Interest Group Chapter with a post-graduate education programme.

In my view, the ideal is the latter model and, as time goes by, the shift is likely to be towards this informed and encouraging type of GP and oncologist because that is what patients are saying they want and need.

QUALITY, SAFETY AND EFFICACY

When it comes to efficacy, we are interested in evidence for the potential for effects on cancer progression and survival and possible symptom relief.

Looking at safety, we want to know about the risk of direct adverse effects and the risk of interactions with conventional treatments.

When it comes to herbs, supplements and other biological agents we also need information about the quality, potency and doses of ingredients.

As evidence becomes stronger and more accessible to practising GPs through our conventional conduits of information, such as our journals and continuing medical education programmes, the consensus will shift on whether a particular therapy may be reasonably recommended, accepted or discouraged on the basis of quality, safety and efficacy.

INTEGRATIVE MEDICINE

"Integrative Medicine is the practice of medicine that reaffirms the importance of the relationship between practitioner and patient, focuses on the whole person, is informed by evidence, and makes use of all appropriate therapeutic approaches, healthcare professionals and disciplines to achieve optimal health and healing".[6]

The widespread interest in the community and the medical profession in complementary therapies has led me and many colleagues inevitably down a professional path of integrative medicine.

What is integrative medicine?

Firstly, what is it NOT? Integrative medicine is not "alternative medicine", and it is not "complementary medicine".

Integrative medicine is founded in high-quality conventional medicine first and foremost. But this philosophy of medicine widens the scope of clinical practice to embrace non-conventional treatments from different philosophies and health-care systems.

There is an out-dated concept of "non-conventional" treatments being synonymous with "unproven", but there is growth in evidence for treatments that fall outside the basic training and expertise of most Western-trained medical practitioners.

There is also an argument I hear often that once something is "proven" then it becomes mainstream and therefore not "complementary". This is also a specious line of reasoning, because there is usually a significant lag time between publication of evidence, mainstream acceptance and adoption of a treatment into commonly accepted therapeutic guidelines.

Integrative medicine has emerged as a response to patients with cancer seeking out adjunctive treatments outside conventional cancer treatment but wanting informed medical advice and supervision of their plan. This is not a small fringe group.

Primary care physicians in Australia and elsewhere are integrating a range of complementary therapies into their practices, either by delivering the therapy themselves, or by referring patients to practitioners (see Table 1).

A recent National Prescribing Service survey[7] indicated that approximately 30% of GPs in Australia identify themselves as practising integrative medicine, by combining orthodox with complementary therapies.

The therapies most integrated tend to be those that the doctor believes are based on good evidence and/or are safest.[8] Four therapies with particularly high referral rates are acupuncture, meditation, hypnosis and chiropractic. Herbal medicine, naturopathy and osteopathy also have referral rates of close to 30%. In terms of doctors practising complementary therapies, vitamin therapy is most frequently used, followed by acupuncture, meditation and hypnosis. Despite the increasing prevalence of use of CAM,

Table 1. Rates of practice and referral for complementary therapies by Australian GPs.

	Ever referred (%)	Have practised (%)
Acupuncture	89.6	19.0
Meditation	79.6	15.3
Hypnosis	81.6	8.7
Chiropractic	68.5	5.0
Herbal medicine	29.1	4.8
Naturopathy	29.7	3.2
Vitamin therapy	16.9	25.1
Homeopathy	19.2	2.5
Osteopathy	29.6	2.8
Aromatherapy	17.5	1.1
Spiritual healing	19.5	2.1
Reflexology	10.1	0.5

Source: Pirotta *et al.*[10]

medical education has been slow to incorporate these topics into the curriculum.[9] A survey of Australian GPs in 2005 found that over 75% of GPs said they formally refer their patients for these therapies.

There is a hierarchy of acceptance when it comes to doctors feeling comfortable with discussing or recommending CAM treatments. Partly this is due to varying levels of knowledge, partly it is due to actual and perceived levels of published evidence and partly it is due to the doctor's perception of safety.

By way of illustration, in my conversations with colleagues there seems to be little discomfort with support groups, sensible dietary modification, massage therapy, yoga, exercise and psychological and mind–body therapies.

Acupuncture in trained hands has increasingly become recognised as a safe and effective treatment for side-effects such as chemotherapy-associated nausea.

Where we start running into difficulty with consensus on safety is in the types, combinations and doses of nutritional supplementation, herbal products and other biological agents.

Australian GPs believe the risks of complementary therapies are seen to mainly arise from incorrect, inadequate or delayed diagnoses and interactions between complementary medications and pharmaceuticals, rather than the specific risks of the therapies themselves.[11]

The best currently available (although not infallible) arbiter is scientific evidence, but cultural and social context is also an important variable.

For example, at least 85% of doctors in Germany also practise herbal medicine.[12] Here, the prevailing consumer culture, the medical establishment and the regulatory framework for the practice of herbal medicine within medical practice are synchronous.

MOTIVATION FOR DOCTORS TO DEVELOP EXPERTISE IN COMPLEMENTARY THERAPIES

No practitioner can expect to be a master of every modality of health-care, but the GP of the future is going to need to be at least familiar with many different kinds of therapies their patients with cancer are interested in or engaging in. There are several reasons for this.

Doctors will have a range of motivations for developing an interest in complementary therapies in cancer treatment.

There is a professional "duty-of-care" imperative. Fully informed consent means just that: patients being fully informed of the potential benefits and risks of the many treatment options available to them. This will usually involve various combinations of surgery, chemotherapy and radiotherapy. But it must also consider mind–body therapies such as mindfulness or counselling, physical therapies like massage, acupuncture, herbal medicine, nutritional medicine and more.

What patients will not accept is blocking of discussion of these other treatments, blanket refusal of support for any kind of adjunctive treatment or demeaning of their choices.

There is definitely a growing acceptance that times are changing. This awareness is driven by the questions our patients ask, observing the outcomes for patients who explore options outside their conventional oncology treatments and messages from the medical and general media.

Professional curiosity is another driver.

One of my patients is a young mother in her thirties who was diagnosed with breast cancer. She undertook surgery, radiotherapy and chemotherapy. She also explored and adopted a range of adjunctive treatments throughout her conventional treatment schedule. I remarked that she seemed to tolerate treatment extremely well compared with some other patients I had observed going through similar treatment without adjunctive therapies.

I asked her for details of what she had been doing.

Her reply was thought-provoking. She said that her oncologist had made a similar remark about how well she seemed to have tolerated the chemotherapy, but that the oncologist had not asked the next question … what did you do differently that other patients did not do?

Another motivator is to expand the medical skill set, so that we have a wider range of effective options for patients. Doctors are required to undergo continuing medical education. If we develop an interest in adjunctive cancer care, then it is possible to increase the medical skill set by focusing education or self-directed learning in that area.

There is a growing awareness of herb–drug, herb–supplement or supplement–drug interactions and doctors who are looking after patients with cancer are acutely aware of the need to ensure not only that adverse interactions are avoided, but that potentially beneficial interactions can be exploited.

It is common to hear of patients with cancer being told to "stop everything" while they are having chemotherapy. This is confusing for patients who are aware that any action they take could have serious, even life-threatening implications, but where there is evidence for a reasonable expectation of benefit then patients are being disadvantaged. An example would be the use of glutamine mouth rinse and swallow to reduce mucosal ulceration from cytotoxic chemotherapy.[13]

A very strong motivator for my medical colleagues, and I include myself in this, is that we hate to look stupid or ill-informed in our patients' eyes or in the opinion of our colleagues. There was a time where doctors who embraced CAM were considered a bit "left-of-centre". However, the pendulum has swung in the other direction, so that doctors who appear to have no knowledge or interest in CAM in the face of substantial evidence are considered "Luddites".

Then there is the substantial group of doctors who change their mode of practice as a result of an epiphany arising from a health crisis in themselves, or a loved one. There is nothing quite like personal experience to focus you on solutions that sit "outside the square".

Motivations for GPs to develop expertise in complementary therapies

- Acknowledgement that times are changing
- Professional curiosity
- Enlarge their skill set
- Desire to avoid adverse reactions and drug interactions
- Response to patient queries and demands
- Not wanting to look stupid or ill-informed
- A personal health-related epiphany

THE PRIMARY CARE TEAM

General practice is central to the primary care landscape in Australia, yet there are many other participants in the delivery of primary health-care to patients in the community, particularly in an integrative model of care.

In an ideal world patients would have advice from their GP, specialists and natural therapies practitioners in a co-ordinated management plan.

The integrative health model can work in a number of ways. The first is the "bolt-on" model, where an allied health practitioner such as a naturopath or traditional Chinese medicine (TCM) practitioner works in a medical clinic with a group of doctors. Alternatively, a doctor with an interest in a form of CAM might be the medical person in a team of allied health practitioners.

The second type of integrative model is a virtual team. This might take the form of a doctor working solo or in a group practice, who finds allied and complementary health practitioners with appropriate qualifications in the general geographic area of their practice, and refers patients depending on their health needs.

In some cases the CAM practitioner knows doctors who are happy to work co-operatively with them and will recommend a doctor to their patients for medical advice. For this model to work safely, active communication between practitioners is a non-negotiable necessity.

A patient-held record is one method I use to encourage information exchange.

This is a file with a copy of all the patient's test results and investigations, and a list of every medication, supplement they are taking and treatment they are undertaking. This file then travels with them to any consultation.

But to be truly integrative, the third and only genuinely "integrated" integrative practice model is one where practitioners of different persuasions work under the same roof with an integrated records system and an active communication between practitioners about a patient's progress and treatments. Each practitioner has access to patient notes about what treatment has been advised by other practitioners, so the risk of interactions or duplication is reduced. A true integrative practice requires the practitioners to meet regularly to discuss the latest research, to discuss treatment protocols and case studies.

One of the impediments for doctors working in multi-disciplinary practices or virtual teams in the community cross-referring with practitioners such as TCM practitioners or naturopaths is the lack of a consistent accreditation process for courses, or registration for practitioners.

With the vicarious liability considerations under medical negligence laws, doctors are understandably cautious about making professional referral to naturopaths without there being a registration process. In 2012 TCM practitioners will undergo national registration. The National Herbalists Association of Australia is also in favour of a national registration process for appropriately qualified practitioners.[14]

SELF-PRESCRIBING

One of the groups I worry about is the uniformed or underinformed self-prescribers. These are the patients who hear from a friend or read in a magazine that there is this wonderful natural product they should be taking and it worked wonders for someone they knew. There is a perception that "natural" products are inherently safe, and with easy accessibility to ingestible herbs and supplements in pharmacies, supermarkets and via the Internet, patients who self-prescribe without sufficient knowledge or advice are taking an unacceptable risk. There is a strong case for the development of accurate consumer medicines information in relation to non-prescription items, particularly with cancer patients, who are likely to be undergoing several types of high-risk medical or surgical interventions.

In many cases, patients are using CAM treatments (either self-prescribed, or recommended by CAM practitioners, or concerned friends and relatives) that may affect their conventional medical treatments.

A recent example is a patient who had developed polycythaemia ... too many red blood cells. Her pharmaceutical treatment was hydroxyurea. But that wasn't working as it should. Her dose was increased. Nothing happened. She came to see me for an opinion. We discovered that she was taking slippery elm to help her bowels. It can, at least theoretically, reduce absorption of some drugs. She had not thought it significant enough to report to her haematologist. We decided she would stop it to see what happened. Her red cells dropped rapidly and her dose of medication had to be halved.

Self-referral to CAM practitioners is also a common activity amongst cancer patients and it can be quite a process just to find out all of the interventions and sources of advice and treatment a patient has actually accessed, when and what effect they had. There is also a risk that a practitioner in a non-registered modality is not qualified to provide the advice they are giving. This is an unacceptable public health risk.

ACCESS AND AFFORDABILITY

One important point about the use of evidence-based CAMs in cancer care in Australia is that, because most therapies are not supported by Medicare or the Pharmaceutical Benefits Scheme, patients need to pay for them out of pocket, with limited subsidies coming from private health insurance for those who have insurance. Even for patients with chronic disease management plans, there is a limit under Medicare of five subsidised visits to allied health practitioners in a whole calendar year. This just doesn't go very far for patients with the acute intense needs of a recent cancer diagnosis.

The tertiary sector is making noises that it is interested in integrative cancer concepts but, realistically, it is unlikely that subsidised services would be available for all patients when and for as long as they needed those services. Some integrative medicine advice or interventions cost little. These might include support groups, meditation classes, walking regularly or adopting sound nutrition. Other interventions are more therapist-intensive or expensive such as massage therapy or herb/vitamin therapies. This leads to an issue of affordability. For some patients, this places complementary therapies in the luxury category.

Additionally, goods and services tax (GST) is applied to CAMs and not to pharmaceutical products. This is another added cost to the consumer. Maybe some of the millions the Federal Government collects in GST from CAMs could be applied to financial support for complementary/integrative medicine research, which is grossly underfunded in comparison with pharmaceutical research.

It is essential that patients with cancer can turn to their GP for information about evidence-based medical and adjunctive treatments that may help relieve their symptoms, prevent or mitigate the side-effects of oncology treatments, accelerate rehabilitation and increase survival.

It is equally important for the GP to act as a filter for patients who are emotionally vulnerable and looking for answers to direct them away from potentially harmful or expensive therapies with little or no likelihood of benefit.

The integrative model of health-care in Australia could be described as a "work in progress". The change has started in the primary care sector and is largely undeveloped in the private and public hospital sectors. Professional education, research, statutory regulation and community awareness must continue to be on the agenda for change.

REFERENCES

1. Boon HS, Olatunde F, Zick SM. Trends in complementary/alternative medicine use by breast cancer survivors: comparing survey data from 1998 and 2005. *BMC Women's Health* 7:4. http://www.biomedcentral.com/1472-6874/7/4 (2007) [Accessed 7 March 2011].
2. Lafferty WE, *et al.* The use of complementary and alternative medical providers by insured cancer patients in Washington State. *Cancer* **100**: 1522–1530 (2004).

3. Paltiel O, *et al*. Determinants of the use of complementary therapies by patients with cancer. *J Clin Oncol* **19**(9):2439–2448 (2001).
4. Simes, Lee. Medical observer blog, 8th March, 3:05pm (2010).
5. Cohen MM, Penman S, Pirotta M, *et al*. The integration of complementary therapies in Australian general practice: results of a national survey. *J Altern Complement Med* **11**(6):995–1004 (2005).
6. Developed and adopted by The Consortium of Academic Centers for Integrative Medicine, May 2004. Edited May 2009 and November 2009.
7. Brown J, Morgan T, Adams J, *et al*. *Complementary Medicines Information Use and Needs of Health Professionals: General Practitioners and Pharmacists*. National Prescribing Service, Sydney (2008). http://www.nps.org.au/research_and_evaluation/research/current_research/complementary_medicines/complementary_medicines_report [Accessed 7 March 2011].
8. Cohen MM, Penman S, Pirotta M, *et al*. The integration of complementary therapies in Australian general practice: results of a national survey. *J Altern Complement Med* **11**(6):995–1004 (2005).
9. Phelps KL, Hassed C. *General Practice: The Integrative Approach*, Elsevier, London (2010).
10. Pirotta MV, Cohen MM, Kotsirilos V, *et al*. Complementary therapies: have they become accepted in general practice? *Med J Aust* **172**(3): 105–109 (2007).
11. Cohen M, *et al*. The integration of complementary therapies in Australian general practice: results of a national survey. *J Altern Complement Med* **11**(6):995–1004 (2005).
12. Himmel W, Schulte M, Kochen M. Complementary medicine: are patients' being met by their general practitioners? *Br J Gen Pract* **43**: 232–235 (1993).
13. Anderson PM, Schroeder G, Skubitz KM. Oral glutamine reduces the duration and severity of stomatitis after cytotoxic cancer chemotherapy. *Cancer* **83**(7):1433–1439 (1998).
14. http://www.nhaa.org.au/index.php?option=com_content&view=article&id=282:national-herbalists-support-call-forregistration&catid=73:media&Itemid=265

14

Complementary and Alternative Medicine: The Perspective of a Medical Oncologist

Ray Lowenthal

ABSTRACT

Complementary and alternative medicine (CAM) treatments for cancer have become popular in recent years, but in general do not have the support of the medical profession. The main reason for this lack of support is the paucity or absence of high-quality scientific evidence of their efficacy and safety. Furthermore, the use of CAM is often based on premises that are open to question, such as: Is everything natural harmless? What constitutes evidence? Can the mind control cancer? Are vitamins risk-free? Can boosting the immune system control cancer? Can dietary changes influence cancer outcome? These and other pertinent issues relating to CAM are explored. Despite caveats that arise from questioning CAM in this way, some forms seem indeed to be safe and may be helpful as complementary, but not as alternative, treatments; they include meditation, massage and music therapy. The development of 'integrated cancer centres' that offer certain types of CAM based on evidence, along with standard scientifically proven anticancer treatments, is welcomed.

Keywords: Complementary and Alternative Medicines; Evidence; Integrated Cancer Centres; Medical Oncologist.

When Woody Allen was asked what he would like people to say at his funeral, he is reported to have quipped 'Look — he's still breathing!'. This remark illustrates the attitude most of us have to death, we'd rather it would go away. Even in today's realistic 'in your face' age, it's understandably difficult for many to accept the inevitable. If we have a potentially fatal illness and someone tells us that it can be cured or alleviated by a simple 'natural' remedy, no wonder such a remedy is often taken up with gusto.

Surveys show that cancer is the most feared disease in our community and for good reason; despite many treatment advances, it has recently overtaken cardiovascular disease as our most common cause of death. (This is partly due to improvements in prevention and treatment of heart disease, and partly the ageing of the population, cancer being predominantly a disease of older persons.) Even for cancers with high cure rates (such as childhood leukaemia, early breast cancer, testicular cancer) there are no guarantees. Furthermore, current societal attitudes that call for health professionals to be completely frank and honest with their patients, mean that cancer patients are clear about the uncertainties of diagnosis, treatment and prognosis. Thus it should come as no surprise that many cancer patients look beyond orthodox ('allopathic') medicine to improve their chances.

My aim in this essay is to look at both sides of the argument concerning the potential value of complementary and alternative medicines (CAMs) from the point of view of a practising medical oncologist who deals every day with patients with cancer in all its stages, from early and newly diagnosed to advanced and life-shortening. I particularly wish to draw attention to certain misconceptions that have favoured CAM's popularity. For convenience I will use the term CAM to embrace a wide range of 'treatments'; not to restrict the term's usage to herbs and medications, but also to include physical measures, such as massage and acupuncture. My aim though is a positive one; not just to give warning about the potential dangers of uninformed use of CAMs, but also to point to those CAMs that may well be helpful and safe.

Table 1. Recommended authoritative websites giving CAM information.

www.mskcc.org/aboutherbs
www.quackwatch.com
www.nccam.nih.gov
www.naturaldatabase.com
www.cancer.org

When writing on this topic two decades ago, it was fair to say that, for most forms of CAM used for cancer, evidence of either benefit or harm was completely lacking. Increasing appreciation of the topic's importance, though, means that now we have scientific assessments of at least some forms of CAM, recognising nonetheless that much more research is needed. The results of the assessments that have been performed are now widely available on the Internet and in publications[1] (see Table 1). For example, we now know that high-dose vitamin C is useless both for prevention and treatment of cancer, but probably reasonably harmless.[2,3] On the other hand, Laetrile (an extract of apricot kernels that has enjoyed considerable support over a long period) is useless as an anticancer treatment and potentially harmful.[4–6] The herb comfrey, once recommended as a CAM for cancer, is itself carcinogenic.[7]

In contrast to these herbs and medicaments which seem not to be useful, research has indicated that meditation or mind–body therapy of various types has potential benefits.[8–10] Medical acupuncture may relieve nausea and vomiting[11] and perhaps vasomotor symptoms of menopause,[12] although such claims are disputed.[13,14] The evidence for use of acupuncture for pain relief also remains uncertain, despite widespread belief in its value.[15]

On the other hand, some folk-remedies may indeed be effective. Recent placebo-controlled studies of ginger have shown some benefit in managing nausea and vomiting of pregnancy and in the post-operative setting.[16,17] Its value for chemotherapy-induced nausea and vomiting is the subject of a large ongoing clinical trial[18] although another recently published trial indicated it was of no additional benefit when given with standard antinausea medication.[19]

IS EVERYTHING NATURAL HARMLESS?

There is much mythology about the supposed harmlessness of 'natural' products. Those who subscribe to this view — and there must be many, judging by the ubiquitousness of the word 'natural' on labels of supermarket products — have not given the matter much thought. Tobacco after all is just as natural as ginger. Alcohol is as natural as cranberry juice. The stalks of the rhubarb plant when cooked make a delicious desserts yet this same plant's leaves are poisonous to humans. It's evident that the one part of the plant is as natural as the other. Indeed, the 'poisonous' properties of some natural products have been harnessed in appropriately small doses as medicinals, a few even as anticancer agents. The Madagascan periwinkle, for example, is the source of chemotherapeutic drugs that have been in use for over 50 years, including vincristine and vinblastine, the so-called vinca alkaloids which have been part of the combination of drugs that has led to the modern-day successes in the cure of childhood leukaemia and other cancers.[20] Other natural sources of drugs used in cancer therapeutics include the yew tree (docetaxel, paclitaxel), opium poppy and mandrake plant (epipodophyllotoxins). It's of interest that the latter was used as a folk-remedy by the American Indians. Some very effective anticancer agents are derived from moulds and again could be described as 'natural' in the same way as penicillin, also derived from a mould, is natural. They include doxorubicin and related drugs that are key ingredients of the chemotherapy cocktails used so successfully to cure certain lymphomas and widely used with considerable efficacy for malignancies of other types, including breast cancer.

Thus, to equate CAM with 'natural' and therefore harmless, and orthodox medical treatments as 'not natural', is disingenuous at best, and misleading or deceptive at worst. Those who promote 'natural' treatments as 'alternatives' to proven medical treatments may be genuinely misled, or in some cases peddlers of fraudulent and bogus treatments. Sadly there are many out there who are amoral in their pursuit of riches and quite happy to take large sums from desperate cancer patients. The advent of the Internet has given these wicked people a new forum, enabling them to reach into the homes of the distressed and despairing. It makes me so sad when a patient tells me they wish to forego a recommended scientifically-proven treatment for some beautiful-sounding quasi-scientific 'natural' baloney.

WHAT IS EVIDENCE?

Elsewhere in this tome is a detailed discussion of the meaning of the word 'evidence' and what constitutes it. A brief description is warranted here, though, as the question of evidence goes to the philosophical heart of the attitude of scientific oncology to CAM. To someone scientifically trained there is basically only one high standard of evidence and that is scientific evidence, by which I mean (to state the blindingly obvious) evidence that is 'evident' — i.e. that can be seen or derived from experiment or observation. In clinical medicine the gold standard is evidence derived from properly constituted clinical trials. Clinical trials are experiments using human subjects that aim to improve treatment outcomes. Because of clinical trials the cure rate for childhood leukaemia has risen from zero 60 years ago to 80% now. How was this achieved? To determine whether one treatment is better or worse than another, the two must be directly compared. This can be done by having two groups of patients that so far as possible are the same (same diagnosis, same stage of disease, same average age, same proportion of men and women, and so on), and giving one group treatment A and the other treatment B. After a certain pre-defined period the outcomes are compared (proportion in remission, proportion still alive, incidence of side-effects and so on). To minimise the risk of bias in the allocation of patients to either group (in other words to ensure that the disease attributes in the two groups are properly balanced), the allocation is done 'randomly' or by chance; these days by computer, but akin to tossing a coin. If feasible, neither the patients nor their doctors should know if they are taking A or B (i.e. the drug administration is 'double blind'). There should be a sufficient number of patients in the trial, so that statistically speaking one can have confidence in the result.

The description in the paragraph above is of a so-called phase III controlled, randomised, blinded trial, the highest standard of evidence. Many, but admittedly not all, of the medications that oncologists recommend have been tested in this way. Very few

CAMs have been. Here's the contrast and the concern. Just because someone has an idea that a certain treatment might be effective doesn't necessarily mean it will be — it must be tested. There are many examples in orthodox cancer treatment where good ideas proved false when tested in this way. A case in point is: the many types of melanoma vaccine that have seemed promising in preliminary studies (phase I and II), but which failed to live up to their promise when adequately tested in phase III trials. Another example relates to the question of dosage; it is often thought that if a certain dose of a drug or a combination is helpful, a bigger dose would be better. Phase III trials have indeed proven this to be the case for some cancers (e.g. relapsed lymphomas), but not so for others (e.g. breast cancer). When confronted with high-quality evidence giving such results, oncologists are prepared to discard an inferior treatment for the better one, or the less toxic. Good evidence like this is largely lacking for CAMs, but where it is available we often find that many CAM practitioners, sadly, are not swayed by the results of modern research. They may prefer to rely on the 'wisdom of the ancients' or some other lesser form of so-called evidence.

THE MIND–BODY RELATIONSHIP

To my mind, one of the most pernicious myths regarding CAM is the idea that one can prevent or control cancer by thought processes — the 'mind–body' concept taken to an unjustified extreme. One only has to see cancer in the operating theatre or in the mortuary to realise how forlorn a hope this is (sadly). Unfortunately this idea leads patients to blame themselves if they cannot maintain a so-called positive attitude, or if the disease recurs (relapses) despite their best mental efforts. Scientifically speaking, whether depressed cancer patients have poorer outcomes remains uncertain and controversial.[21] However, generally speaking, good evidence has been available for some time that various psychological attitudes do not determine or influence cancer outcomes.[22,23] Even more destructive is the idea that bad or negative thoughts have somehow been responsible for bringing on the cancer in the first place — in other words that patients have caused their own cancer by not having sufficient beautiful thoughts, or perhaps through being depressed. Despite a widespread belief that stressful life events subsequently increase the rate of development of cancer, the results of studies are far from conclusive.[21]

This is not in any way to dismiss the concept that psychological support is helpful for patients with a cancer diagnosis. On the contrary, psychological support is extremely useful in aiding patients to get through what is undoubtedly one of the most difficult periods of their lives. The recognition of the importance of such support has spawned a whole field of scientific study, known as psycho-oncology. Most oncology units in Australia either operate support groups themselves, or have links to non-government organisations such as the state and territory Cancer Councils that do so.

A fascinating recent book by American author Barbara Ehrenreich shatters the myth of positive thinking and exposes it as faux science.[24] Ehererreich, already a prominent author, was shaken to investigate the positive-thinking industry when she developed breast cancer herself and was inundated with advice to "smile or die". Her views, that attitude has little if anything to do with subsequent survival after a diagnosis of cancer, are supported by a number of research studies.[22,23]

ARE VITAMINS HARMLESS?

Patients often say regarding one or other proposed CAMs that 'at least it can't do any harm, can it?' I have already dealt with the myth of 'natural' equating to 'harmless'. However, some substances are so widely used and so generally considered harmless that it might seem almost sacrilegious to question their safety. Consider, for example, vitamins. Many in the population take daily vitamin supplements; the proportion in Australia is reckoned to be about 25% and it is even higher in the USA. They do this in the hope or belief that so doing will improve general health and encourage longevity. Cancer patients too hope to improve their general health or perhaps boost their 'immune system'. However, evidence that otherwise healthy persons on a good mixed diet can improve their well-being by taking daily multi-vitamins is sadly lacking. (There may be special circumstances where some vitamin supplements are useful, for example supplementary vitamin D for populations living at high latitudes, where the residents are unlikely to receive adequate sunlight in the winter to convert vitamin D precursors in the skin to the active form.) For cancer patients there is no evidence of benefit from multi-vitamins, and there is more than a hint that high doses of certain vitamins may actually be harmful. In a famous large experiment carried out in Finland, thousands of smokers were randomly allocated to beta-carotene (a form of vitamin A), vitamin E or placebo. The hypothesis was that the vitamins would act as antioxidants and reduce the rate the smokers developed lung cancer. Unexpectedly, not only was the rate of cancer not lower in those receiving the active agents, it was actually higher![25] An analogous lack of benefit and potential harm has been found in similar studies of gastrointestinal cancer[26] — although one large trial from China has shown some potential benefit, when used in a population where nutritional deficiencies were commonly encountered.[27] More recently a large Swedish study found that women taking multi-vitamins were more likely to develop breast cancer than women not taking multi-vitamins.[28] These adverse findings initially startled the researchers. However, ask yourself this: what is the normal role of vitamins? Although the answer of course differs between the various vitamins, as a generalisation one could describe the action of vitamins as to encourage cell growth and division. But isn't this the last thing one would want to do to a cancer? The point is, no treatment can be assumed to be either beneficial or harmless until it is fully tested in a properly controlled, randomised study. Because such trials are generally lacking for CAMs it's on the whole impossible to guarantee that a particular form of CAM is harmless.

THE IMMUNE SYSTEM AND CANCER

What about the immune system? Many patients hope to defeat their cancer by 'boosting the immune system'. So is an inadequate immune system responsible either for causing the cancer or failing to control it? Unfortunately this is another myth that has not stood the test of time. The idea arose during the 1960s and 1970s and was particularly promoted by Australian Nobel laureate Sir Frank Macfarlane Burnet who developed the idea of 'immune surveillance'. The concept was that cancer cells arise constantly but are generally destroyed by an intact immune system before they can take hold. If this theory were true, patients with illnesses that suppress the immune system should have high rates of cancer. In fact it is not so. HIV/AIDS patients, for example, whose immune systems are severely depressed and who, as a consequence, are inundated with life-threatening infections, do not have a greatly increased rate of the *general* run of cancer types. They do, however, get a few special cancers (Kaposi's sarcoma, lymphomas) that are due, or thought to be due, to viral infections.[29]

Thus, 'boosting the immune system' even if it were possible, is unlikely to be helpful in reducing the rate of cancer development or the growth of cancer once it appears. At any rate I know of no way of boosting the immune system generally apart from eating well. Vaccines will of course boost specific immunity against particular organisms (but not general immunity). Vaccines to boost specific anticancer immunity have been widely tested, for no cancer more so than malignant melanoma. Much early promise has not borne fruit when subjected to phase III trials and there is no cancer vaccine in current general use for treatment of established cancers, although trials continue. (I must here make the distinction with cancer prevention, where recent work has clearly shown a significant benefit for papilloma vaccines in the prevention of cervical cancer in women and for the hepatitis B vaccine preventing chronic hepatitis B and liver cancer.)

Indeed, one might even postulate that 'boosting the immune system' could be potentially harmful if it actually worked. Lymphomas, for example, are cancers of lymphocytes, the soldier cells of the immune system. Boosting them might speed the growth of lymphoma, at least in theory. This is another warning that no treatment can be accepted unless it is properly tested.

DIET AND CANCER

Can dietary changes influence cancer outcome? Of all the CAMs, this is the one most commonly followed by cancer patients. The variety of dietary changes recommended is legion. Some changes to diet are almost universally made by newly diagnosed patients, given that the diagnosis of any serious illness prompts most to question how they live their lives. First we should ask whether there is any scientific basis for altering diet when one has a diagnosis of cancer. There is of course good evidence that one's habitual diet can quite strongly influence the risk of development of certain cancers. A diet rich in fruit and vegetables, for instance, is associated with a lower risk of bowel cancer than a diet poor in those items. Vegetarians have lower rates of many cancers than the general population. But that is not to say that once cancer has already developed dietary changes may influence the outcome. There is precious little evidence for that. However, one can hardly argue with the general proposition that a 'healthy' diet is likely to be good for everyone, including those already diagnosed with cancer.

Where one takes issue is with the various fad diets. Amongst those proposed in recent times are veganism, 'white food' diets, diets consisting solely or largely of fruit juices, and diets from which various substances are forbidden, such as mushrooms. Such radical changes in diet run the risks of being unbalanced (lacking in important dietary components such as protein) and of causing weight loss over and above that already caused by the cancer itself. My recommendation is to obtain good advice from a qualified dietician, before embarking on major dietary changes.

EXOTICA

There is a tendency to regard anything that has allegedly come from some exotic far-away place as likely to have magical properties. In this category we have Romanian pills, Mongolian tea, Hungarian 'Avemar', Japanese nutrients, the 'Swiss diet' and Tahitian Noni juice. All of these were amongst the many suggestions made by the general public to the former Premier of Tasmania, Jim Bacon, when in 2004 he announced publicly that he had developed inoperable lung cancer.[30] Often the word is that the inhabitants of such places live uncannily long and healthy lives, the explanation for which is said to be the use of a particular plant or diet. Many such items or dietary components, if not available at the local 'health food store', can no doubt be purchased through the Internet.

Another danger arises in the use of enemas. Their popularity seems based on the concept that cancer is a 'dirty' disease and that one should rid the body of 'toxins', though what these toxins are is rarely stated and never proven. Although an occasional enema may be useful if one is suffering from severe constipation, frequent use of enemas is potentially dangerous, with well-documented risks of infection and disturbances of salt and water balance,[31–33] and of no proven benefit in the treatment of cancer.

CONCLUSION

For those contemplating CAM treatments as complements to the recommendations of their medical practitioners, I strongly advise not only discussing this with the relevant specialists and general practitioners, but also consulting one or more of a multitude of authoritative books and websites (see Table 1). There one can find scientifically based information, so far as it exists, on hundreds of CAMs.

THE FUTURE

What should be the approach of the oncology community to CAMs? Recognising that many patients understandably are interested in pursuing CAM of one form or another, the concept of 'integrative oncology' has arisen. As discussed elsewhere in this book, integrative oncology strives to make certain 'complementary' treatments available to cancer patients, along with the orthodox, in the one institution. The CAMs that are acceptable are those for which at least some evidence of benefit exists, and which are unlikely to be harmful. One of the best known of such services has been set up by Dr Barrie Cassileth at the famous New York hospital, the Memorial Sloan-Kettering Cancer Center. Her philosophy provides access to qualified masseurs, exercise classes, medical acupuncture, dietary advice and psychological support amongst other services, but no herbs outside clinical trials.[34] In this regard her Department of Integrative Oncology has a keen interest in traditional Chinese medicine and conducts formal randomised studies of Chinese herbal remedies, as well as of acupuncture and other complementary treatments.[35] In Australia Dr David Joske has set up a similar service at the Sir Charles Gairdner Cancer Centre in Perth, W.A., with a rule of 'no ingestibles' (see Chapter 9 in this book).[36] Music therapy is available at the Peter MacCallum Cancer

Institute, Melbourne.[37] Taking the scientific approach to CAM has proved popular with patients and with funding bodies.

So, where to from here? It's evident that many cancer patients are not satisfied with orthodox medical treatments alone. For many reasons, including the need many patients feel to be actively involved in their treatment rather than merely passive recipients, they are looking at CAMs of various forms. The physicians and nurses of our oncology departments must accommodate these desires, but in ways that encourage use of proven treatments with minimal potential for harm. The drive to establish 'integrated oncology centres' with strict adherence to scientific evidence is one way this can be achieved.

REFERENCES

1. Ernst E. A primer of complementary and alternative medicine commonly used by cancer patients. *Med J Aust* **174**:88–92 (2001).
2. Gaziano JM, Glynn RJ, Christen WG, *et al.* Vitamins E and C in the prevention of prostate and total cancer in men: the Physicians' Health Study II randomized controlled trial. *JAMA* **301**:52–62 (2009).
3. Creagan ET, Moertel CG, O'Fallon JR, *et al.* Failure of high-dose vitamin C (ascorbic acid) therapy to benefit patients with advanced cancer. A controlled trial. *N Engl J Med* **301**:687–690 (1979).
4. Ellison NM, Byar DP, Newell GR. Special report on Laetrile: the NCI Laetrile Review. Results of the National Cancer Institute's retrospective Laetrile analysis. *N Engl J Med* **299**:549–552 (1978).
5. Milazzo S, Lejeune S, Ernst E. Laetrile for cancer: a systematic review of the clinical evidence. *Support Care Cancer* **15**:583–595 (2007).
6. Unproven methods of cancer management. Laetrile. *CA Cancer J Clin* **41**:187–192 (1991).
7. Hirono I, Mori H, Haga M. Carcinogenic activity of Symphytum officinale. *J Natl Cancer Inst* **61**:865–869 (1978).
8. Nidich SI, Fields JZ, Rainforth MV, *et al.* A randomized controlled trial of the effects of transcendental meditation on quality of life in older breast cancer patients. *Integr Cancer Ther* **8**:228–234 (2009).
9. Speca M, Carlson LE, Goodey E, *et al.* A randomized, wait-list controlled clinical trial: the effect of a mindfulness meditation-based stress reduction program on mood and symptoms of stress in cancer outpatients. *Psychosom Med* **62**:613–622 (2000).

10. Targ EF, Levine EG. The efficacy of a mind-body-spirit group for women with breast cancer: a randomized controlled trial. *Gen Hosp Psychiatry* **24**: 238–248 (2002).
11. Shen J, Wenger N, Glaspy J, *et al.* Electroacupuncture for control of myeloablative chemotherapy-induced emesis: a randomized controlled trial. *JAMA* **284**:2755–2761 (2000).
12. Walker EM, Rodriguez AI, Kohn B, *et al.* Acupuncture versus venlafaxine for the management of vasomotor symptoms in patients with hormone receptor-positive breast cancer: a randomized controlled trial. *J Clin Oncol* **28**:634–640 (2010).
13. Lee MS, Kim KH, Choi SM, *et al.* Acupuncture for treating hot flashes in breast cancer patients: a systematic review. *Breast Cancer Res Treat* **115**:497–503 (2009).
14. Lee MS, Shin BC, Ernst E. Acupuncture for treating menopausal hot flushes: a systematic review. *Climacteric* **12**:16–25 (2009).
15. Ernst E. Integrated medicine revisited. *Focus Altern Complement Therap* **13**:73–74 (2008).
16. Ozgoli G, Goli M, Simbar M. Effects of ginger capsules on pregnancy, nausea, and vomiting. *J Altern Complement Med* **15**: 243–246 (2009).
17. Nanthakomon T, Pongrojpaw D. The efficacy of ginger in prevention of postoperative nausea and vomiting after major gynecologic surgery. *J Med Assoc Thai* **89**(suppl 4):S130–S136 (2006).
18. Hickok JT, Roscoe JA, Morrow GR, *et al.* A phase II/III randomized, placebo-controlled, double-blind clinical trial of ginger (Zingiber officinale) for nausea caused by chemotherapy for cancer: a currently accruing URCC CCOP cancer control study. *Support Cancer Ther* **4**: 247–250 (2007).
19. Zick SM, Ruffin MT, Lee J, *et al.* Phase II trial of encapsulated ginger as a treatment for chemotherapy-induced nausea and vomiting. *Support Care Cancer* **17**:563–572 (2009).
20. Seam P, Janik JE, Longo DL, *et al.* Role of chemotherapy in Hodgkin's lymphoma. *Cancer J* **15**:150–154 (2009).
21. Fox BH. The role of psychological factors in cancer incidence and prognosis. *Oncology* (*Williston Park*) **9**:245–253; discussion 253–256 (1995).
22. Cassileth BR, Lusk EJ, Miller DS, *et al.* Psychosocial correlates of survival in advanced malignant disease? *N Engl J Med* **312**:1551–1555 (1985).
23. Cassileth BR, Walsh WP, Lusk EJ. Psychosocial correlates of cancer survival: a subsequent report 3 to 8 years after cancer diagnosis. *J Clin Oncol* **6**:1753–1759 (1988).

24. Ehrenreich B. *Smile or Die: How Positive Thinking Fooled America and the World*, Granta Books, London (2010).
25. The Alpha-Tocopherol Beta Carotene Cancer Prevention Study Group. The effect of vitamin E and beta carotene on the incidence of lung cancer and other cancers in male smokers. *N Engl J Med* **330**: 1029–1035 (1994).
26. Bjelakovic G, Nikolova D, Simonetti RG, *et al*. Systematic review: primary and secondary prevention of gastrointestinal cancers with antioxidant supplements. *Aliment Pharmacol Ther* **28**:689–703 (2008).
27. Qiao YL, Dawsey SM, Kamangar F, *et al*. Total and cancer mortality after supplementation with vitamins and minerals: follow-up of the Linxian General Population Nutrition Intervention Trial. *J Natl Cancer Inst* **101**:507–518 (2009).
28. Larsson SC, Akesson A, Bergkvist L, *et al*. Multivitamin use and breast cancer incidence in a prospective cohort of Swedish women. *Am J Clin Nutr* **91**:1268–1272 (2010).
29. Caceres W, Cruz-Amy M, Diaz-Melendez V. AIDS-related malignancies: revisited. *P R Health Sci J* **29**:70–75 (2010).
30. Lowenthal RM. Public illness: how the community recommended complementary and alternative medicine for a prominent politician with cancer. *Med J Aust* **183**:576–579 (2005).
31. Eisele JW, Reay DT. Deaths related to coffee enemas. *JAMA* **244**: 1608–1609 (1980).
32. Keum B, Jeen YT, Park SC, *et al*. Proctocolitis caused by coffee enemas. [letter]. *Am J Gastroenterol* **105**:229–230 (2010).
33. Margolin KA, Green MR. Polymicrobial enteric septicemia from coffee enemas. *West J Med* **140**:460 (1984).
34. Wesa K, Gubili J, Cassileth B. Integrative oncology: complementary therapies for cancer survivors. *Hematol Oncol Clin North Am* **22**: 343–353, viii (2008).
35. Cassileth BR, Rizvi N, Deng G, *et al*. Safety and pharmacokinetic trial of docetaxel plus an Astragalus-based herbal formula for non-small cell lung cancer patients. *Cancer Chemother Pharmacol* **65**:67–71 (2009).
36. Joske DJ, Rao A, Kristjanson L. Critical review of complementary therapies in haemato-oncology. *Intern Med J* **36**:579–586 (2006).
37. O'Callaghan C. Clinical issues: music therapy in an adult cancer inpatient treatment setting. *J Soc Integr Oncol* **4**:57–61 (2006).

15

Complementary and Alternative (or Unproven) Therapies: Perspectives of a Surgeon

Tom Reeve

ABSTRACT

Currently more than half of all Australians use one or more complementary and alternative medicine (CAM) items year by year. At the same time, sales of CAM materials exceed the cost of conventional medicines. So well established is CAM culture, that it is time medical and surgical professionals took more notice of its extensive role in medical care. At this time there is strong interest in having all conventional medical activity evidence-based. Although CAM has been the subject of many randomised controlled trials, and some have been accepted into integrated practice, most lack the rigour in their development to render them acceptable in day-to-day practice. It is suggested that, in spite of these observations, the continued pressure arising from increasing usage of CAM therapies, together with patients' expectations, should be given greater consideration in integration with conventional medicine, while ensuring maintenance of standards. This will not be an easy task. As CAM usage may result in deleterious outcomes, it is imperative that its use is elicited when taking a patient's history. The consultation should be conducted in an atmosphere of mutual respect and understanding, to discourage the patient from withholding information. When possible, clinicians should be apprised of CAM agents that have adverse interactions with standard treatments and of CAM agents that may be dangerous. As CAM is now clearly established in the public domain, it would seem that appropriate steps should be taken to educate clinicians in CAM, by introducing changes to undergraduate curricula. Such a move may lead to better understanding at medical and community level.

Keywords: CAM; Conventional Medicine; Evidence-Based; Patient Expectation; Randomised Controlled Trials.

INTRODUCTION

Medicine is the art or science of restoring or preserving health using drugs or curative substances. **Surgery** has the same aim using manual or instrumental interventions, as well as curative substances to achieve a satisfactory outcome.

Although science-based medical care has developed as the predominant basis of medical practice in Western countries, a fair number of the population bypass it and seek their treatment in non-conventional areas known broadly as complementary and alternative medicine (CAM).[1]

The Clinical Oncological Society of Australia defines the broad spectrum of activities covered by the acronym CAM as follows.[2]

Complementary Medicine

Complementary medicine is any intervention that is used in conjunction with standard Western health practices.

Integrative Medicine

Integrative medicine is an approach that combines the best of standard Western health interventions and the best of complementary medicines, based on evidence.[3] For example, the use of a course of relaxation therapy in conjunction with standard radiotherapy or chemotherapy regimens to reduce stress or anxiety.

Alternative Medicine

Alternative medicine is an intervention or product offered as an alternative treatment to standard Western medical practices.

This chapter does not address Chinese herbal or traditional medicine, or ayurvedic medicine.

COMMENTS ON DEFINITIONS

Most alternative therapies fall into the unproven category (scientifically) and it would seem that their continued use relies on the many years of perception of "satisfactory" if unsubstantiated clinical outcomes.

Complementary therapies are advertised and available for the broadest possible spectrum of diseases; however, cancer treatments have been studied more intensively in recent times. The Benheim Integrated Medicine Center, Memorial Sloan-Kettering[4,5] Cancer Center (MSKCC) provides comprehensive information in the field and its website provides an excellent insight into herbs and integrated medicine. Other high-quality units continue to be developed and their websites are valuable sources of current information.[6–8] These units are unique in that they study their therapeutic programmes at a high level, to explore and evaluate the capacity of specific complementary therapies to modify the symptomatology that can be associated with cancer or with cancer treatments. The MSKCC unit also investigates botanicals for any potential antitumour effects. This unit provides evidence-based information on complementary, but not alternative, therapies.[4]

BACKGROUND FROM THE DIFFIDENT SURGEON

Surgeons are consulted in reference to a wide range of diseases in the course of their training and practice and have learned to manage clinical problems effectively by surgical means. However, in some conditions, conventional treatments do not always provide the high-level outcome that patients, their families and their community expect of modern medical care. When anticipated outcomes are not met, patients and carers give consideration to other approaches to management, particularly if the patient has malignant disease and indeed any disease.[9] This, as might be expected, is a time when complementary and alternative therapies may be chosen as a form of treatment. Complementary therapies have been carefully evaluated, some by randomised trials, and found to make a contribution to the quality of life (QoL) both physically and emotionally for many patients with serious illness.[3,4] These therapies appear, on available evidence, to be a safer approach than unproven remedies if an approach other than conventional therapy is being sought.[10] The careful interpolation of complementary therapy in a sound medical environment with ethical approval, appropriate investigation and careful monitoring of outcomes is an accepted way to probe the further promotion of such activity. Such an approach could assist the move towards further integrating conventional and complementary therapies.[10,11]

Although the availability of a wide range of options can be readily "surfed" on the Internet or obtained by exploring community channels, e.g. a best friend or well-meaning neighbour, some caution needs to be observed in both taking and implementing the advice so received.[10,11] This level of uncertainty does not exist in relation to conventional practice, where professionals are rigorously tested and approved, as are the materials they use. The Australian Government has examined complementary medicine activity under the Therapeutic Goods Act of 1989, which came into effect in 1991, and the "Complementary Medicine in the Australian Health System" Report of 2003.[12] In this report there is significant encouragement for innovation, research and data protection. The aim was to meet the standards of the National Medicines Policy.[13]

This report notes that, at the time of its publication, Australian production of CAM was AUD $800 million and 20% of this was exported; "more and more Australians are looking for positive health and lifestyle outcomes through the use of complementary medicine". The majority of alternative (complementary) medicine users appear to be doing so, not so much as a result of being dissatisfied with conventional medicine, but more because they find these health-care alternatives to be more congruent with their own values, beliefs and philosophical orientation towards health and life.[12,14]

Astin *et al.*,[15] in a review of incorporation of CAM into mainstream practice, demonstrated that doctors were referring patients for CAM or incorporating better known forms of CAM into their practice. In this study, data varied somewhat, based on regional differences and some complicating problems. The authors asked for national representative samples and more vigorous surveys to improve studies. They also promoted outcome studies to give physicians direction and help them make decisions based on evidence, "rather than regional economic and cultural norms".

WHAT HAPPENED BEFORE CAM MOVED UPMARKET?

As a surgeon who trained in the 1950s and 1960s, I was fully aware that medical practice that strayed outside the boundaries of "convention" was alternative, the term "complementary" was only aborning and "integrated" medicine was yet to be conceived. At that time neither alternative nor complementary medicine received anything other than short shrift by practising surgeons. In my experience the treatments were regarded with suspicion as being fraudulent, mindless or dangerous and to be avoided. The use of unproven drugs, herbs or untested mechanical interference in patient care was essentially forbidden in teaching hospitals, and numbers of doctors claimed that many results were based on myth. Although these censorious restrictions were nominally in place, there was a very wide range of "patent" medicines as they were called, used in the community; many were frequently given iconic status and often entitled "Grandma's remedies".

Although a number have disappeared over the years many remain, and of course there are others stepping up to take their place.

When I was child in the 1920s–1930s, Grandma still had significant control over "inner health". This could be achieved most effectively by weekly cleansing of the bowel, usually every Friday night. Senna leaves were infused overnight and the tea resulting from the infusion was dispensed to the family. It was an effective inner cleanser. It is noted that the same term is being promoted on television now, with a new agent.

Castor oil in a threatening blue bottle was a worthy weekly substitute for senna tea. It was usually cunningly camouflaged with orange juice — senna was preferred by the children in my neighbourhood. The blue castor oil bottles are now valued antiques.

There was also an extensive range of ointments, liniments, rubs, potions, embrocations, salves, pills, tablets, draughts, tonics and poultices. Almost all were directed at a specific ailment although some had a more "shotgun" application.

WHY EMBRACE CAM — ARE PATIENTS DRIVING THE AGENDA?

That CAM therapies have become more widely used over the last 30 years is a given. Australia has not been immune to this activity, as noted by the Expert Committee on Complementary Medicine in the Australian Health System;[12] repeat studies in South Australia demonstrate continuing use of complementary, alternative and integrated medicine by over 50% (52.2%) of the population in 2004.[16]

Wider use of CAM combined with its social and political acceptance in the USA has led the Institute of Medicine to further its work on understanding the science and the implications for policy.[17] Cohen[18] states that up to 60% of Australians use/take natural supplements and may continue their use in hospital without advising their doctor. He also noted that, in a Victorian study, 40% of patients "undergoing cardiac surgery were also taking undisclosed supplements", clearly continuance of this dangerous practice should be addressed.

These various changes in community attitudes have been in part in response to long-standing clinical practices — a number of which persist. When I commenced clinical practice in academic outpatients, consultation was relatively swift, the surgeon conveyed the decisions regarding treatment to the patient and the patient was expected to go to the desk and follow admission and other instructions. No questions or refusals were expected. Refusal might mean transfer to another surgeon and/or facility and there was only limited discussion. The process was directive and frequently paternalistic.

Over time, however, community changes have occurred; there is more education about medical matters and radio doctors, television programmes and health advocate organisations have informed patients of their right to ask questions, express options and exercise choice.

These healthy directions have continued and, although the outcomes are yet to be optimised, the long term will see an increase in meaningful discussion between doctor (surgeon) and patient, almost certainly to their mutual advantage.

This trend towards a greater voice for the patient will almost certainly apply to CAM and, in fact in the USA, some health maintenance organisations have already embraced CAM, because of market demand, but the insurance industry is concerned at the lack of information on sound research into clinical activity, cost-effectiveness and standards of practice with CAM.[19]

A study by Barnes *et al.*[20] suggested that the more accepted forms of CAM are those used by individuals as part of self-care, in the belief that combined with conventional care it would help in their case (54.9%) and further noted that more than half (50.1%) used CAM as an interesting treatment to try, rather than because of cost-efficiency.

It would seem that CAM of itself is seen as a conglomerate of natural agents that are perceived as being natural and safer than conventional medicine. In a series of studies the appeal of CAM and the positive perception of CAM, as against conventional treatment, was the perception of the latter's invasiveness;[21] surgeons therefore do not appear welcome. This view is held even though the effectiveness of many CAM programmes has not been determined. When effective elements of CAM are elucidated, those that are distinguishable from conventional therapy and validated might well be incorporated into integrated interventions. There have also been some other views and studies to be noted.[9]

In general, the reasons for the use of CAM therapies are "locked in" to communal views that various agents can "tone up" various body systems and maintain general health.

A recent systematic review in cancer patients,[22] largely mirrored the above reasons, with a perceived beneficial response from CAM (38%), a desire for control (17%), a last resort when conventional therapy had failed (10%), and looking for and finding hope (10%). It also supported decision-seeking strategies in determining the use of CAM.

It has been suggested that chronic symptoms, and the perception that side-effects of conventional therapy may be difficult to tolerate (e.g. alopecia), can have effects on patient choice. It is also likely that limitations of conventional treatments may lead to choice of CAM therapies.[9]

The fall in CAM dollar expenditure in Australia between 2000 and 2004 from $2.3 billion to $1.8 billion may relate to the expense involved and non-government funding.[12]

The mindset of CAM users may also differ from those following a conventional path, with a prospective study involving 111 men[23] noting that those who used CAM were more uncertain about prostate cancer and its treatment than those men who chose to follow the conventional therapy route.

Overall, it would seem that the public has made its own decisions regarding CAM use and these decisions will need to be acknowledged and respected if a full understanding and benefit flowing from CAMs is to be achieved.

WHAT CAM THERAPIES ARE AVAILABLE?

When CAM is reviewed one encounters a significant number of modalities, which do not have any unifying bonds, but provide a broad menu from which to choose.

This list is not exhaustive.[24]

- Acupuncture
- Massage and touch therapies, including therapeutic touch
- Religion — spiritual healing
- Relaxation
- Osteopathy
- Colour therapy
- Psychological therapy including: counselling, group therapy, meditation
- Herbal medicine
- Iridology
- Chiropractic
- Reflexology
- Hypnosis
- Dietary modifications, vitamins — nutritional therapy
- Homeopathy
- Meditation

- Systematic administration of plant and animal extracts, hormonal materials
- Non-invasive medical devices or procedures
- Aroma therapy
- Yoga

This daunting list of therapies for patients requires great care in selection if initiated by the surgeon or a diplomatic non-confronting and non-judgemental and understanding discussion if initiated by the patient.[25,26]

It is a sound maxim that conventional health professionals should not participate in the use of unproven treatments, but be able and prepared to be supportive of the patient using them, provided there is no clear contraindication to the CAM employed.

So the surgeon is ducking and weaving to be supportive and yet avoids using any of the specific CAM approaches.

However, as already stated, there are strong movements being established to oversee the introduction or quasi-cooperation of medical professionals in complementary or integrative medicine.[9]

HOW ARE THESE MODALITIES RELATED TO SURGICAL PRACTICE? WHAT SPECIAL SKILLS ARE RELATED TO THEIR UTILITY FOR THE SURGEON?

The increase in the use of CAMs seems to have become a clear part of the community's behaviour in terms of their attitude towards consulting conventional medical professionals. In a recent report,[27] on a study of more than 1,000 people who accessed health information online in the previous month (November 2009), it was found that 27% (Australians) of those "searching for information felt they were able to diagnose and treat an ailment without the need of a health professional". If this trend continues, it is clear that self-diagnosis will encourage a wider use of unproven therapies and this should alert doctors to be more careful in relation to history-taking, to ensure that they elucidate a patient's current medications, and ensure that they volunteer any treatment that is self-chosen.[25,26]

These findings further alerted me to take more interest in complementary therapy, both in the sense of monitoring any patient's self-therapy and ensuring its safety, as well as being as certain as possible that I was not causing an egregious error by overlooking possible dangerous and/or adverse drug interactions.

It has become an imperative to review the Cochrane Library[28] from time to time, to alert oneself to new reviews and randomised controlled trials (RCTs) on CAM. Unfortunately, to date only 20% of 67 RCTs currently recorded yielded a finding that would suggest further trials to allow integration to be explored, but the activity recorded by the Library helps surgeons (and others) to keep abreast of positive and negative findings.

There is now a clear message for all health professionals in clinical practice that they should question all patients carefully as to their current medications and, if using CAMs, whether they are proposing to introduce other items into their medication menu. The consultation and direct questioning should be carried out in a professional manner, being supportive, understanding and non-judgemental. Such an approach should help to avoid possible adverse interactions with CAM agents.[25,26]

FREQUENTLY ASKED QUESTIONS IN RELATION TO CAM[4]

Is There an Evidence Base to Support CAM Clinical Practice?

The use of CAM agents arises from community interest and their ultimate application is based on community choice. The controls that oversee their development and manufacture are neither as rigorous nor stringent as those that the Government applies to conventional medicine. It would appear that purchasers/users are interested in outcomes to a greater degree than levels of evidence.[21]

Although CAM is apparently becoming more popular with clinicians[9,14,15,21,22] there does not appear to have been a parallel level of activity to improve the evidence base for CAM. This is probably due to factors that do not normally impinge on conventional practice. From a methodological point of view, CAMs differ from conventional treatment in that, rather than choosing from a conventional reservoir of appropriate therapies, CAMs are based on individually tailored treatment, so making the patient a special individualised recipient of the proposed therapy ("a cornerstone of the CAM philosophy").[10,29] This fact limits CAM practitioners, if not precluding them, from freely adopting RCTs, at best there is limited cooperation. A major factor has been that, where evidence-based CAM treatments have been reviewed, the situations where CAMs have been promoted have often been found to be based on poor-quality RCTs. Frequently these have almost passed their use by date. For example, 30 similar observations were made in relation to clinical trials of meditation in health-care where, in spite of "statistically significant improvement in the methodological quality over time calls are being made to vigorously improve trial design, execution and reporting of results".[30] There remain recruitment difficulties and difficulties in deciding on appropriate end-points, outcome measures and placebos.[29]

Clinicians have been reticent in resolving many of these issues in spite of a continuous rise in patient interest and, in view of this, there is an increasing need for integration of CAM and conventional medical systems, so meeting patient's expectations and needs, while meeting accepted standards of scientifically-based medical practice.[28]

These activities will need funding, establishing research priorities and obtaining ethics approval[29] and ensuring the same rigorous safety checks required of conventional comparators.

The perceptions that relate to evidence and research are difficult in Australia where, increasingly, doctors are trained to determine the evidentiary level and quality of either individual or multiple treatments when applied clinically.

However, there are always doctors who are scanning the horizon for new cutting-edge treatments that can be integrated into medical care.

There is not the same alacrity in Australia to embrace some of the CAM treatments that are being promoted in other countries; these may involve approaches that go significantly beyond mainstream in surgery, radiotherapy, chemotherapy and hormone therapy and, as might be expected, focus on malignant disease.

An article in the *Weekend Australian*[31] was written to coincide with turning the first sod of a new comprehensive Cancer Centre in Sydney that follows the advocacy of the late Christopher O'Brien, a surgeon who promoted comprehensive (including integrated) cancer care. The author of the article reports on a wide range of treatments reported in December at a meeting of cancer specialists in Vienna. A major report addresses laser needles (red, green, blue and infrared) in a range of cancers, muscle and bone, and also addresses migraine problems. The laser needles are inserted intravenously through a cannula without causing pain or discomfort. The effects vary according to wavelength and are said to boost the immune system, some promote healing and some assist in breaking down cancer cells and make treatments like chemotherapy more effective. These needles are to commence trials in the USA very soon.

The trace mineral selenium is reported in one study to reduce diarrhoea after radiotherapy for endometrial cancer.

A great number of these studies are being undertaken in Europe and have not yet reached Australia, where there is understandable caution about using treatments not comprehensively trialled.

However, Australian medical groups, including oncologists, have been busy establishing priorities to guide their research efforts. Funding to continue investigation of therapies and high-quality products and services will be provided by the National Institute of Complementary Medicine (NICM),[7] National Health and Medical Research Council (NHMRC) and New South Wales (NSW) Cancer Institute.[30]

It is clearly important that local research efforts be maintained and that embracing overseas advances, when they meet appropriate standards, should continue, and the process should be expedited wherever possible: *"integrated cancer services will not achieve their potential in Australia if they simply bring existing treatments under one roof"* (Avni Sali, President, Australian Integrative Medicine Association).[30]

Evidentiary endorsement can follow appropriate local research and assist in furthering the processes that can integrate conventional and CAM therapies.

Attitude of Medical (Surgical) Practitioners to CAM and Education Directed to CAM

It would appear that doctors feel they are not required to have a wide knowledge of non-traditional or CAM medicines, although, many doctors voluntarily educate themselves in the CAM area and are pleased to discuss this with their patients.[9,32]

An important exploratory qualitative study was evaluated in the UK.[32] The study was small, directed towards general practice with eight participants and the ninth was a homeopathic doctor working in a hospital and receiving referrals from primary care. The study revealed, as perhaps might be expected, that CAM has champions, doubters and detractors.

The author of the study was able to identify five key themes that appear important if CAM is to receive a wider welcome.

1. A doctor's personal experience of conventional medicine and CAM shapes their views on CAM.
2. Doctor/patient communication about CAM and patient disclosure.
3. Perceptions of the evidence base for CAM.
4. Doctor's information and training needs regarding CAM.
5. The role of CAM within the National Health Service (NHS).

Doctors also wish for wider identification and separation of CAM that is effective or ineffective, and those that may be acceptable to doctors. It was not seen that CAM would be widely incorporated into the NHS, yet some elements may indeed improve the overall quality of case management and enrich the doctor's practice.

It appears clear for this and other studies that medical graduates should have an understanding and working knowledge of CAM if they are to "mix" it with their patients. Some universities have already recognised the level of the population use of CAM and included its study in their curriculum, and this move should probably be expanded to others, but would require significant awareness not to introduce overload for undergraduates.[33]

CAM and the Consultation

In the past, when a surgeon took a patient's history, it was usual to ask about other forms of medication or treatment; the question was posed expecting answers that related to conventional therapies. Until recent times, unless the surgeon had some inkling, non-conventional therapies, where involved, would not have been considered worthy of a question.[25]

Times are changing and reports indicate that more than 50% of Australians are, or have been, associated with a CAM therapy.[16] This in effect means that half our consultations may be with people using CAM. Some of these people may be using CAMs that may interact adversely with conventional therapy. It is imperative that the surgeon elucidates if such is the case and achieve sound risk management. Although patients are seeking to discuss CAM more openly, surgeons should become more aware of the role of CAM in surgical practice.[25,26]

In summary, it is clearly important that each and every patient be carefully questioned about current medication or proposed usage of CAM treatments in a supportive, understanding and non-judgemental way, to protect patients' self-esteem and be more likely to avoid adverse reactions between conventional and CAM therapies.[25,26]

Can CAM be Useful in Surgical Practice (The Surgeon's Acceptance of CAM)?

With a clear rise in the interest in and use of CAM, whether for specific reasons as noted by Verhoef[22] in patients with cancer or just as something else to try,[20,34] whatever the motivation, the increase in numbers of users is impressive and it becomes prescient to recognise the "desire" of the patient to use CAM. Whatever its source, this desire may be valuable to both patient and surgeon in setting boundaries for their further interaction.

The consultation is usually the initial phase of interaction and represents a special occasion for both surgeon and patient. It is a time when both evaluate each other and its success is important to smoothly progress a treatment programme. On welcoming the patient to the office a number of critical events follow, the surgeon notes the patient's mien, the strength of the handshake, the degree of physical activity and ease in rising from a chair and progressing across a room and the bodily appearance. These attributes are quickly assessed by both participants and special features may well lead to special questions and observations during the consultation. This is a time when the level of comfort developed between the participants will determine the ease and veracity of information that flows between them.

Where will Complementary Medicine Fit in This Scenario?

Initially, when the history-taking is occurring, is the time to determine whether CAM is being utilised by the patient, the reason for it and its extent and safety should be determined. Towards the end of the consultation it may be appropriate to make a series of suggestions, some of which will relate to CAM.[25,26]

The time has probably arrived when the bias inherited and entertained by the surgeon should be radically reviewed and the optimal information available melded into surgical practice.

What Complementary Items could have a Significant Place in Surgical Practice?

The elements that contribute to bodily habitus are frequently discussed at consultation and whereas past discussions may have been a little cursory e.g. diet — "push yourself away from the table three times a day before meals", they can be modified to a fuller discussion or lead to referral for more advice.

Diet

Diet is one of the most discussed items in daily conversation. It is a feature of hundreds of articles by supposed gurus in print and visual media — all with a new message. In a country where quality and enjoyable food abounds, common sense in relation to food intake is sometimes lacking. Surgeons prefer their patients to be optimally nourished if possible when evaluating them for diagnosis or operation. A "healthy diet" underpins a healthy body and supports it through its daily vicissitudes or injury and infection. The NHMRC has issued dietary guidelines for Australian adults.[35] The guidelines promote a variety of vegetables, fruits and wholegrain cereals, while advising a reduction in intake and careful watch on the levels of salt, sugar and saturated fats and alcohol that the adult ingests. Promotion of the guidelines is sound health policy in which the surgeon can take a part.

In a community advised to avoid excessive exposure to sunlight, the advice does not mean its complete exclusion. Exposure of the face and arms for 10 minutes a day in summer before 10:00 am or after 2:00 pm (this holds in winter in the north, but 30–50 minutes is required in the south) is required to maintain adequate vitamin D levels.[36]

Extra vitamins and minerals are unnecessary, and excess of either may be counterproductive to health,[37] however, appropriate fibre intake is a valuable part of diet and is to be encouraged.

Promoting special aspects of food for prevention of illness is also on the horizon — lycopene (the antioxidant compound that gives tomatoes their colour) and other carotenoid-bearing foods, although not as good a source of antioxidants as tomatoes, may prove useful in a preventive diet. Cooked tomatoes, sauce and paste contain more lycopene than fresh tomatoes. The US Food and Drug Administration in an evidence-based review found "limited evidence to support an association between tomato consumption and reduced risks of prostate, ovarian, gastric and pancreatic cancers".[38] For defined clinical problems, e.g. diabetes, referral for medical and/or diabetic or nutritional advice would be appropriate. Using diet in a clinical sense is different to using diet to maintain health.

Over and above all this discussion, a timely and friendly warning to keep weight in check and avoid obesity and its possible unpleasant outcomes would be a worthwhile path to walk.

Physical Activity and Exercise

It would seem responsible for surgeons to ensure that patients meet exercise requirements to assist in burning up the kilojoules/calories they ingest. Although a 30 minute walk three times a week is suggested, it might be better to suggest that it be additional to the usual routine and this would rarely be excessive. Aerobic exercises produce a response of "huff and puff" but can help further in maintaining cardiovascular health.

When muscle mass decreases, resistance exercise under expert supervision may help to maintain or increase muscle mass and strengthen bones, of particular value in the diminishing strength associated with ageing, particularly when induced by androgen withdrawal.[39]

Relaxation

Many times a consultation with a surgeon can leave a patient feeling "uptight" and the surgeon should attempt to defuse that state — a careful question and answer may go a long way towards achieving this. Advice could extend to:

- "taking a walk when tense". Move outside yourself and notice other things and people;
- find "relaxed surroundings and just muse or read"; and
- take a tepid bath and "blank out" until the feeling of relaxation takes over.

These approaches and advice are simple and may help resolve feelings of tension.[1]

Meditation

This is another approach to equanimity. Randomised trials have been done in this area,[1,40] but have not been of sufficient rigour to verify strong benefit. It has long been held — by the Dalai Lama and others — that meditation has a direct effect on the brain.[41] Laboratory work suggests that currently used technology may be able to produce some of the beneficial effects of meditation. This area is perhaps outside the scope of the surgeon, impacting as it may on religious and other beliefs and lifestyles.

A recommendation to review information on Google may provide new and enriching insights for the patient, provided they are viewed in perspective and checked when next seeing the doctor.

Music

Music has been studied in depth as an aid to patient well-being in terminal cancer in a rigorous RCT evaluating the QOL, which demonstrated a higher level for those receiving music therapy. This increased over time on receiving more music therapy and control patients experienced a lower QOL. There were no significant differences between groups in relation to physical function or length of life.[42]

As a surgeon I have found these findings to be anecdotally confirmed on a number of occasions and endorse its use.

Recently, a note from a surgeon friend undergoing radio-chemotherapy for head and neck cancer indicated that he found music a valuable adjunct to his care. "Let us be thankful for the amazing qualities of music! Every day that I was covered with the mask and bolted to the table for radiation treatments, I choreographed the session to the music of a selected composer. I was able to transport my mind to a better and more peaceful place of this and to be less fearful and more relaxed in a stressful situation. Behold, the power of song". (J. Bonnet, personal communication.) These few words further empower the employment of this modality.

Acupuncture

It is usual to advise acupuncture to reduce post-operative and post-chemotherapy nausea or vomiting and it can prove useful for post-operative pain, particularly as outlined by the NIH Consensus statement.[43]

Counselling and Support Groups

The surgeon may find that the opportunity for patients to discuss their problems with others who have similar problems is of significance and worthy of referral as appropriate. In Australia, support groups have developed a significant reputation in the field of prostate cancer.[1,44] They can help to reduce stress and improve self-esteem.

Massage

Massage and touch therapies have been used by people undergoing cancer treatment and reports suggest that they can reduce "pain, fatigue, anxiety, depression and nausea".[1] The reduction of discomfort is noted in practice.

Herbal Medicine

Surgeons should not endorse herbal medicine,[4] but accept its use by patients if there is no distinct contradiction to or distinctly adverse drug interaction from the treatment, e.g. homeopathy and other surgeons may use these rather than those outlined here.[4] Recent studies have shown that, with a number of herbal remedies "there may be a risk of heavy metal content", there should be an awareness that herbal remedies may play a part in cases with unexpected surgical or medical outcomes. The extent of the role of cases presenting to forensic facilities is yet, however, to be determined".[45]

CONCLUSION

CAM is now very much with us.

To use CAM would appear to give people more options in relation to their medical care and allow a greater measure of self-esteem to emerge.

Commencing undergraduate programmes in relation to CAM would appear a worthwhile initiative.[33]

Surgeons would be wise to have a sensitive antenna to their patients' wishes and work with them towards more satisfactory outcomes from their mutual interaction.

REFERENCES

1. Cancer Council NSW. *Understanding Complementary Therapies (A Guide for People with Cancer, their Families and Friends)* (2008).
2. http://www.cosa.org.au/members-area/group-resources/cit/cit-toolkit/definitions.html [Accessed 10 January 2011].
3. Institute of Medicine. *Complementary and Alternative Medicine in the United States*, National Academic Press, Washington (2005).
4. Memorial Sloan-Kettering Cancer Center. *About Herbs — Botanicals and Other Products: About This Resource.* http://www.mskcc.org/mskcc/print60783.cfm [Accessed 1 January 2010].
5. Memorial Sloan-Kettering Cancer Center. *What is the Difference Between Integrative, Complementary and Alternative Medicine?* http://www.mkscc.org/mkscc/print1985cfm [Accessed 31 December 2009].

6. NCCAM — National Centre for Complementary and Alternative Medicine. Washington DC. http://www.nccam.nih.gov or www.google.com.au/(search nccam) [Accessed 1 January 2010].
7. National Institute of Clinical Medicine (NICM). Canberra, ACT, Australia. http://www.nicm.edu.au [Accessed 1 January 2010].
8. MD Anderson Cancer Center HT. *Cancer Treatment and Cancer Research*. www.mdanderson.org.au [Accessed 1 January 2010).
9. Lewith G, Robinson N. Complementary and alternative medicine: what the public want and how it may be delivered safely and effectively. *J R Soc Med* **102**:411–414 (2009).
10. Rosenthal DS, Dean-Clower E. Integrative medicine in hematology/oncology: benefits, ethical considerations, and controversies. *Hematol Am Soc Hematol Educ Program* 491–497 (2005).
11. Ernst E, Cassileth BR. How useful are unconventional cancer treatments? *Eur J Cancer* **35**:1608–1613 (1999).
12. *Complementary Medicine in the Australian Health System*. 2003. http://www.tga.au/docs/pdf/cmreportspdf [Accessed 11 December 2009].
13. National Medicines Policy. http://www.health.gov.au/internet/main/publishingusf/content/National+Medicines+Policy [Accessed 26 January 2010].
14. Astin JA. Why patients use alternative medicine: results of a national study. *JAMA* **279**:1548–1553 (1998).
15. Astin JA, Marie A, Pelletier KR, *et al*. A review of the incorporation of complementary and alternative medicine by mainstream physicians. *Arch Intern Med* **158**:2303–2310 (1998).
16. MacLennan AH, Myers SP, Taylor AW. The continuing use of complementary and alternative medicine in South Australia: costs and beliefs in 2004. *Med J Aust* **184**:27–31 (2006).
17. *Use of Complementary and Alternative Medicine (CAM) by the American Public*. http://www.iom.edu/cn/Activities/PublicHealth/CAM use apx [Accessed 12 October 2009].
18. Cohen M. *Call for Hospitals to Acknowledge Alternative Medicine*. http//www.medicalsearch.com.au/News/call-for-hospitals-to-acknowledge-alternative-medicine. [Accessed 11 November 2009].
19. Pelletier KR, Astin JA. Integration and reimbursement of complementary and alternative medicine by managed care and insurance providers: 2000 update and cohort analysis. *Altern Ther Health Med* **8**:38–39 (2002).

20. Barnes PM, Powell-Griner E, McFann K, *et al.* Complementary and alternative medicine use among adults: United States, 2002. *Adv Data* **343**:1–19 (2004).
21. Swartzman LC, Harshman RA, Burkell J, *et al.* What accounts for the appeal of complementary/alternative medicine, and what makes complementary/alternative medicine "alternative"? *Med Decis Making* **22**:431–450 (2002).
22. Verhoef MJ, Balneaves LG, Boon HS, *et al.* Reasons for and characteristics associated with complementary and alternative medicine use among adult cancer patients: a systematic review. *Integr Cancer Ther* **4**:274–286 (2005).
23. Steginga SK, Occhipinti S, Gardiner RA, *et al.* A prospective study of the use of alternative therapies by men with localized prostate cancer. *Patient Educ Couns* **55**:70–77 (2004).
24. Zollman C, Vickers A. ABC of complementary medicine: complementary medicine and the doctor. *BMJ* **319**(7224):1558–1561 (1999).
25. Schofield P, Diggens J, Charleson C, *et al.* Effectively discussing complementary and alternative medicine in a conventional oncology setting: communication recommendations for clinicians. *Patient Educ Couns* **79**:143–151 (2010).
26. Eisenberg DM, Kessler RC, Foster C, *et al.* Unconventional medicine in the United States. Prevalence, costs, and patterns of use. *N Engl J Med* **328**:246–252 (1993).
27. Lunn S. *The Australian*, Dec. 7, p. 3 (2009).
28. Cochrane Library — search complementary medicine. http://www.interscience.wiley.intersciencewiley.com/cochrane-search-fs.html?mode=start search&product-windows internet explorer [Accessed 7 January 2009].
29. Robotin MC, Penman AG. Integrating complementary therapies into mainstream cancer care: which way forward? *Med J Aust* **185**:377–379 (2006).
30. Clarke SJ. *Complementary Therapies.* Incite — Journal of the Cancer Institute of NSW. http://wwwincite.cancerinstitute.org.au/articles/complementary_therapies.apsx [Accessed 20 October 2009].
31. *Tess Livingstone. A Suitable Case for Treatment. Weekend Australian*, Jan. 9, p. 2 *Inquirer* (2010).
32. Maha N, Shaw A. Academic doctors' views of complementary and alternative medicine (CAM) and its role within the NHS: an exploratory qualitative study. *BMC Complement Altern Med* **7**:17 (2007).

33. Rampes H, Sharples F, Maragh S, *et al.* Introducing complementary medicine into the medical curriculum. *J R Soc Med* **90**:19–22 (1997).
34. Nahin RL, Pontzer CH, Chesney MA. Racing toward the integration of complementary and alternative medicine: a marathon or a sprint? *Health Aff (Millwood)* **24**:991–993 (2005).
35. National Health and Medical Research Council. *Dietary Guidelines for Australian Adults*, NHMRC, Canberra, ACT (2003).
36. Berwick M, Kesler D. Ultraviolet radiation exposure, vitamin D, and cancer. *Photochem Photobiol* **81**:1261–1266 (2005).
37. Ma RW, Chapman K. A systematic review of the effect of diet in prostate cancer prevention and treatment. *J Hum Nutr Diet* **22**(3):187–199 (2009).
38. Kavanaugh CJ, Trumbo PR, Ellwood KC. The U.S. Food and Drug Administration's evidence-based review for qualified health claims: tomatoes, lycopene, and cancer. *J Natl Cancer Inst* **99**:1074–1085 (2007).
39. Galvao DA, Taaffe DR, Spry N, *et al.* Combined resistance and aerobic exercise program reverses muscle loss in men undergoing androgen suppression therapy for prostate cancer without bone metastases: a randomized controlled trial. *J Clin Oncol* **28**:340–347 (2010).
40. Ospina MB, Bond K, Karkhaneh M *et al.* Clinical trials of meditation practices in health care: characteristics and quality. *J Altern Complement Med* **14**:1199–1213 (2008).
41. Reiner PB. Meditation on demand. *Sci Am Mind*, 65–67 (2009).
42. Hilliard RE. The effects of music therapy on the quality and length of life of people diagnosed with terminal cancer. *J Music Ther* **40**:113–137 (2003).
43. NIH Consensus Statement. *Acupuncture*. Nov. 3–5, **15**(5):1–34 (1997).
44. *Support groups*. http//en wikipedia org/wiki/support_groups [Accessed 6 February 2010].
45. Byard RW. A review of the potential forensic significance of traditional herbal medicines. *J Forensic Sci* **55**:89–92 (2010).

16

Mind over Medicine: Revealing the Blame Game

Deborah Gray

"I knew I'd be fine. The goddess always looks after me".

My beautiful friend's big brown eyes were luminescent as she spoke about her sunset run along the black volcanic-rock beaches of Maui.

"I was swimming as the sun started to go down over the horizon. The transparent turquoise ocean lapping around me was suddenly lashed with bolts of orange and pink sun-fire".

"I felt that sunset go through me like lightning. I just felt so alive and full of energy that I started to run like a wild colt out of the water and along the beach. For a split second I worried about tripping over the rocks or cutting my toes on the shards of lava stone. But I was so connected, so 'one' with that fiery Hawaiian goddess energy that I just knew I could run as fast and as freely as I wanted to anywhere over the old volcanic sea bed in complete safety — and be completely fine".

And of course she was. Athena Starwoman looked more than fine. Perched on a chaise lounge in a private suite of her favourite Sydney hotel — the Ritz Carlton, Double Bay. Nearing 58 years of age, her dainty feet, and long brown legs still incredibly slim and shapely, were living proof. Her toes perfectly manicured — not a blemish or molten rock scar in sight.

I loved Athena's stories about her adventures around the world — she was always regaling us, her friends, with exciting and funny stories about her trips to far-away and exotic locations. She travelled constantly to remote retreats. A lot of them health resorts. They were places to go chill out from all her hard work as a writer and speaker. Not just as a vacation, but these trips were also a precious time to maintain her deeply spiritual and almost palpable connection to Mother Earth. Nature. Or as she liked to call it 'The Goddess'.

LIVING THE BIG TRUTH

Athena's very magical connection to all the natural environments, including the stars, the oceans and the earth, her innate spirituality along with her thirst for knowledge were incredibly inspirational to everyone she came in contact with. Not only because she wrote so successfully about these very things, but because this was really who she was — inside and out. It was simply her complete reason to exit. It was her Big Truth. And for as long as I knew her, she tried to live that truth every day of her life.

Her belief in herself and her ability to get things done through her own ideas and her own power of mind were also an integral part of her daily life and work.

Well why not? That's how Athena Starwoman had built a small empire. Her unwavering focus to follow her own ideas and dreams — step by mindful step. From modest beginnings in the 1960s as an unknown Melbourne schoolgirl — all the way to worldwide renown and material success. She did this virtually unaided and under her own steam from day one. She was not often encouraged or helped in her endeavours either — in fact up until the 1980s when Athena became a worldwide force in astrology, she always joked that she was often dismissed back in the early days as nothing more than a mild eccentric. Always being advised by various friends and work colleagues to 'tone it down' a bit. Now in the first decade of the new millennium most of those old colleagues were vying along with scores of others for media interviews as well as offering her more writing projects than she could deal with.

When she changed her name from Susan to 'Athena' in the early 1970s it was basically because she thought the name Athena would be a better fit for her work as an astrologer. She later added the last name Starwoman after a meditation training session in the USA with a Native American medicine-man who kept calling her 'that star woman' (because he couldn't remember her real name). When she arrived back in Sydney from California a year or two later, most of her friends and family thought she had made a big mistake by taking on such a hippy dippy moniker, but again she proved everyone wrong. And with her sheer force of personality and media savvy, turned her flower-power pseudonym into a clever branding coup.

Athena Starwoman. A name that was unforgettable. Entirely suited to what she did and who she was. Nowadays famous people all over the world use their names as their marketing brands which they zealously protect and market across all forms of media, fashion and products. And like Athena, if the name they were born with doesn't suit that process, they simply choose one that does.

Athena was ahead of her time in many ways, but she was lucky enough to live through to an age where not only her name but her ideas and writings were eventually celebrated and respected as being among the world's best of her genre. She wrote the book (both metaphorically and literally) and much more, on not only astrology but also power of mind techniques. Even the way she lived, her own dream-come-true materially yet spiritually aware lifestyle was inspirational to hundreds of thousands of people around the world.

If anyone on this earth could create a successful life, build wealth and spiritual awareness, find a perfect soulmate and stave off the threat of physical ailments using the power of positive thinking — it would certainly be Athena.

To most of us four out of five of these achievements would be miraculous. But sitting with her that sunny afternoon back in December 2003 neither of us entertained any kind of thought that she would not live long enough to experience another Australian summer.

SOULMATE SISTERS

November 2004, I sat in the downstairs room of Athena's split-level apartment on Queensland's sparkling Gold Coast, having a light dinner and watching reruns of *'Sex in the City'* together with my best friend. Her big brown eyes were just as luminous and the soul within them just as inspirational as ever, but now her already slim body was so fragile she looked like a tiny porcelain figurine. So delicate and fragile that I had to be careful not to touch her hand too firmly in fear of breaking it. We laughed and cried together all that night watching episode after episode of Carrie and her irreplaceable girlfriends going through their trials and tribulations in New York City. It was so special to each of us because Athena and I had both lived in New York at around the same time for years in the 1980s and 1990s. We'd already been good friends in Australia, but our chance meeting up on the other side of the world in Manhattan had led to us to becoming even closer. We had so much in common, both expat Australians living in the Big Apple, both with a similar approach to life and its mysteries. Eventually we started developing projects together and became co-authors on several self-help and magical books, many of which became international best-sellers, translated into 11 different languages around the world. Living in New York had bonded us as sister soulmates forever.

Now we were both back in Australia. I was back living in Sydney with my partner and she was here in what was meant to be her ultimate dream apartment overlooking the Pacific Ocean.

Knowing Athena as such a unique personality, combined with her phenomenal success as a manifester of dreams, it was always destined that this experience, along with every other time spent with her, could never be anything but memorable to the nth degree.

THE GODDESS VERSUS THE GP

Athena's personal choice of breast cancer treatment was to opt for 'non' treatment. Think it away. Build on self-belief. And absolutely stay away from standard medicines at all costs. When she had told me some months before that she had felt a lump and suspected very strongly it could be breast cancer, no amount of talking her into trying more than herbal detoxes and meditations could convince her to change her mind. It was unthinkable to me that she was so sure that standard medicine would be 'worse than the disease'. I was to find out later that this is not so uncommon a reaction amongst women as one would think.

I'll never know if Athena had chosen standard medical treatment in time, whether she would have been cured of breast cancer, or if it would have helped her live any longer than she did.

But what I'm sure of is that when it was much too late to switch over to a medical treatment, when the cancer had spread too far to operate or treat with chemotherapy or radiation, it was then that Athena deeply regretted that she had not given herself at least a chance to try another form of treatment.

As we talked about her life and her illness during her last weeks she told me that she had lived her whole life with the belief that the mind can do anything, achieve anything, including heal the body. And the proof was that it worked so brilliantly, for the majority of her life, time after time.

"Deborah, I've created a great life for myself using those exact techniques. I really was convinced that if anyone could do it — it would be me. That I should have been able to use my training, and my positive mindset to kick this disease. But what I didn't do is give myself a 'plan B', an alternative just in case I needed to. I regret that now and I think it was a mistake that has cost me precious time before I was ready to go. My body is fading in front of my eyes and it's too late for me to try anything else to give it a fighting chance. What I wanted least of all, I still have to do and there's nothing I can do to avoid it. No matter how strong my mind and will still is, I now couldn't bear living without constant drugs — if only to dull the unbearable pain. I never wanted any kind of drugs or strong medicines. I never wanted to even take an aspirin for a headache. And the terrible irony is that the pain is so bad that I cannot bear one more moment awake without this morphine drip. My spirit and mind are still as strong as ever, but I was a fool to think I have total control over my whole body. I know now that no one does".

All the psychic therapists, the natural healers she had seen, all the websites, videos and self-help books she'd read over those past months. Thousands of words and vision from 'masters' of the alternative health industry giving support to the millions on how cancer can and should be treated completely drug-free. But we both came to see a very big flaw in that advice and a very important point of simple logic. No-one either I or Athena had met in the alternative health industry had spoken clearly and openly on the fact that, if one does get to the terminal stage, some kind of drugs and medical intervention, at the very least powerful opiates, are unavoidable.

It's totally inhuman and a 'dark-ages' mentality to think any human would have to live through that kind of pain unaided by the best of modern medical care. Athena and I talked at length about the fact that if eventually a person is going to have to put some very powerful (and to some minds toxic) drugs through their body anyway — then many would probably take a second look at the possibility of other kinds of powerful (and in some minds toxic) drugs or other standard medical interventions beforehand. Drugs and treatments that don't just dull the pain but might just give you some months or even years to live. Or at the very least the knowledge you'd called on everything available. And possibly give you some precious grains of hope for a bit more time.

It's natural for human beings to fight for life. Even for just another six days, weeks or months, most people would give anything.

No human being should be left to handle this level of pain without some kind of medical help — and the worst part is that when Athena was finally willing to get help from a cancer specialist, all they could truthfully offer her at that stage were painkillers. "I don't know if it would have really helped" she told me, "but at least I'd know that I had tried everything I could".

It was too late for Athena to try out any kind of equally powerful drugs or medical treatment that might just give her some more time. But she wanted to assure me that if she had her time back again then she would try out everything under the Sun and the Stars. Including surgery, chemotherapy, radiation and all the others while still keeping helpful natural techniques and of course plenty of mind power and positive thinking.

To date there is not a lot in the new-age industry and not much either from standard medical practitioners on how to combine these two fields of health therapies. Athena blamed herself for not knowing where to research more and hated having to wonder what would have happened if she'd known that in the end medical help and actual hospitalisation is more than likely unavoidable, especially during the palliative care stage. When patients truly need and deserve round-the-clock medical care and nursing. But she had the courage to admit to those regrets and disappointment, she did that with her usual strength of mind and character then she eventually put even those last regrets aside to try and move on to face her passing with some peace of mind and connection with her spirit.

THE SECRET BLAME GAME

She had suspected for a long time that she might be fighting cancer, but only sought medical help when she was knocked off her feet by the pain. By then, once she'd been told by the doctors that she had only a few months to live, she didn't want anyone to know. She wanted her illness to be kept a secret. I was one of only a couple of friends and family she told. At one stage she thought of herself as a failure, for succumbing to illness when her life's work was about positive energy and well-being. This was additionally painful for her and made her illness I think even harder for her to bear. But despite these times of regret and unhappiness, at no stage did I hear anything but great courage and absolute bravery from her. And kindness when she spoke about everyone she'd loved and been close to. She just couldn't bear to speak on the phone or let anyone directly see her like this, because she said that she didn't know what she could say, how she could explain how such a thing could happen. In a terrible way, I think she almost blamed herself for getting sick. She was a great believer in the 'law of attraction'. *What you think you become*. And she, like thousands of others from the baby boomer generation and beyond, had read a lot of those countless self-help books which attempt to align illness and maladies of different parts of the body with various psychological misalignments.

Seeing the emotional pain and conflicts she was going through at a time when she really needed comfort and hope, started to open my eyes as to how prevalent and basically unhelpful these kinds of self-help books are. The blame for everything is squarely put on the sufferer or the victim's shoulders.

If Athena had survived her breast cancer a while longer, she would be up there now with the rest of the world's most famous masters of positive thinking, she would have probably been alongside her husband espousing the secret of the 'laws of attraction'.

But she didn't survive. Athena could master the so-called 'law of attraction'; she definitely was a master of positive thinking but it was not enough to win this battle of life and death. She regretted not trying standard treatments earlier, before it was too late, but eventually using her remaining inner strength and showing incredible bravery, she used her intelligence and clarity to instead work her way through to the other side of that regret. I believe she found her peace through that same courage of her conviction. A few months after being diagnosed with advanced breast cancer Athena Starwoman passed away dearly loved and still dearly missed by those close to her as well as her fans and readers from around the world.

As her friend and colleague I don't wish to impart any absolutes on the do's and don'ts of mind power or complementary therapies. But I know how I feel when I still see so many alternative therapists and 'experts' in the media marketing countless books and videos about the 'laws of attraction' and positive thinking as a cure all for every illness out there. I look at it from the depth of experience as at the least naively insincere with very little merit or tangible proof; at worst a dangerous manipulation of so many millions of open-minded people.

Doesn't the general public deserve to be given better researched material and all the current facts as they are now known within both the alternative and standard medical industry? We need a more balanced point of view. The doctors and practitioners of standard medicines and the alternative, complementary industry need to start building bridges. The fear and misunderstandings between the different industries are not working. The public wants and needs more. A lot of women I now discuss these kinds of treatment choices with, either socially or through my website mailing lists, have a lot of fear and mistrust of standard medicine and doctors. And there are quite a few I've met since this experience who tell me than they would do exactly the same thing, primarily because they are convinced that 'the cure is worse than the disease'. Where this antidoctor and antimedicine certainty comes from is a very complex issue, and a subject that really needs a whole book's worth of research in itself. But on the whole, most women and men

I bring this issue up with would prefer to have both complementary and standard medicines to choose from. Some way to effectively merge the best of the two in a way that would be medically feasible. Which could include meditation, positive thinking exercises, as well as a healthier diet regimen, and whatever herbal or natural tonics they might be allowed to include in their therapies. Most people I've spoken to want to have the ability to do both if the need arises. Anyone should have access to as much information as possible to help them make a truly informed choice. Whether that is between using standard medical or alternative treatments, or a combination of both is always going to be a personal choice. I don't advocate laws or regulations to take that natural right away or to stand on a soap box arguing that all natural therapies and positive thinking are useless. Because I don't believe that either. I've followed an instinctual and holistic way of life and work from which I've enjoyed many direct benefits. And it's now common knowledge that eating well, staying away from toxins like smoking and too much alcohol, basically following a more natural way of life with exercise and rest is very beneficial to both the body and mind, not to mention the accepted 'placebo' effect which is really 'positive thinking' under another name.

There is no absolute wrong or right decision when it comes to what treatments we personally choose to try to cure us or even how we choose to leave this planet. Every adult has the right in our free society to make that decision themselves. Anyone who's been through a loved one dying of cancer knows how painful for them and heartbreaking for everyone around them the experience is. There's nothing I feel I could add to anyone's knowledge of that kind of experience and probably very little I could personally write that would truly alleviate anyone else's suffering and grief either. But perhaps revealing this story, and sharing this painful process can produce some small seeds of understanding and hard-earned life experience that no amount of new age philosophising, religious theorising or standard medical know-how can replace. For Athena that would be a fitting addition to her inspirational legacy.

Personally, those seeds have grown into deep roots that have spread out and cracked open my own core beliefs, forcing me to look at a whole range of new territories. The experience and the regret my friend went through had broken my heart, smashed around my spirit and forced me, sometimes kicking and screaming, to face up to a very different and hopefully more balanced way of looking at life in general. It was a complete epiphany. A mammoth life lesson, where I also learnt to accept the fact that I, along with most others, know very little about the truly mysterious and miraculous ways of life and death. It's the great paradox isn't it? Spend most of your life studying the metaphysical mysteries to realise that even most of the greatest philosophers in known history eventually came to the same conclusion — that when it comes to the truly miraculous ways of life and death, we know almost nothing.

But perhaps it's a tiny minuscule more than the last. All a matter of opinion, really. Accept it and move on to how you may truly touch others for the better. With compassion and empathy for other human beings — working hard to be free and independent and try to leave something positive behind for the next generation. I hope that this contribution is at least some kind of helpful insight into the current 'alternative versus standard' debate which may also add to the knowledge bank of this and other generations to come.

17

Barriers to Conducting Complementary and Alternative Medicine Clinical Trials

Byeongsang Oh and Haryana M. Dhillon

ABSTRACT

Complementary and alternative medicine (CAM) is widely available and used frequently by cancer patients and the general public in Australia. This high usage occurs despite limited evidence for the safety and efficacy of CAM being available to cancer patients, the general public and health-care providers, including CAM practitioners. In order to protect cancer patients and the general public against the harmful use of CAM, comprehensive and rigorous research into CAM is required. It is possible that the appropriate use of CAM may improve the over all well-being of patients, as well as ameliorating the impact of specific illnesses. In this chapter, we discuss the complexity of CAM research, barriers to conducting clinical trials of CAM, practical issues to consider when planning and conducting CAM clinical trials and make some practical suggestions for CAM researchers.

Keywords: CAMs; Research; Clinical Trials.

INTRODUCTION

The use of complementary and alternative medicine (CAM) by cancer patients has begun to be incorporated into routine cancer care in the USA and Australia.[1,2] Most adult cancer patients in the USA[3] and about 65% of adults with cancer in Australia use CAM at least once after the diagnosis of cancer.[4,5] However, it is difficult to advise patients on the effective and safe use of CAM in the context of conventional Western medicine with the limited evidence currently available. Most CAM practitioners rely on information derived from their CAM training and experience when treating patients, rather than on the results of clinical trials. Consequently, in recent years there have been policy changes in the USA and Australia to encourage the development of an evidence base for CAM.

In response to the growing high consumer demand for CAM and concerns regarding the safety and efficacy of CAM, the US Congress established the National Center for Complementary and Alternative Medicine (NCCAM) in 1998, to conduct research into CAM practices.[6]

Meanwhile in the UK the "Foundation of Integrated Medicine" was formed in 1999 and recently renamed "The Prince of Wales Foundation for Integrated Health".[7] This organisation aims to promote the use of evidence-based CAM therapy in the conventional medicine practice environment. In Australia, the National Institute for Complementary Medicine (NICM) was established to support CAM research in 2007 and the National Health and Medical Research Council (NHMRC) announced a special call for CAM research applications in 2007 that allocated 5 million dollars for CAM research for the first time.[8] The response and number of submissions received in response to this special funding round were much larger than expected, indicating that researchers are interested and willing to undertake high-quality CAM research if funding is available. As a result of these initiatives, there has been a substantial increase in the amount and quality of CAM research and CAM papers published in high-impact medical journals.[1,9–11] Nevertheless, compared with other fields of study, research funding and the number of CAM researchers in Australia remain small compared with the USA and UK, whereas the number of general practitioners practising CAM and the number of CAM practitioners have increased in response to growing consumer demand.[12,13]

The conduct of high-quality research requires thoughtful and rigorous research design and the use of appropriate methodology; this is no different in CAM research. A multi-disciplinary approach to the design and planning of CAM research is essential. The multi-disciplinary team should include a CAM practitioner experienced in delivering the type of CAM under investigation, health-care professionals and a biostatistician, from the beginning. Many of the previously reported CAM clinical trials were designed and conducted either by CAM practitioners alone, conventional health professionals or academic researchers, with no single group having the skills required to design and conduct such studies.

It is important to understand that the paradigm of illness and treatment used by CAM practitioners is a cornerstone in the development of high-quality CAM research. For Western health professionals, recognising that CAM practitioners operate using different paradigms of diagnosis and treatment is important in developing a shared language, to support the development of the CAM research project. For example, CAM diagnosis generally uses terms such as "disharmony" and/or "imbalance" of organ function caused by disruption of emotion and unbalanced lifestyle rather than specific physiological symptoms of organ dysfunction with an external cause such as bacterial or viral infection. In conventional medicine, and particularly the modern specialist system, the diagnostic emphasis is more specific to individual organs or body parts using pathological tests and other medical diagnostic tools such as X-ray, ultrasound, PET, or MRI. A further complication is the difficulty of translating CAM terminology into scientific English, as CAM practice is based on concepts and terms that have no equivalent translation or conceptualisation in Western scientific thinking, and language communication can be difficult. For example, the term "Qi" used in Chinese medicine, translates as "life force energy", a concept that has not been fully incorporated into Western medical models; it is not measurable or quantifiable with current diagnostic tools and tests. In terms of treatment strategy, generally conventional medicine focuses on treating individual organs, body parts or body systems and predicting specific responses to treatments. However, CAM treatment emphasises emotion and balance in body function as a whole system, with the expectation that treatment efficacy is slow, occurring over extended durations without undesirable side-effects.

CAM research methodology has become increasingly complicated, particularly as conventional and CAM researchers have begun to work more closely together. We now see efforts to ensure the reproducibility of CAM interventions and quality assurance of their delivery. To do this effectively it is critical to understand the differences between CAM and conventional medicine and build a bridge between the two approaches. For this reason, the NCCAM and the NHMRC also encouraged collaborative CAM projects.

The purpose of this chapter is to discuss the barriers to CAM research and provide some suggestions to future CAM researchers based on earlier studies of CAM in the context of cancer care at university teaching hospitals.

DISCREPANCIES OF CAM DEFINITIONS

Complementary medicine (CM) is used in conjunction with conventional medicine; for an intervention to be considered as CM it is expected that it will have scientific evidence to support its efficacy and safety.[14] Alternative medicine (AM) is defined as an intervention used in place of conventional medicine. AMs rarely have scientific evidence to support their use, and may be used by people instead of conventional medicine.[14] Important concerns arise regarding the potential harm of AM, particularly in cases where people with cancer choose to use AM while delaying or stopping conventional medicine.

In the literature the term CAM (often referred to as unproven therapies, alternative therapy, unorthodox therapies and CM) is used frequently, even though there is a distinction between CM and AM. Many of these practices are considered CAM even if contextually used only as complementary therapies. Nonetheless, the term CAM is still widely used.

Formulating a definition of CAM is difficult, as the term encompasses a variety of therapies, remedies, nutrition and dietary supplements, as well as lifestyle changes including exercise, prayer and spiritual practice.[15] The concept of CAM also changes over time, as some practices and techniques become accepted into mainstream medicine. Inclusion of therapies under the term CAM depends in part on the practitioner, scientific proof of their benefits and mechanisms, and government regulation. For example, as there is scientific proof of the benefits and mechanisms of meditation and acupuncture, if these treatments are conducted by a medical practitioner, they are considered as mainstream medicine and no longer CAM.[16] Another example is Chinese medicine; both the Chinese and Korean governments' health regulations consider Chinese medicine to be as therapeutically valid as Western medicine. Chinese medicine is not considered as CAM within these countries, but rather as another form of mainstream medicine.[17]

The definitions and terms used to describe CAM differ between organizations. The World Health Organization (WHO) developed a global strategy on traditional medicine (TM) and CAM in 2003. According to the WHO, TM refers to health traditions, including belief systems, used for therapeutic practice mostly in developing countries and by some indigenous people in developed countries.[18] In contrast, CAM refers to a broad set of health-care practices that are not part of a country's own tradition and are not integrated into the dominant health-care system.[19] Despite some differences in definition between TM and CAM, these terms are often used interchangeably, such that CAM becomes "TM/CAM".[20] NCCAM in the USA defines CAM as "a group of diverse medical and health care systems, practices, and products that are not presently considered to be part of conventional medicine".[21]

DIVERSITY OF CAM THERAPIES

A major concern in CAM research is that most studies consider CAM therapies as a unified system, despite the enormous diversity of therapies included under this label. NCCAM distinguishes between CAM in five domains:

- **biologically–based treatments** such as herbal medicine and nutritional supplements;
- **mind–body-based treatments** including meditation and relaxation;

- **manipulative treatments** including massage, chiropractic and reflexology;
- **energy medicine** such as acupuncture, qigong and therapeutic touch; and
- **whole medical systems** such as traditional Chinese medicine, ayurveda and homeopathy.

In contrast, the Cancer Institute of New South Wales groups CAM into six domains:

- **nutritional and dietary therapy**;
- **herbal therapy**;
- **mind–body therapy**;
- **energy therapy**;
- **manipulative and body-based therapy**; and
- **traditional whole medical systems**.

Whichever classification system is used, some CAM therapies fall between the boundaries of these domains. A comparison of the CAM classifications discussed above is shown in Table 1.

In other studies the relatively simple division of CAM into biological and non-biological therapies was used, based on the report that oncologists were more concerned about biologically-based CAM than non-biologically-based CAM.[22]

DISCREPANCIES OF PARADIGMS BETWEEN CAM AND CONVENTIONAL MEDICINE

The existing paradigm of conventional medicine, a reductionist view of the patient, was developed in the 17th century derived from Cartesian dualism (which postulates that the mind and body are separate entities).[23] The modern scientific biomedical model began to replace early Western medical traditions, such as herbalism and bleeding, based on the Greek "four humours" theory, under the influence of Cartesian dualism. In the biomedical model, healing has been viewed through the mechanism of cause and effect.

In contrast, most CAM kept the traditional "holistic or humanistic care" approach, which integrates mind, body and soul. Today, CAM practitioners consider the entire person, including physical,

Table 1. Comparison of CAM classifications.

WHO	NCCAM	Cancer institute of NSW
Used very broad concept of CAM and did not classify CAM domains	Classified CAM into five domains	Classified CAM into six domains
Traditional medicine	Whole medical systems: built upon complete systems of theory and practice such as homeopathy, naturopathy, traditional Chinese medicine and ayurveda	Traditional whole medicine systems: naturopathy, homeopathy, ayurveda, traditional Chinese medicine
Complementary and alternative medicine	Biologically-based practices: substances found in nature, such as herbs, foods, and vitamins, include dietary supplements, herbal products, shark, etc.	Nutritional and dietary approaches: supplements, Gerson diet, macrobiotic diet, coenzyme Q10, omega-3 fish oils, shark cartilage, etc.
		Herbal supplements: ginseng, black cohosh, red clover, etc.
	Mind–body medicine: a variety of techniques designed to enhance the minds capacity to affect bodily function and symptoms. Meditation, prayer, mental healing, art, music or dance	Mind–body therapies: imagery, psychotherapy, meditation, spiritual healing, prayer, hypnosis
	Manipulative and body-based practices: based on manipulation. They include acupuncture, chiropractic, osteopathy, massage and naturopathy	Manipulative and body-based therapies: acupuncture, massage, reflexology, chiropractic
	Energy medicine: involve the use of energy fields (qigong, reiki and therapeutic touch) including bio-electromagnetic-based therapies (pulse field, magnetic fields, etc.)	Energy medicine: reiki, therapeutic touch, qigong. Bio-electromagnetic-based therapies are not included in this domain

mental, emotional and environmental aspects, during diagnosis and treatment. For this reason, most CAM therapies are also known as "preventative medicine". Recently, as more clinicians have investigated and seen the effectiveness of some CAM therapies in relieving side-effects of conventional anticancer treatments and their ability to improve well-being of cancer patients, they have become more open to incorporating those with an evidence base in their practice. A recent study suggested that 64% of US medical schools and most UK medical schools introduced CAM courses into the medical school curriculum.[24] As a result, future doctors will be more familiar with CAM and expected to integrate CAM into their medical practice.

LACK OF EVIDENCE-BASED CAM RESEARCH

Lack of research into the safety and efficacy of CAM has been identified as a major barrier to integration of conventional and CAM practice.[25] Most CAM therapies have evolved within traditional cultures and ancient philosophies, having been practised for many centuries. Their safety and efficacy has been most commonly supported by historical anecdotal data, case studies and observational studies. The relatively recent practice of evidence-based medicine is based on the randomised controlled trial (RCT). This methodology was introduced to review new drugs for safety and efficacy by the Food and Drug Administration in the USA in 1938.[26] Since then, the RCT has been generally accepted as the gold standard for testing the safety and efficacy of conventional medicine.[27]

A major barrier to the conduct of RCTs of CAM interventions is their complexity and the difficulty with which blinding of treatments can be achieved. The holistic, person-centred nature of many CAM therapies involves the tailoring of therapy to the individual person's needs and symptoms, making it difficult to standardize treatments and test across large groups of patients. One of the main criticisms of the RCT design is that the results apply to populations and that interpreting them to apply to individual patients is complex. Predicting patients who will be responders or non-responders within a population for which a treatment is known to be effective is very difficult. This approach is at odds with the philosophy of CAM, which focuses on individuals and personalised treatments.[28]

However, the RCT remains the most robust approach to testing the safety and efficacy of CAM interventions.

Lately, in recognition of the limitation of the RCT design and development of genome technology, the concept of personalized cancer care, treatment tailored to an individual that ultimately helps to improve health outcomes, is gaining traction in the medical community. Personalized care was introduced a theme of the American Society of Clinical Oncology Annual Meeting in 2009.

Furthermore, with understanding of the complexity of evidence-based CAM research, whole system research (WSR) CAM guidelines were developed by a Canadian CAM research team.[29] The WSR CAM guidelines suggest the integration of multiple designs and methods, including quantitative methods, qualitative research and case studies to develop innovative CAM designs, suitable to each CAM intervention.

EVALUATING THE OUTCOME

Evaluating the efficacy and safety of CAM interventions and products with double-blind RCT methods requires validated, reliable and relevant outcome measurements. In determining the efficacy and safety of a CAM intervention it is essential that the tools used are sensitive enough to detect the subtle effects of CAM interventions. Most of the effects of CAM are more diffuse and subtle than those associated with conventional medicines. Verhoef *et al.*[30] reported that the most commonly identified barrier to CAM research was the fact that appropriate and relevant outcome measures do not exist, and current available conventional medical research measurement tools have not yet been developed to address the unique process, context and outcomes of CAM interventions.

As research has focussed more on the patient-centred outcomes associated with both conventional and CAM interventions, a range of measurement tools assessing patient-reported outcomes have been developed and implemented within the health and social science disciplines, providing standardised approaches to the assessment of these patient-reported outcomes.[31] Despite the development of patient-centred outcome measurement tools, there is a growing recognition by CAM practitioners and researchers that outcome measurement tools suitable for assessment of CAM interventions need to be developed, as those currently available may not be sufficient to fully assess the observed treatment. In some forms of CAM, traditional criteria such as symptom relief, cure or survival may not be appropriate as endpoints. Rather they wish to evaluate outcomes in terms of alterations in energy, emotional balance, healing, ability to cope with disease, well-being and prevention of disease in the long term than an immediate response.

Moreover, when CAM researchers decide to use currently available outcome measurement instruments developed for conventional medical research, selecting an appropriate outcome measurement tool that is sensitive enough to detect the efficacy of CAM interventions is essential. For example, in measuring quality of life (QOL) of cancer patients, the Functional Assessment of Cancer Therapy-General (FACT-G) questionnaire is more sensitive to detect certain dimensions of QOL and requires smaller sample sizes to meet statistical power than the European Organization for Research and Treatment of Core Cancer Quality of Life (EORTC QLQ C-30). There is a clear need to develop measurement tools that can evaluate the outcome of CAM interventions.

A stepped approach to the development of CAM research, as suggested by Verhoef *et al.*,[29] offers a high likelihood of identifying and systematically evaluating potentially useful CAMs. It is based on the concept of "whole systems research" in which both qualitative and quantitative research methods are used to study the interventions' effectiveness along with the process, context, outcomes and philosophy. Acknowledging the philosophical foundations of particular CAM supports better theoretical models of how they work and may lead to improved integration of CAM theories and conventional mechanistic approaches, it will certainly contribute to the development of approaches to assessing CAM.

In studying a CAM that has not previously been researched, researchers need to start with small qualitative studies in patients with clearly documented medical and psychosocial histories and belief systems, to develop an understanding of the possible effects of CAM (similar to case studies or series). Using the findings from qualitative studies guides how to deliver and evaluate an intervention and in which populations. Determining the appropriate target group for treatment is similar to the approaches emerging for optimal use of targeted, biological agents in people with specific genetic mutations.

Recently, the National Institute of Health (NIH) in the USA recommended a Three-arm design for CAM studies (intervention arm, placebo control arm and usual care control arm) instead of the two arms used in conventional medicine (intervention arm and placebo control arm). The Three-arm design will improve the evaluation of CAM but will add significantly increased financial costs of running research projects. Where blinding of treatments is not possible, this must be acknowledged and the inclusion of an attention-control group (in addition to standard care alone) needs to be considered. Improving the rationale for a CAM intervention with rigorous qualitative data supporting it and incorporating relevant control groups will result in a vastly improved evidence base for CAMs and their interactions with conventional therapies.

LIMITED RESEARCH FUNDING FOR CAM RESEARCH

At present, CAM research is at a disadvantage in competing successfully for general research funding, mainly due to insufficient interest by researchers and sponsors. Unlike conventional medicine, most CAM interventions (except some herbal products) are not easy to patent, limiting the potential to generate a return on investment for commercial sponsors. Furthermore, in Australia most herbal interventions are marketed as foods, without making claims of efficacy for specific diseases. As a result, there is little incentive for companies marketing these formulations to conduct rigorous, clinical research to test their effectiveness. For this reason, it is difficult to obtain commercially interested sponsors for CAM research. Thus, given the widespread use of CAM and their potential interactions with conventional therapies delivered in the public health system, public funding for CAM is imperative.

In recent years, more funds from major funding agencies have become available for research into CAM. It is estimated that the National Health Service allocated 0.08% of its research budget to CAM research in the UK.[7] In 2005, the National Center of Complementary and Alternative Medicine (NCCAM) in the US budgeted $123 million for CAM research. Australia also allocated

$5 million for CAM research in 2007, but specific CAM funding has not been repeated, and the response to this funding round in 2007 demonstrated the inadequacy of funding for CAM research. To date, the number of research projects testing CAM interventions awarded by the NHMRC have been very small compared with the number of biomedical projects funded. The perceived lack of rigour in CAM research projects is a common problem for CAM projects. For example, they may be criticized for not being adequately controlled, lack of placebo for the intervention, non-standardization of treatment or limited supporting data. Further, reviewers often request scientific literature on safety and efficacy of CAM interventions to support the funding application. As, in most instances, safety data for CAM interventions are not available, it may be sensible to incorporate a staged approach to CAM research. This would establish the safety of a CAM intervention in the context of conventional medicines, before a large-scale clinical trial is commenced.

Several actions are required to secure research funding. Firstly, the design of CAM research needs to be improved and it is recommended that the research team be multi-disciplinary, including CAM practitioners, conventional health professionals and academic researchers. Secondly, the process of assessment of CAM research applications needs to be revised. The inclusion of an additional panel member who has CAM research experience on CAM review committees would add to the knowledge base of these committees. This approach has been taken by NCCAM in the USA. Ideally, given that the CAM therapy market in Australia is worth millions of dollars annually, prioritizing and quarantining a proportion of public research funds for CAM research seems reasonable.

ETHICS APPROVAL FOR CAM RESEARCH

All research including CAM clinical trials requires approval by the appropriate regulatory and ethical authorities before participants can be recruited into a study. Most practitioners, unless involved in clinical research, have little experience with the ethics approval processes, which varies between hospitals and States. In Australian public hospitals, research is approved by Health Research Ethics

Committees, which are charged with the responsibility of patient protection. This requires a comprehensive review of the research project, including the scientific validity. Clear and concise justification of the rationale for the CAM intervention including any supporting pre-clinical or epidemiological data is required; the critical criterion is to demonstrate that the potential benefits of the intervention and study outweigh the potential harms.

In relation to scientifically rigorous CAM clinical trial design, Miller *et al.*[32] argue that, in general, research on CAM should adhere to the same ethical requirements as for all clinical research, and specifically that randomized, placebo-controlled clinical trials should be used for assessing the efficacy of CAM treatments whenever possible. It is appropriate to adapt double-blind controlled RCTs with biological CAM such as herb and nutrition supplements. Nevertheless, practical and ethical constraints make it impossible in some cases to use placebo controls and double-blind controls with non-biological CAM intervention (e.g. meditation, Yoga, relaxation and Qigong). If it is not possible to use a placebo or blind a particular intervention, it is best to explain why this is the case, rather than to fail to mention that it has been considered and discounted.

Practical Issues to Consider in Conducting CAM Clinical Trials

CAM Practitioner Qualifications and Skills

The qualifications and skills of CAM practitioners are important in CAM research. CAM practitioner qualifications vary from certificates resulting from completing a weekend workshop course (e.g. Reiki, therapeutic touch and hypnosis) to bachelor degrees from accredited universities (e.g. acupuncture, Chinese medicine and naturopathy). Due to the lack of government regulation of CAM qualifications it is difficult to compare the skills of CAM practitioners. A notable exception is the state of Victoria, where the Chinese Medicine Registration Board of Victoria regulates acupuncturist and Chinese medicine practitioner registration.

In biological CAM, the practitioner's experience can influence the outcome of interventions. The diagnosis and treatment strategy of disease can be different between individual CAM practitioners even within the same CAM modalities (e.g. a Chinese herbal prescription can apply to multiple diseases and a variety of symptoms can be treated with the same prescription).

In the case of non-biological CAM, the CAM practitioner's skills and experience have the potential to influence the outcome of CAM interventions more than with biological CAM. The therapist effect is of concern for many conventional approaches to person-centred interventions targeting behaviour change. For example, in chiropractic and massage therapies the practitioner's skills and experience in dealing with specific patient populations are important in delivering appropriate care, in addition to the practical aspects of their education and training. A system for accrediting and registering CAM practitioners is needed. Public access to registered practitioners is essential in assisting the general public to identify those practitioners who are qualified to deliver care safely. It would also assist researchers to identify CAM practitioners for potential research collaborations.

Support CAM Research Within the Conventional Health-care System

As CAM therapies are widely used by specific patient groups and the general public, the potential risk of their interaction with conventional medicines makes them an important issue for the public health system. Whether appropriate or not, research into new drugs and other conventional approaches to health-care is prioritised above CAM research. Recognition of the widespread use of some CAM interventions and the importance of addressing their safety and efficacy are key components to creating a supportive environment for conducting CAM clinical research.

The majority of hospital staff are very supportive of CAM clinical trials, despite perceiving themselves as lacking time and being overburdened. The main reasons given for not supporting CAM trials were to protect their patients from unproven therapy and negative views on CAM. Ensuring the rigour of the methodological approach and engaging with health professionals early will contribute to the successful conduct of the CAM research study. As with any research, it is important to have clinicians championing the study, promoting it to their colleagues and supporting the research team.

The logistics of delivering CAM therapy in the conventional hospital setting can be challenging and may limit the implementation of CAM supported by evidence. For example, in running a medical Qigong programme (traditional Chinese medicine treatment involving gentle exercise and meditation), we experienced difficulties in identifying suitable space and suitable times to run the programme. However, with persistence these difficulties were overcome and clinicians, hearing positive reports from their patients, became increasingly supportive of the programme. We have had similar experiences in running acupuncture studies, having to adapt delivery of treatment to suites that were set up to deliver chemotherapy rather than acupuncture.

Ideally, future development of cancer treatment centres will include integrated facilities for CAM treatment delivery during the full disease trajectory and for the increasing number of cancer survivors. Providing access to CAM therapy in the conventional health-care system can support and promote an evidence-based approach to implementing CAM therapy, with those treatments offered having an evidence base or being researched within the centre prior to full implementation.

Competition for Recruitment

The problem of competing trials is common to all clinical research. Within any given teaching hospital it is likely that there will be a number of clinical trials that are available for patients to take part in. In general, anticancer treatment trials will take priority over all others, and some studies will specifically exclude participation in more than one study. Where there are competing trials, one pragmatic approach is to develop a hierarchy of clinical trial presentation. For example, for a patient with advanced lung cancer, a treatment trial of a new biologic agent may be the first trial the patient is introduced to, and they may then go on to be approached about a medical Qi Gong study. It is also important to determine at what point in a patient's disease trajectory the trial needs to be introduced. For example, a treatment trial may need to be introduced before patients are offered any treatment, whereas a study of a herbal formulation may not need to be introduced until after conventional anticancer treatment has begun.

Motivation of CAM Research Team

Training and motivating CAM research team members are also essential for the CAM clinical trial, just as in trials of non-CAM therapies. In our previous study, research assistants who had less motivation for CAM research recruited fewer participants than those who were interested in CAM research. Motivating research staff with CAM education may improve recruitment of participants for the CAM clinical trials when large sample sizes are required.

RECOMMENDATIONS

To expand and facilitate the development of an evidence base for CAM interventions we recommend the following.

- Developing specially tailored CAM research training.[33]
- Setting up CAM research teams in collaboration with health-care professionals is essential in addition to biostatisticians and experienced CAM researchers.
- Encouraging multi-disciplinary CAM research teams to apply for research funding from public agencies such as NHMRC, NIH, NCCAM and NICM.
- Applying for alternative sources of research funding from private and public institutions.
- Encouraging collaboration of CAM research with international institutions as well as national institutions.
- Encouraging research directed at long-term outcomes and supportive care, areas that have limited control or treatment options by conventional medical care and that offer the possibility of low-cost and preventative health-care management.
- Developing appropriate CAM research outcome measurements (qualitative and/or quantitative approach) based on consumers' needs and demands considering the limitations of randomized clinical trials.
- Registering CAM studies with the clinical trial registry to avoid duplication of efforts wherever possible.

CONCLUSION

The use of CAM by cancer patients and the general public continues to grow despite the limited scientific information about CAM. In response to increased CAM use, Western governments have recognized the need for CAM research and allocated research funding specifically for this purpose. The implications and feasibility of a double-blind RCT methodology for the assessment of CAM interventions continue to be debated. The complexity of CAM research design has been recognized, but there is no single agreed approach to overcoming methodological challenges. Innovative approach to CAM research design are needed. The assessment of CAM projects, coupled with improvements in the justification and rationale for them, is needed. Finally, long-term support for CAM research from government agencies is essential to drive investigations into the safety, efficacy and effectiveness of CAM in order to protect cancer patients and the general public from harmful CAM use. Only when this evidence is available will it be possible to develop evidence-based guidelines regarding the appropriate use of CAM interventions and integrate this evidence with conventional medicine within the health-care system.

REFERENCES

1. Oh B, *et al*. Impact of medical Qigong on quality of life, fatigue, mood and inflammation in cancer patients: a randomized controlled trial. *Ann Oncol* **21**:608–614 (2010).
2. American Health Association. More hospitals offering CAM services, *Health Forum Rep* (2008).
3. Richardson MA, *et al*. Complementary/alternative medicine use in a comprehensive cancer center and the implications for oncology. *J Clin Oncol* **18**:2505–2514 (2000).
4. Oh B, *et al*. Patient-doctor communication: the use of complementary and alternative medicine by adult patients with cancer. *J Soc Integr Oncol* **8**:56–64 (2010).
5. Miller M, *et al*. The use of unproven methods of treatment by cancer patients. Frequency, expectations and cost. *Support Care Cancer* **6**:337–347 (1998).

6. Berman J, Chesney MA. Complementary and alternative medicine in 2006: optimising the dose of the intervention. *Med J Aust* **183**:574–575 (2005).
7. Ernst E, Schmidt K, Wider B. CAM research in Britain: the last 10 years. *Complement Ther Clin Pract* **11**:17–20 (2005).
8. National Health and Medical Research Council. Complementary and Alternative Medicine Special Call for Research Applications (2007) [Accessed 7 December 2009]. http://www.nhmrc.gov.au/funding/funded/historical/cam.htm
9. Demark-Wahnefried W, *et al.* Lifestyle intervention development study to improve physical function in older adults with cancer: outcomes from project LEAD. *J Clin Oncol* **24**:3465–3473 (2006).
10. Moadel AB, *et al.* Randomized controlled trial of yoga among a multiethnic sample of breast cancer patients: effects on quality of life. *J Clin Oncol* **25**:4387–4395 (2007).
11. Lautenschlager NT, *et al.* Effect of physical activity on cognitive function in older adults at risk for Alzheimer disease: a randomized trial. *JAMA* **300**:1027–1037 (2008).
12. Owen D, Lewith GT. Teaching integrated care: CAM familiarisation courses [see comment]. *Med J Aust* **181**:276–278 (2004).
13. Easthope G, Beilby JJ, Gill GF, *et al.* Acupuncture in Australian general practice: practitioners characteristics. *Med J Aust* **196**:197–200 (1998).
14. Cassileth BR. Complementary and alternative cancer medicine. *J Clin Oncol* **17**(suppl 1):44–52 (1999).
15. Davidson R, *et al.* Psychological characteristics of cancer patients who use complementary therapies. *Psycho-Oncology* **14**:187–195 (2005).
16. Jacobs GD. The physiology of mind body interactions: the stress response and the relaxation response. *J Alternat Complement Med* **7**(suppl 1):83–92 (2001).
17. Robinson N. Integrated traditional Chinese medicine. *Complement Ther Clin Pract* **12**(2):132–140 (2006).
18. Bodeker G, Kronenberg F. A public health agenda for traditional, complementary, and alternative medicine. *Am J Pub Health* **92**:1582–1591 (2002).
19. WHO. *National Policy on Traditional Medicine and Regulation of Herbal Medicines: Report of a WHO Global Survey*, Geneva, WHO (2005).
20. Cornelio D, Warber S. Social construction of CAM. *Mol Intervent* **3**:182–185 (2003).

21. NIH. *CAM Basics* (2007) http://nccam.nih.gov/health/whatiscam/ [Accessed 20 June 2008].
22. Girgis A, Adams J, Sibbritt D. The use of complementary and alternative therapies by patients with cancer. *Oncol Res* **15**:281–289 (2005).
23. Switankowsky I. Dualism and its importance for medicine. *Theor Med Bioethics* **21**:567–580 (2000).
24. Wetzel MS, Eisenberg DM, Kaptchuk TJ. Courses involving complementary and alternative medicine at US medical schools [see comment]. *JAMA* **280**:784–787 (1998).
25. Boon H, Verhoef M. Building complementary and alternative health care research capacity: workshop report. *Complement Ther Med* **10**:49–51 (2002).
26. Walker LG, Anderson J. Testing complementary and alternative therapies within a research protocol. *Eur J Cancer* **35**:1614–1618 (1999).
27. Meldrum ML. A brief history of the randomised controlled trial: from oranges and lemons to the gold standard. *Hematol/Oncol Clin North Am* **14**:745–760 (2000).
28. Hart A, Sutton CJ. n-of-1 trials and their combination: suitable approaches for CAM research? *Complement Ther Med* **11**:213–214 (2003).
29. Verhoef MJ, Vanderheyden LC, Fonnebo V. A whole systems research approach to cancer care: why do we need it and how do we get started? *Integr Cancer Ther* **5**:287–292 (2006).
30. Verhoef M, *et al.* Evaluating complementary and alternative medicine interventions: in search of appropriate patient-centered outcome measures. *BMC Complement Altern Med* **6**:38 (2006).
31. Bowling A. *Measuring Health: A Review of Quality of Life Measurement Scales*, 3rd edn, Open University Press, Maidenhead, Berks (2005).
32. Miller FG, *et al.* Ethical issues concerning research in complementary and alternative medicine. *JAMA* **291**:599–604 (2004).
33. Witt CM, Linde K. The need for CAM research training. *Forsch Komplement/Res Complement Med* **15**:69–70 (2008).

18

Teaching Complementary and Alternative Medicines to Medical Students

Craig Hassed

ABSTRACT

Considering the prevalence of use of complementary and alternative medicine (CAM) in the community and the growing evidence base for effectiveness, medical students need to develop informed and balanced attitudes, skills and knowledge about this field that are going to prepare them adequately for future medical practice. However, the teaching of CAM content in conventional medical curricula has tended to be tokenistic and piecemeal at best or, at worst, totally absent. Where it does appear, CAM content is often marginalised rather than being seen as an integral part of the core knowledge and skills required of a well-rounded and informed doctor. This is problematic for a number of reasons including that the new graduate is less aware of which therapies are potentially useful or harmful and is therefore less able to help patients make informed and safe decisions regarding this aspect of their health-care. It can also potentially impede the therapeutic relationship and communication between doctor and patient especially if a patient has a disposition towards using CAM.

This chapter will review some of the background issues regarding the teaching of CAM in medical education and make some suggestions about what should be minimal content in modern medical curricula. At a minimum, this content should include teaching on the common CAM modalities, ethics, economics of CAM, evidence, safety and risks including interactions, clinical applications, clinical skills in history-taking and communication around CAM, and how to find and assess further information. Rather than being taught as a separate discipline, CAM is best integrated into the wider curriculum and grounded in a philosophy of medical education based upon integrative medicine principles.

Keywords: CAMS; Curriculum; Integrative Medicine; Medical Students; Teaching.

INTRODUCTION

Why spend time studying complementary and alternative medicine (CAM) in already overcrowded medical courses? There are a number of possible answers to that question, some of which will be examined in this chapter, and many other answers will be explored in greater depth in other chapters. To set a context, however, some points are worth mentioning here. One answer is that CAM holds a mirror up to conventional medical education and practice. It helps a medical student to develop critical reflection, which is surely a core skill that any medical educator would wish to see among medical graduates. Exploring CAM helps a student to be reflective about issues such as:

- what constitutes modern medicine;
- clinical research, critical appraisal and evidence-based medicine;
- community attitudes to health and illness;
- health economics and resource allocation;
- communication and the doctor–patient relationship; and
- interprofessional education, practice and ethics.

Although many medical students feel the need and have the interest to know more about CAM, many feel that their medical education does not prepare them adequately in this area.[1] Considering why people are using CAM may be useful in telling us something about the real or perceived deficiencies of orthodox medicine such as:

- dissatisfaction with the medical profession, particularly its perceived lack of humanity;[2]
- the time and nature of the consultations with CAM practitioners;
- orthodox medicine has difficulty in successfully managing many chronic diseases and diseases associated with ageing;
- the desire for increased access to information and autonomy, along with a reduced tolerance of paternalism;[3]
- concerns about the expense, invasiveness or overuse of pharmaceuticals in orthodox medicine;
- the rise of the consumer movement and post-modernism;[4] and
- people finding that CAM is effective for improving well-being, managing symptoms or altering the course of disease progression.[5]

CAM use is common among patients with specific illnesses like cancer,[6] HIV and multiple sclerosis (MS)[7] with approximately two-thirds of such patients using them. CAM users are more often younger, female, better educated and from higher socio-economic groups. Thus, more people are wishing to look for a wider range of management strategies, to consult varying information sources, and also to make up their own minds about which treatments to use. Another reason for the modern graduate to know more about CAM is because of the increasing levels of referral and use among medical practitioners. For example, among Australian general practitioners approximately 90% have referred patients to CAM practitioners and over one in five practise the common modalities like prescribing vitamins and supplements, administering acupuncture or teaching meditation and relaxation therapies.[8,9] As such, CAM is a reality which the orthodox medical profession cannot afford to ignore and if it attempts to do so it is more likely to marginalise itself, rather than CAM. It would be far better for the medical profession to take a leadership role in helping to ensure quality training, research, standards and ethics.

THE DEFINITION AND AIMS OF MODERN MEDICINE

At first glance the answer to the question, 'what is the aim of medical education?' might seem too obvious to mention. The obvious answer would be 'to train doctors'. 'But what', one might then ask, 'do doctors need to know in order to be adequately trained?' 'They need to know about modern, orthodox medicine'. This is where the apparently simple question begins to become more complicated. 'What, then, is the definition of modern, orthodox medicine and what does it include and what is excluded from it? And what is the aim of modern medicine?' Let us look briefly at each of these questions because one's responses might help to better delineate what should be included in medical education.

Defining Orthodox and Unorthodox Medicine

The definition of orthodox or conventional medical practice has rather blurry edges that are constantly moving. These edges also vary widely, not only from one country to another, but from one hospital or medical practice to another, and even between clinicians working within the same hospital or clinic. If one tries to define 'conventional' or 'orthodox' medicine, as various national medical councils have attempted to do,[10] the most common definition is that orthodox medicine is scientific and evidence-based. Unorthodox medicine — which includes both CAM — is by definition unscientific and not evidence-based. Although this definition might be accurate much of the time, it does not take too long to see that many things done in orthodox medicine are not based upon sound evidence, but upon convention or tradition.

Another prominent factor influencing medical practice is the marketing influence of the pharmaceutical industry. The consistent and widespread publication bias in favour of pharmaceuticals makes it both easy for clinicians to make decisions that are influenced by such bias and for patients to become justifiably disillusioned with modern medicine and so look for alternative models of health-care. Not to help our medical undergraduates to be aware of such issues does our profession no credit, nor does it adequately prepare them for the realities they will one day have to deal with.

The resistance to change and adopting new evidence when conventional medical therapies are shown not to be effective, or have costs and side-effects that outweigh their benefits, are to a significant degree testament to the power of patient expectation, advertising from the pharmaceutical industry, and the tendency for beliefs and behaviours to become fixed and unquestioned. Examples could include that most prescriptions for antibiotics have little scientific rationale for their use. Consider also the heavy promotion, high expense, toxicity and hasty uptake of many new cancer drugs,[11] or the lack of placebo trials supporting many commonly used surgical practices such as arthroscopy and knee debridement for osteoarthritis and chronic knee pain.[12,13] Even the evidence base that well-intentioned clinicians are using to help patients make informed decisions demonstrates a heavy publication bias in favour of the drugs, suggesting that most industry-led pharmaceutical research is motivated by marketing rather than science.

Then, of course, there is a range of unorthodox therapies that have gathering evidence supporting their use. Many of these have better safety profiles than commonly used conventional treatments. Examples could include St. John's wort for depression,[14] Co-enzyme Q10 for hypertension,[15] acupuncture for pain relief,[16] and saw palmetto for benign prostatic hypertrophy[17,18] to name a few. A case could be made that these therapies should be considered as first-line treatments or as reasonable options when considering potential approaches to managing a given condition. For example, omega-3 fatty acids have been found to be more effective for managing hyperlipidaemia[19] than any pharmaceutical. They also have beneficial side-effects and lower cost. Unfortunately, prescribing most of these therapies is unlikely to be taught within medical curricula or discussed by clinicians in bedside teaching as valid treatment options. If the lecturer or clinician does not know about them, then they are unlikely to mention them and may even dismiss them out of hand.

Thus, using evidence as the defining line between orthodox and unorthodox treatments is often true but also often fallacious. Examples have been given to make a point, but the point from an educator's perspective is not to have students believing that all CAMs are helpful or safe, but rather to help students to walk that fine line between healthy scepticism and open-mindedness to new ways of thinking. In a sense, the issue is about training questioning minds in such a way that transcends any artificial distinction we might draw between orthodox and unorthodox philosophies or treatments.

Science, Scepticism and Human Psychology

At times one might wonder whether orthodox medicine is all that it believes itself to be. 'Science' is done by scientists, and scientists, being human, imply that science is as much about people and human psychology as it is about objective scientific facts. Probably a more accurate and practical definition of orthodox medicine is that it is what most doctors believe or do in practice and unorthodox medicine is what doctors don't generally believe or do in practice.

Part of the problem may be that, consciously or unconsciously, medical educators often draw arbitrary, unhelpful and rigid boundary lines within our thinking with the result being that all too often things that fall within the boundary are accepted unquestioningly — i.e. there is a lack of healthy scepticism — and things that fall outside the boundary are rejected out of hand — i.e. they often suffer from a form of unhealthy scepticism. It can foster a kind of war-like mentality which closes down dialogue and where health-care professionals from various persuasions become combatants rather than colleagues. Potential informative discussions potentially become acrimonious debates. Objectivity and truth are most imperilled in such circumstances. Caught in this war are patients and their families who are then pressured to take sides. They may receive too much conflicting advice and may cease to communicate with their doctors about the management decisions they are making.

The implications for medical education are that teachers need to be informed, need to refer to up-to-date evidence with an open mind, and would do well not to draw artificial and unhelpful boundaries rather than just be interested in what works, what is safest, what is most economical, and what fits with the patient's preferences.

Integrative Medicine

To an extent, CAM is a term that may be becoming limited or perhaps even obsolete. The more useful term is integrative medicine (IM).

IM refers to a holistic philosophy and way of practising medicine that includes orthodox medical practice but also places a greater emphasis on wellness, the integration of lifestyle factors, and the use of CAM where it is safe, ethical and supported by evidence. In many ways, IM is not alternative practice, but *is* best practice. Naturally, the approach to any given health issue will be guided by evidence, practitioner experience and, importantly, patient preferences. In the IM model CAM does not sit outside or compete with orthodox medical practice, but rather various modalities are interconnected and complementary. For example, this is the approach that is being investigated as the way of the future for health-care in the USA,[20] as well as the approach taken by the Royal Australian College of General Practitioners (RACGP),[21] and it is the model that has been introduced into the curriculum at Monash University.[22] It is likely that this more integrated approach offers the best opportunity to break down unnecessary and artificial barriers, and to cease fighting unhelpful turf wars.

If one says that the aim of modern medicine is to treat illness — i.e. the practice of medicine based on the illness model — then which treatment modalities are included and which excluded, and how would one decide where to draw that arbitrary boundary line? As has been mentioned, medical educators struggle to draw clear distinctions between what would be considered orthodox and unorthodox medical practice. There often arises a legitimate criticism that modern medicine in its practice and funding has for too long underrecognised the importance of the holistic perspective, lifestyle issues and the prevention of illness. It would seem that the greatest aspiration of modern medicine is merely to help a person over the line from having demonstrable symptoms and illness to no longer having demonstrable symptoms or illness — which does not mean that the illness is not still there, nor that the person is well. Many practitioners and patients may argue that orthodox medicine largely ignores the importance of higher order wellness.

It is for the reasons of preferring a holistic or wellness approach, or in order to receive lifestyle advice and counselling, that many people seek out CAM practitioners.[23] Surely these are services that the orthodox practitioner and health-care system should be providing. This is not an argument for a different health-care system, but rather an argument for a significant renovation of the health-care we are currently delivering. The deficiency in modern health-care, whether it be real or perceived, needs to be addressed and all the better if it can be addressed early in the educative process.

The Aim of Medical Education

The aim of medical education necessarily follows from defining the aim of medical practice — although one could also argue that medical education also prepares one for careers that are not primarily clinically focused such as researchers, pathologists, medical administrators or medical educators. If, generally speaking, the aim of medical education is to produce a well-rounded, generic doctor, who understands both the prevention and treatment of illness, and if the future of modern medicine is to be able to span both illness and wellness, then some significant changes need to be made to the way that most medical courses approach CAM teaching. Consider the following issues.

- Approximately two-thirds of the population in most developed countries use one form or other of CAM whether they be administered by a medical or non-medical practitioner or, as is commonly the case, these therapies are self-administered.
- Some CAMs may provide useful therapies either aimed at cure, slowing the progression of the illness, ameliorating symptoms, or possibly producing higher level well-being. As such, a doctor needs the knowledge and skills to sort the wheat from the chaff and administer or recommend the CAMs that are safe and effective.
- CAM could potentially interact, for better or for worse, with orthodox therapies. As such, a doctor needs to routinely ask patients about them and know where to find out reliably which ones interact with which medicines.
- Patients may be making decisions about which orthodox medical treatments to use, or whether to use them at all. Such decisions can be significantly affected by their use of CAM. Apart from having implications for educating patients, it is also difficult to individualise treatments to a given patient without knowing about their views and preferences.
- When a doctor is asked a question about CAM, currently the doctor is not likely to know the answer. A blanket response of warning

against the use of CAM, or a derisory remark that they are all ineffective, is likely to be unconvincing and uninformed. Interestingly, two-thirds of the bold statements made by medical experts in grand rounds are contrary to or are unsupported by evidence.[24] Hence, we may not pause to reflect before we speak as often as we should. In orthodox medicine we need to be as rigorous with our attention to evidence as we demand from CAM advocates.
- The significant and legitimate concerns about the motives and influence of the pharmaceutical industry on the community and the medical profession[25] cannot be ignored, as they may be driving more people to use CAM in what they perceive to be a more wholesome and unbiased form of health-care delivery.

Considering that the majority of patients do not wish to turn against conventional medicine when they adopt CAM, the majority would feel comforted to speak with their medical practitioners about these matters if such conversations could be opened up in a respectful way. The fact that the general public are, by and large, using these therapies on a widespread basis, and the variety of ways that they can impact upon health, one could consider that a modern and well-trained generic doctor must be informed about this field of health-care.

WHAT IS CURRENTLY BEING TAUGHT ON CAM?

Most medical courses tend to either ignore issues related to CAM altogether or marginalise it. For example, data from the USA,[26] Europe,[27] and Japan[28] indicate that medical schools vary widely in their approach and content as far as teaching CAM is concerned. Many courses do not teach content on CAM at all, whereas others have compulsory familiarisation subjects. In Canada a useful initiative has attempted to provide standards and consistency in CAM teaching.[29] More information about the Canadian national initiative to integrate CAM in undergraduate medical education programmes can be found on the associated website.[30] NCCAM had set up a previous initiative in the USA aimed at enhancing education in this area.[31] In Australia most medical schools teach less than five hours of content on CAM, mostly related to generic issues rather than clinical applications.[32]

When practitioners go out to search for CAM courses themselves, they may find a mixed bag in terms of quality. Much of the educational content on CAM in 'evidence-based' CAM courses is of questionable quality and often not based upon an objective assessment of the evidence.[33] It behooves a medical educator to refer to the best evidence available, to teach in an objective and unbiased manner and to help students to navigate their way through the maze of information and misinformation available.

WHAT SHOULD A CAM CURRICULUM COVER?

Although each individual medical school will vary in terms of content, time dedicated to CAM teaching, and method of delivery, it is not too early to suggest that any up-to-date and comprehensive medical curriculum needs to include CAM content. At the very least, a range of generic issues need to be covered and, one would suggest, a number of clinical issues should also be covered. Although one could make a case for all students needing to know about the applications of those CAMs that have good evidence supporting their use, detailed knowledge of any particular modality will probably always remain outside the brief of medical curricula. For example, it is not expected that students will graduate being skilled acupuncturists or herbalists, although they might be expected to know some common and clinically important examples of current or potential use, the indications for the use of these treatments and any major contraindications or interactions. Electives and post-graduate training for interested students and doctors may be the best means to learn about any particular modality in more detail.

On the one hand we need to be open to many of the things that significantly affect health, but are much undervalued in medical education, practice and resource allocation. On the other hand we need to discourage the use and promotion of those health-care practices and therapies that do not work, particularly when they have significant side-effects and are expensive. Therapies in this latter category have significant potential to prey upon the concerns of uninformed and vulnerable patients. This responsibility is not one that a medical student's education can afford to ignore.

Content for a CAM Curriculum

The following are proposed as the bare minimum for a medical curriculum to cover in relation to CAM teaching.

1. Generic issues
   a. The history of CAM
   b. Modern attitudes towards and usage patterns of CAM in the community
   c. International and cultural perspectives on CAM
   d. Terms and definitions
   e. CAM modalities and classifications
   f. The commonly used CAMs
   g. The ethics and medico-legal issues of CAM use
   h. The economics of CAM
2. Research and evidence in CAM
   a. Research issues and challenges in CAM
   b. Current state of the CAM evidence base
   c. Levels of evidence for effectiveness and safety of various CAM modalities
      i. Effective and safe
      ii. Doubtful efficacy, but safe
      iii. Effective, but questionable safety
      iv. Ineffective and unsafe
3. Clinical issues
   a. Communication with patients and CAM practitioners
   b. History-taking
   c. The doctor–patient relationship
   d. Safety and interactions
   e. Clinical decision-making involving CAM
4. Information sources and appraisal
   a. Textbooks
   b. Data bases
   c. Journals
   d. Websites
   e. Further education

The aim of such a component of the medical course should not necessarily be to extensively train a doctor in any given therapy, nor to turn a medical practitioner into a CAM practitioner, but rather to give an overview of the main issues and how to proceed in making decisions with patients about where such therapies might fit into the management plan and where to find further information. It would be fair to say that if there is good evidence supporting the benefits and safety of any particular therapy, be it complementary or conventional, that therapy should be considered and recommended, or at very least discussed as one of the possible treatment options and the benefits and risk of its use discussed, as they would be with any other treatment. Even if doctors do not feel adequately trained to administer a CAM treatment themselves, or to field questions about it, they should still know that it exists and where the patient could go in order to find out that information. The doctor may play an important role in helping a patient to interpret information that they have found for themselves. Indeed, the student or clinician should be trained to follow up on patient questions and inquiries regarding CAM as a part of their commitment to life-long learning.

Personal Reflections on Teaching CAM to Medical Students

As an educator I have an interest in developing a questioning attitude amongst the medical students I teach. This attitude is a balance between open-mindedness and critical thinking. Unfortunately, I do not believe that until now the orthodox medical education system has done this job well. All too often the area has been dominated by the apathy of many educators regarding CAMs and the vocal, unreflective and rigid scepticism of a few.

In my experience, the majority of medical students are open to and interested in CAMs, but more in an IM model, rather than CAM as a different health-care system. To teach it effectively, one needs to be focused on evidence and avoid taking sides, or inculcate divisive attitudes. Encouraging students to cultivate a healthy scepticism, not just about CAM, but about the whole of their medical education is, I believe, a life-long skill and attitude that will stand the students in good stead and guard against fixed beliefs and closed minds for the rest of their careers. I believe it is not the job of the educator to attempt to make the students' minds up for them, but to help them find a way to approach the subject for the benefit of themselves as clinicians, and for their patients.

CONCLUSION

If medical education does not come to terms with the necessity of teaching about CAM within an IM framework we not only risk providing an incomplete curriculum taught in a disintegrated framework, but we also miss an outstanding opportunity to teach specific and relevant content while honing generic skills in critical reflection. CAM can be used as a way to train astute and thoughtful clinicians who, like able-bodied seamen, learn to navigate their way through waters which, although little explored and potentially leading to fertile new lands, are often shrouded in the mists of uncertainty and blown by the winds of controversy.

REFERENCES

1. Clement YN, Williams AF, Khan K, *et al.* A gap between acceptance and knowledge of herbal remedies by physicians: the need for educational intervention. *BMC Complement Altern Med* **5**:20 (2005).
2. Weatherall D. The inhumanity of medicine: time to stop and think. *BMJ* **309**:1671–1672 (1994).
3. Jonas W. Alternative medicine — learning from the past, examining the present, advancing to the future. *JAMA* **280**:1616–1618 (1998).
4. Coulter I, Willis E. The rise and rise of complementary and alternative medicine: a sociological perspective. *Med J Aust* **180**:587–589 (2004).
5. Astin J. Why patients use alternative medicine: results of a national study. *JAMA* **279**:1548–1553 (1998).
6. Gage H, Storey L, McDowell C, *et al.* Integrated care: utilisation of complementary and alternative medicine within a conventional cancer treatment centre. *Complement Ther Med* **17**:84–91 (2009).
7. Leong EM, Semple SJ, Angley M, *et al.* Complementary and alternative medicines and dietary interventions in multiple sclerosis: what is being used in South Australia and why? *Complement Ther Med* **17**:216–223 (2009).

8. Pirotta MV, Cohen MM, Kotsirilos V, *et al*. Complementary therapies: have they become accepted in general practice? *Med J Aust* **172**:105–109 (2000).
9. Cohen M, Penman S, Pirotta M, *et al*. The integration of complementary therapies in Australian general practice: results of a national survey. *J Altern Complement Med* **11**:995–1004 (2005).
10. www.amc.org.au/images/publications/MedEd-Complementary Medicine2000.pdf.
11. Morgan G, Ward R, Barton M. The contribution of cytotoxic chemotherapy to 5-year survival in adult malignancies. *Clin Oncol (R Coll Radiol)* **16**:549–560 (2004).
12. Kettunen JA, Harilainen A, Sandelin J, *et al*. Knee arthroscopy and exercise versus exercise only for chronic patellofemoral pain syndrome: a randomized controlled trial. *BMC Med* **5**:38 (2007).
13. Nutton RW. Is arthroscopic surgery a beneficial treatment for knee osteoarthritis? *Nat Clin Pract Rheumatol* **5**:122–123 (2009).
14. Morgan AJ, Jorm AF. *Ann Gen Psychiatry* **7**:13 (2008).
15. Ho MJ, Bellusci A, Wright JM. Blood pressure lowering efficacy of coenzyme Q10 for primary hypertension. *Cochrane Database Syst Rev* Oct **7**(4):CD007435 (2009).
16. Lin JG, Chen WL. Review: acupuncture analgesia in clinical trials. *Am J Chin Med* **37**:1–18 (2009).
17. Beckman TJ, Mynderse LA. Evaluation and medical management of benign prostatic hyperplasia. *Mayo Clin Proc* **80**:1356–1362 (2005).
18. Boyle P, Robertson C, Lowe F, *et al*. Meta-analysis of clinical trials of Permixon in the treatment of symptomatic benign prostatic hyperplasia. *Urology* **55**:533–539 (2000).
19. Studer M, Briel M, Leimenstoll B, *et al*. Effect of different antilipidemic agents and diets on mortality: a systematic review. *Arch Intern Med* **165**:725–730 (2005).
20. http://www.help.senate.gov/Hearings/2009_02_26/2009_02_26.html.
21. RACGP and AIMA http://www.racgp.org.au/policy/complementary_medicine.pdf [Accessed 4 March 2011].
22. Hassed CS. Bringing holism into mainstream biomedical education. *J Altern Complement Med* **10**:405–407 (2004).
23. Astin J. Why patients use alternative medicine: results of a national study. *JAMA* **279**:1548–1553 (1998).

24. Linthorst G, Daniels J, Van Westerloo D. The majority of bold statements expressed during grand rounds lack scientific merit. *Med Edu* **41**:965–967 (2007).
25. Friedman LS, Richter ED. Relationship between conflict of interest and research results. *J Gen Intern Med* **19**:51–56 (2004).
26. Brokaw J, Tunnicliff G, Raess B, *et al*. The teaching of complementary and alternative medicine in U.S. medical schools: a survey of course directors. *Acad Med* **77**:876–881 (2002).
27. Barberis L, Schiavone M, Zicca A, *et al*. Unconventional medicine teaching at the universities of the European Union. *J Altern Complement Med* **7**:337–343 (2001).
28. Tsuruoka K, Tsuruoka Y, Kajii E. Complementary medicine education in Japanese medical schools: a survey. *Complement Therap Med* **9**:28–33 (2001).
29. Verhoef MJ, Brundin-Mather R. A national approach to teaching complementary and alternative medicine in Canadian medical schools: The CAM in UME project. *Proc West Pharmacol Soc* **50**:168–173 (2007).
30. The CAM in UME project. http://www.caminume.ca [Accessed 4 March 2011].
31. Haramati A, Lumpkin MD. Complementary and alternative medicine: opportunities for education and research. *Exp Biol Med (Maywood)* **229**:695–697 (2004).
32. Pirotta M, Hassed C, Kotsirilos V, *et al*. Teaching CAM in our medical schools — is it time to bite the bullet? *Focus Health Prof Edu Multidisc J* **9**:6–22 (2007).
33. Marcus DM, McCullough L. An evaluation of the evidence in "evidence-based" integrative medicine programs. *Acad Med* **84**:1229–1234 (2009).

19

The Consumer Experience — Case Studies of Complementary Therapy Use Among People Diagnosed with Cancer

Vivienne O'Callaghan

ABSTRACT

As part of the development of Cancer Council New South Wales' publication of the book *Understanding Complementary Therapies*,[1] the author gathered anecdotal evidence about the use of complementary therapies by people with cancer in Australia. This information gave Cancer Council a glimpse into the reasons why some people chose to use these therapies, what benefits they hoped to gain from them and whether or not these benefits materialised. We were also interested to know whether consumers were talking to their clinicians about using complementary therapies and the attitudes their conventional health practitioners had towards complementary therapies. This background work resulted in Cancer Council obtaining a number of case studies, some of which were published in the book, to give readers an understanding of other people's experiences with complementary therapies. Although only a small sample of people contributed their thoughts, the data collected show that complementary therapies are used by a wide range of people of different ages, genders, social backgrounds and cancer types, although there is a clear leaning towards women with breast cancer. This chapter gives an overview of the different perspectives that consumers have when it comes to thinking about — and using — complementary therapies for cancer.

Keywords: Anecdotes; Cancer; Complementary Therapies; Understanding.

OBTAINING THE STORIES

We sent out an email via Cancer Council's support group network, inviting interested people to share their stories about using any type of complementary therapy during or after cancer treatment. The same request was made to some complementary therapist networks, so that practitioners who had treated cancer patients could either talk about their experiences themselves or put clients in touch with Cancer Council.

We defined complementary therapies as any natural therapy or practice that was used — or could be used — in conjunction with conventional medical treatment for cancer. These included different holistic health-care systems, such as traditional Chinese medicine (TCM), naturopathy and ayurvedic medicine; body-based practices such as massage, aromatherapy and acupuncture; biological-based therapies, such as herbal medicine and nutrition; mind–body techniques including meditation, counselling, music therapy or art therapy; and other therapies that are said to work on a vibrational or energetic level, and which don't fit easily into the above categories, such as homeopathy or flower remedies.

In all, 21 people offered their stories and insights as consumers of complementary therapies. Of these, the author interviewed eight people, two sent through detailed written notes about their experiences, and a further 11 people shared (in writing) some personal thoughts about the key advantages they derived from using their nominated complementary therapy. Some names published here have been changed to protect the contributors' privacy.

AN OVERVIEW OF THE RESPONDENTS AND THE THERAPIES USED

The gender breakdown of contributors was 15 women to six men. Twelve of those women had been diagnosed with breast cancer, with one woman also having a later diagnosis of non-Hodgkin's lymphoma. The other cancer types represented were lung (2), non-Hodgkin's lymphoma (1), [a]prostate (2), bowel (1), kidney (1), thyroid (1) and skin (1).

At the time of sharing their stories, most people had completed their treatment and were in remission. Three people had advanced cancer, one of whom died before the *Understanding Complementary Therapies* book was published.

For privacy reasons, we did not ask the contributors' age, but from their stories, it was clear that the majority were in their 40s or 50s. Two women with breast cancer were in their 30s. Seventeen people lived in metropolitan areas, whereas four were from rural areas. About half the people indicated their job type. Of those, the majority were professionals or white collar workers, one was a farmer, one worked in a pub and one did home duties.

The therapies people tried were TCM, naturopathy, Western herbal medicine, homeopathy, flower remedies, meditation, relaxation, art therapy, shiatsu, acupuncture, qi gong, tai chi, aromatherapy and remedial massage. Although no-one specifically saw a nutritionist, many people also mentioned that they had changed their diet for the better, with their dietary advice coming from either their TCM therapist or naturopath, or, in one case, a shiatsu practitioner who was also a teacher of macrobiotics.

THE EXPERIENCES OF THE WOMEN WITH BREAST CANCER

Although contacting Cancer Council was a matter of individual motivation, it was interesting that the majority of contributors were women and, of them, most had breast cancer. This anecdotally supports existing Australian research indicating that, among cancer

[a] Not including the woman diagnosed with both breast cancer and non-Hodgkin's lymphoma.

patients, women are more likely than men to use complementary therapies, and that people with breast cancer are some of the highest users of complementary therapies.[2] In the general population, there is also evidence to suggest that women of child-bearing age are more likely to use complementary therapies, with nearly half (49%) reporting its use.[3]

Sarah and Alexandra were both in their early 30s when diagnosed with breast cancer. Both were long-term users of complementary therapies, with Alexandra having a qualification in Western herbal medicine. She self-prescribed herbal medicine and nutritional supplements, whereas Sarah saw a TCM practitioner throughout her cancer treatment.

Alexandra's Story

"I am a young woman with advanced breast cancer and I have used herbs and nutrition for several years. I did a lot of my own research into the use of CAM in cancer treatment. I used andrographis[b] *during chemotherapy for my immune system, and I took glutamine*[c] *religiously to stop any stomach and mouth ulceration. I still got heartburn from time to time but it was only with certain foods such as onions.*

During radiotherapy I started to get some blistering underneath the folds of my breasts, as my skin is fair. I sourced an organic, pure vitamin E cream with nothing else in it, which worked a treat. The sores healed and I did not get any more blistering. I was lucky to have an early appointment for my treatment, so I would go home, shower and then apply the cream. I recommended this to the women in my support group too. They had success with the cream as well — nobody had irritation or burns.

The hardest thing to deal with was my stress and nervous system because I continued to work. So I drank a lot of herbal teas and took nutritional supplements to help me through. There was a clear difference between when I took them and when I didn't!"

---

[b]*Andrographis paniculata* is an Asian herb with anti-inflammatory, antibacterial and antiviral properties.[4]

[c]Glutamine is an amino acid that is also used as a nutritional supplement to help improve immune function and maintain cellular health. It is used by cancer patients with cachexia.[5]

Sarah's Story

"A surgeon looks at your anatomy and is just interested in removing the cancerous growths. An oncologist has a specific treatment programme aimed at killing the cancer cells. Although they were caring people, they weren't looking at the whole picture. It was a great benefit to have someone else look at the big picture. That's what my TCM[d] therapist did for me.

I was 33 when I was diagnosed with breast cancer. My surgeon and oncologist recommended a mastectomy, followed by chemotherapy and hormone-suppressant medication; they were keen to start treatment within the fortnight.

I'd used Chinese herbs and acupuncture for several years for other health issues, including chronic fatigue syndrome and severe period pain. So I really wanted to know whether I could beat the cancer without having to go through conventional treatment. I had heard so much about what chemotherapy does to your body, and I was so used to using natural therapies — and really getting something out of them — that I hoped that my TCM practitioner could help me.

The practitioner, however, encouraged me not to turn my back on Western medicine. And when I asked my oncologist and surgeon what my prognosis was, they said I would probably only live for a couple of years without any intervention, so I really had to reconsider their recommendations. I did get a second opinion, and that confirmed the original diagnosis, so in the end I agreed to have the conventional treatment, but spoke to my oncologist about incorporating TCM into my care.

The oncologist said he couldn't stop me from going down that route, but he asked me to keep my TCM practitioner informed of all the conventional treatment I was going to have. He also insisted that my practitioner use clean, new, disposable needles — rather than reusable needles — during acupuncture to minimise the risk of infection.

I had acupuncture a lot during my cancer journey: the day before my mastectomy to reduce psychological and physical stress; following surgery, in hospital, with the aim of building my blood counts, clearing toxins from my body and restoring my qi (energy); throughout

[d] Traditional Chinese medicine is an ancient system of health originating in Asia, which is underpinned by the idea of qi — or energy flow — and yin and yang (balance). It includes therapies and practices such as herbal medicine and nutrition, acupuncture, acupressure, qi gong and tai chi.[6]

chemotherapy, for nausea and to detoxify my body; during hormone-suppressant treatment, for hot flushes and lethargy; and after my breast reconstruction to reduce swelling.

I also took Chinese herbs, which my TCM practitioner changed depending on what side-effects I had. Most formulas were pre-packaged, such as Run Chang Wan, a traditional laxative formula. [e] *I found this remedy more effective than the Coloxyl tablets I'd been prescribed at the hospital.*

Looking back on my experience of cancer and comparing how I fared to other women in my support group, I'm sure these complementary therapies benefited me. My fingernails did not get discoloured from the chemotherapy, I didn't have withdrawal symptoms when I came off the sleeping pills that were prescribed during chemotherapy, and I haven't had any lymphoedema. These were problems other women were experiencing.

Six years on, I haven't had a cancer recurrence, I've become a mother, and I feel very positive about the future. Now I want to put the cancer behind me and get on with the rest of my life."

Although Sarah had not formally studied complementary therapies as Alexandra had, she was well informed about them as a consumer. She had used various therapies over a long period of time before she was diagnosed with cancer, which meant that, after her diagnosis, she initially put more faith in complementary therapies as a cancer cure than conventional treatment.

It is understandable that if someone has had success with complementary therapies for other ailments and if they strongly believe in the philosophy of healing that underpins natural therapies, they may hope or believe they can achieve the same positive outcomes when treating a disease such as cancer.

To date, there are no known cancer cures from the unadulterated natural medicine spectrum, although there are traditional herbal remedies, such as periwinkle (*Vinca rosea*) and yew (*Taxus brevifolia*), which have had active ingredients isolated and synthesised to make the chemotherapy drugs vincristine (Oncovin) and paclitaxel (Taxol).

A problem with people using natural therapies as alternatives to conventional treatment is that a cure is unlikely and, in their

---

[e] Run Chang Wan is made from peach kernel (*Prunus persica*) and Chinese angelica (*Angelica sinensis*), which are said to lubricate the intestines, and rhubarb (*Rheum officinale*), which has a purgative (laxative) action.

delay to use evidence-based curative treatment, they may lessen the chances of that conventional treatment being effective.

In Sarah's case, her TCM practitioner knew the scope and limitations of the therapy she offered. The practitioner was able to inform Sarah clearly about what TCM could and couldn't do for her. By talking to her oncologist — at her TCM practitioner's request — Sarah was able to weigh up the pros and cons of both kinds of treatment and have a clearer understanding of what refusing conventional treatment would mean for her.

Throughout her treatment and recovery, Sarah's new expectations for TCM were met. Although she realised she couldn't 'beat' cancer through TCM alone, she certainly felt that using Chinese herbs and acupuncture helped her beat the side-effects and make the ride a bit smoother.

Julie — like Sarah — was also familiar with complementary therapies. Making a conscious decision to use them was important to her. She decided to have all the conventional treatment recommended to her, but she was convinced that using natural therapies would benefit her too. She felt that integrating the different therapies was going to offer her the best outcome.

Julie's Story

Julie was 42 when she embarked on the range of treatment for breast cancer: surgery, chemotherapy, radiotherapy and hormone therapy. When she started to experience side-effects from the chemotherapy — mainly severe nausea and terrible digestive disturbances — her GP and oncologist didn't have any effective remedies. So Julie asked about using natural therapies, but they couldn't offer her any advice. She decided to work out for herself what she needed.

The main therapies Julie used were TCM, including acupuncture and shiatsu.[f] She went to a medical doctor who also practised

[f]Shiatsu originates from Japan. It is a form of bodywork (massage) in which pressure points on the body are pressed with fingers, thumbs, elbows, knees, hands and feet. The traditional rationale is that this helps unblock energetic pathways in the body to stimulate one's vital force or the flow of qi.[7]

TCM, as she felt it was important to see someone who could interpret test results, explain how conventional cancer treatments worked and understand how herbs and drugs might react with each other. Julie saw her practitioner every two weeks throughout cancer treatment and continued to see her post-treatment.

Julie's body did not react the same way after every chemotherapy session, so her therapist prescribed individual herbal combinations to address the various side-effects she experienced at different stages of treatment. The main issues were her digestive problems, low blood counts and weak vitality. She felt that the herbs really supported and sustained her. She didn't get any infections at all and was able to keep working two days a week.

Julie also had acupuncture, but the therapy she felt she got the most out of was shiatsu. A few days after her chemotherapy sessions, she saw a shiatsu practitioner who used gentle touch. She said, "Shiatsu helped settle my stomach, improved my appetite, reduced constipation and 'put the pieces back together' that felt fragmented after chemotherapy".

When Julie's treatments were complete, she saw a naturopath for advice on supplements that would help her recovery and improve her general well-being. She started taking vitamin C, a multi-vitamin, antioxidants, flaxseed oil[g] and Ganoderma (reishi) mushroom extract.[h]

At the time of her interview, Julie was 18 months post-diagnosis, in remission, feeling healthy, and back working full-time. Four years later, she is still in remission, and continues to use Chinese herbs, mainly for the hot flushes of menopause, as she's unable to take hormone replacement therapy.

Julie was the only person interviewed who talked about shiatsu. From a physical point of view, her positive experience of this therapy is reflected in a study of shiatsu for patients being treated with chemotherapy in a French hospital. Dominique Chevalier was employed as a physiotherapist in a palliative care unit while also

---

[g]Flaxseed oil has been used since the 1950s as a nutritional supplement for its reputed anticancer action. It also has a history of use for digestive and respiratory problems, arthritis and eczema.[7]

[h]Reishi mushroom is commonly used as an immune stimulant herb by people with cancer or HIV.[9]

studying shiatsu. This gave him the opportunity to work with an oncologist to introduce shiatsu treatments into the hospital. He conducted a study of 16 subjects who received shiatsu soon after having a chemotherapy session.[8]

Chevalier reported that the liver and stomach areas were most significantly affected by the shiatsu, possibly because "the liver [has] a clear association with the storage, distribution and elimination of the toxins inherent in the chemotherapy, and the stomach [relates] to the preoccupation with nausea and vomiting experienced by the patients."

The study showed the patients, as a whole, experienced considerable improvements in nausea, vomiting, constipation and mouth problems, which Julie cited as problems she also suffered from. They also had improvements in other side-effects, such as liver pain, ringing in the ears, fever and fatigue.

Catherine — like Alexandra, Sarah and Julie — also had a long history of using natural therapies. She had a qualification in naturopathy and practised in Western herbal medicine and homeopathy. Catherine rarely visited the doctor, but when she felt pain in her breast and noticed changes to her nipple, she saw her GP. She wanted the least invasive conventional treatment as possible, and she knew from the outset that she would use remedies from the herbal and homeopathic pharmacopoeia that she strongly believed would help her.

Catherine's Story

"I had a core biopsy, which showed a malignancy, so I had a lumpectomy in January. I had always had a high-quality diet and lifestyle, and I took herbal and nutritional supplements for my general well-being. After I was diagnosed, I started to take herbs that would specifically help strengthen and support my body to deal with different aspects of surgery, such as recovering from the anaesthetic and helping my tissue heal.

I remember after the operation, I didn't feel pain but I was really nauseous, so I took a homeopathic remedy called ipecac and an anti-nausea herb called slippery elm to quell this.

Luckily the cancer hadn't spread to my lymph nodes, but the surgeon hadn't got a clear margin, so I had to have a mastectomy in February. I had a lot of pain after this operation, so I took homeopathic remedies in the hospital for pain relief (hypericum) and bruising (arnica). I also had herbs to help heal any scar tissue.

My surgeon and I were really happy with the results, and although chemotherapy was an option, I decided not to have it.

I felt it was important to become informed about the cancer and the different treatments, take control of my own situation and keep up a positive attitude. I recovered more quickly than I or my family and friends expected — I was back working full-time in a couple of months — and I feel really positive about the future."

The other women who were interviewed had never used complementary therapies before being diagnosed with cancer and they found out about them via different avenues — two were encouraged to try TCM by friends, and one went to a naturopath when mainstream medical treatment wasn't able to help her with the side-effects of cancer treatment. Interestingly, more people talked about TCM and its subtherapies, such as tai chi, qi gong and acupuncture, than about Western herbal medicine and naturopathy. None of the people contributing stories were from Asian backgrounds.

For Jann and Rebecca, their introduction to TCM by friends became significant for their overall well-being and — consequently — for the way they came to view complementary therapies in general. Jann discovered qi gong[i] during her cancer journey and found a rewarding spirituality from it. When Rebecca chose to explore TCM, it made her feel empowered at a time when she felt quite powerless. This attitude is one of the key reasons that has been determined for people using complementary therapies during cancer, along with the desire to improve well-being and the ability to develop a strong rapport with a complementary therapist.[6]

Both women still have cancer; Jann was successfully treated for breast cancer but was diagnosed three years later with low-grade non-Hodgkin's lymphoma; Rebecca did go into remission, but eight years later was diagnosed with secondary breast cancer. Jann and Rebecca continue to use TCM as they feel it is tremendously valuable.

---

[i] Qi gong consists of meditation, physical movements and breathing exercises to improve the flow of qi (vital energy) around the body and thus decrease stress and improve well-being.[6]

Jann's Story

"When I got breast cancer, my friend — who really believed in TCM — recommended that I go to see her TCM therapist. The therapist was full of confidence that the herbs and acupuncture he prescribed would help me, and I found that very inspiring.

My oncologist said that using Chinese herbs couldn't hurt, but she did ask that I not take them on the days that I was having chemotherapy, just in case there would be some interaction between the drugs and the herbs. My haematologist has been supportive; he said he thought that the Chinese herbs might help my immune system.

On both occasions — when I was being treated for breast cancer and non-Hodgkin's lymphoma — I felt I coped quite well with the chemotherapy, in regards to nausea, tiredness and general sickness. Although the types of herbs I took changed when I was being treated for the different cancers, generally they were for boosting my immune and nervous systems. Some key herbs were astragalus (Astragalus membranaceus), *ganoderma* (Ganoderma lucidum) *and cordyceps* (Cordyceps sinensis).

Early on during my treatment, I started a qi gong class, which I've continued to this day. Qi gong was very calming and made me more self-aware: I was more aware of the energy in my body. For me it was part of managing the whole of my physical, psychological and spiritual needs. I found it easier to learn than tai chi so I was able to do it at home as well as going to classes.

As I still have non-Hodgkin's lymphoma — which is hard to cure — I'm relying even more strongly on complementary therapies such as TCM and qi gong to support my health."

Rebecca's Story

"I went through treatment for breast cancer at the same time as a friend who also had breast cancer. My friend had a more aggressive cancer and was trying alternative therapies such as vitamin C injections and laetrile therapy.[j]

---

[j]Laetrile is a compound produced from amygdalin, found in apricot kernels, which is used as an alternative anticancer therapy. As there is no scientific evidence for its use and there is a risk of cyanide poisoning when ingesting high quantities, it is illegal in the US.[7] Amygdalin is not allowed in any listed medicine in Australia.[10]

She encouraged me to try traditional Chinese medicine. I had never seen a complementary therapist before, so I had reservations, even though my friend's practitioner was accredited.

But I also wasn't sure about using conventional treatment. I didn't know if I could handle putting myself through the trauma of it all. But I was pressured by my family to do so because I had children. So I had the conventional treatment, but I wanted to do something else that I felt would be positive for myself. That's why I thought I'd try TCM, even though I was dubious about it. By taking that step, I felt it really helped me with the emotional side of things.

My oncologist wasn't supportive of complementary therapies but he didn't say I couldn't use them. My TCM therapist told me that the Chinese herbs would increase the effectiveness of the chemotherapy and I'd have fewer symptoms than expected. That was actually the case for me. I don't know whether it was because I felt empowered about doing something for myself or whether it was actually the herbs. But compared to other people I knew going through the same type of conventional treatment, I felt I was faring pretty well.

My therapist also encouraged me to change my diet: I cut out red meat, sugar, dairy, refined flours and processed foods. I lost some excess weight, felt physically better, and had a lot more energy than other people going through the same kinds of treatment as me.

I don't think anyone should be discouraged from making healthy changes to their diet. I really believe that the body has the best chance of healing itself, as long as you give it the right nutrients — though I don't believe diet alone will cure cancer."

Now coping with the challenges of secondary breast cancer but feeling quite well, Rebecca is embracing complementary therapies again — particularly TCM. She said, "For me, complementary therapies are about the only avenue that offers any hope."

Georgina also placed a lot of hope in complementary therapies when she was suffering from unrelenting side-effects of chemotherapy. Although she was dubious and did not know what to expect from naturopathy, she ended up with the results she was wishing for.

Georgina's Story

Georgina was 52 when she was diagnosed with breast cancer. She was shocked by the diagnosis and felt anxious about chemotherapy and radiotherapy, fearing they wouldn't work. She worried a lot about the future. Plagued with persistent urinary tract infections and never-ending digestive troubles, including alternating bouts of diarrhoea and constipation, and pain and griping in her gut, Georgina sought out the local naturopath. She was nervous about the consultation, however. She made it clear that she didn't want the naturopath to try to treat the cancer and she didn't want to take herbs, as she was afraid they would react with the chemotherapy. Georgina wasn't really sure whether the naturopath could even help.

Because Georgina had so many worries, the naturopath taught her to set aside time each day to work on relaxation and meditation techniques. She learnt how to focus on her breathing and how to do a progressive muscle relaxation, so that her whole body felt more at ease. She started going to a meditation class. These measures helped her feel less frenetic and nervous. She learnt to stop wasting energy on worrying and started to become more at ease with her situation, accepting that she had cancer, but also that she had a good chance of overcoming it.

Georgina was quite lackadaisical about her diet and frequently ate processed, spicy or fried foods. The naturopath felt that this kind of diet wouldn't help her digestive problems, so she recommended that Georgina eat blander foods, such as steamed vegetables, salads and plain rice, which would not irritate her stomach and bowel as much. Georgina also agreed to replace coffee with soothing herbal teas that were calming to both mind and body. She made up blends of dried herbs that had a mild action, such as chamomile, balm and fennel. She did not want to try anything stronger, but found that the teas really assisted her digestion. Georgina also drank aloe vera juice for her digestion, and unsweetened cranberry juice for urinary tract infections.

Within a few weeks, these small changes helped clear up her digestive and urinary complaints and she was able to get through the rest of her conventional treatment without too many problems.

After Georgina finished radiotherapy, she was willing to try some immune-stimulant herbs in tablet form and a multi-vitamin supplement to help boost her overall general health and improve her well-being.

A year later, Georgina was given the all-clear for the cancer, which was an enormous relief. However, she found that her weak point was still her digestive system, so she still occasionally does a gentle detox of her bowel using psyllium husks, and she tries to set aside half a day a week to eat only roughage-filled foods to help keep her regular. Because of the positive changes she experienced, she has remained on her simple, wholesome diet, she continues to drink herbal tea instead of coffee, and she still goes to a regular meditation class.

THE EXPERIENCES OF PEOPLE WITH OTHER TYPES OF CANCER

Typically, the people who did not have breast cancer had not used complementary therapies before their diagnosis, and they started using them for different reasons. Richard was facing a dire prognosis and believed he should harness help from all quarters to give him the best chance of living. Attitude became very important to him. Jack was desperate for an alternative to help relieve symptoms and side-effects that conventional medicines seemed unable to address, so he saw a naturopath. Rodney, who was quite sceptical, learnt about reflexology[k] by chance and ended up finding great benefit in it. Lena had seen a naturopath regularly for massage before being diagnosed with bowel cancer but eventually ended up having naturopathic consultations.

Richard's Story

"I was diagnosed with renal cell carcinoma and had a kidney removed within seven days. At that time, they said I had three months to live. It was a very traumatic period, with many decisions to be made. When I was told there weren't many options, complementary therapies took on a new meaning for me.

I decided that the things I thought that made me ill — my lifestyle, diet, mental attitude and work — needed to be modified if I was to start on the road to recovery. I saw a naturopath, a traditional Chinese medicine practitioner and a psychotherapist. In addition, I had a great team at the

---

[k]Reflexology is a treatment where pressure from hands and fingers is applied to areas of the feet known as reflex points. This is said to balance the flow of energy in the body and relieve a variety of health problems.[7]

hospital and I left there in pretty good physical shape; well, as good as you can be after receiving a 400-mm incision in your abdomen and a kidney removed in a five-hour procedure!

I had regular massages and also saw a physiotherapist. I started qi gong, which was not only great exercise, but gave me some inner strength and a feeling of control over my body. Just by changing my diet, I also started to feel that I had a little control of the situation. I could actually do something positive, and that made a huge difference to my attitude and my confidence.

My mother, brother and sister had all been taken by cancer and passed away relatively quickly and painfully. I had been resigned that this was going to happen to me. But my 'team' made the difference, giving me their expertise and commitment, giving me great alternative viewpoints. Not just with therapies or drugs, but with their thoughts and positive discussions about how they believed that I could recover. The people in my team — the Western doctors, the complementary therapists, my family, friends and work colleagues, through their encouragement, gave me the strength and confidence to continue to be positive and take positive actions. There was a wave of positive energy flowing over me from all these great people!

I appreciate that we all adopt different paths when we learn that we have cancer. I respect the disease and recognise that it is still present in my body and that I am working with it to get better. The chances of it 'going away' are extremely remote, so my philosophy is we have to work together. So I don't hate my cancer, I respect it, as I expect to live with it for a very long time! It has been a great journey — scary and damn frightening at times, but very rewarding as well."

Despite being given a prognosis of three months, four years later, Richard is still doing very well. He believes his attitude and positive thinking have been crucial to his survival.

The scientific jury is still out on whether attitude or positive thinking can affect survival. A study of the emotional well-being of head and neck cancer patients, which was published in the journal *Cancer* determined that "the results add to the weight of the evidence that emotional functioning is not an independent predictor of survival in cancer patients".[11] Another study published in the same journal, which looked at the link between optimism and survival in lung cancer patients showed that "there was no evidence that a high level of optimism prior to treatment enhanced survival [and that] encouraging patients to 'be positive' only may add to the burden of having cancer while providing little benefit".[12]

However, a more recently published study suggested that people with an optimistic disposition had more favourable outcomes than those who were more pessimistic.[13] Jill Jouret says in the *Lancet Oncology*, however, "Although the mind–body–cancer connection is an appealing topic for research, particularly for behavioural scientists, there is little evidence that emotions can affect cancer survival. Patients who receive support such as counselling or guided relaxation might have higher scores on quality-of-life measures, but this has not translated into improved survival."[14]

Jack's Story

Jack was in his late 60s when he was diagnosed with several skin cancers on his face and hands. Over the next five years, he had 45 growths removed through surgery, radiotherapy and cryotherapy (a freezing technique). These procedures left him with scarring and red, dry, scaly, itchy skin.

A year after he was first diagnosed with skin cancer, he developed rheumatoid arthritis for which he was prescribed corticosteroids. Unfortunately, this medication exacerbated the inflamed condition of his skin, so he was taken off the corticosteroids but not prescribed anything else. Frustrated with both his joint pain and the poor appearance of his skin, he decided to see a naturopath for the first time in his life.

Jack's diet was fairly balanced, but he only ate frozen vegetables rather than fresh ones and the naturopath didn't think he was getting enough essential fatty acids. He also drank up to 12 cups of tea a day, along with six cans of beer at night. He didn't drink water.

The naturopath encouraged Jack to eat fresh vegetables and culinary herbs such as parsley and sage, as well as to reduce the amount of tea he was drinking, as large quantities of tea can impair the absorption of vitamins and minerals. She also suggested Jack drink some lemon juice in water to boost his vitamin C levels to help repair skin tissue, and to take apple cider vinegar in water in place of tea to improve his water intake and stimulate his digestion.

Jack also started taking some dietary supplements, including essential fatty acids, vitamin C and tissue salts.[1] He used a pure aloe vera gel on the affected areas of his skin.

Within three weeks, Jack's skin irritation and itchiness had cleared up and his joint pain had started to diminish. Six weeks after seeing the naturopath, the joint pain had completely disappeared, despite having suffered from it for the previous four years. Jack was thrilled with the results, and even though he was already quite fit and healthy for his age, he now feels more robust and also more confident due to the improvement in his skin's appearance.

Like Georgina, Jack was new to natural therapies and had not wanted to try anything too strong. But the fairly simple changes the naturopath suggested resulted in significantly positive outcomes. Yet despite the improvements in his skin and joint pain, Jack was nervous about telling his conventional medical team that he had seen a naturopath. He was only one of two people interviewed by Cancer Council who had not informed their mainstream health practitioners of their complementary therapy use.

On this topic, Jack said, *"I didn't want my doctors to know because I didn't think they'd approve. I was also a bit embarrassed because the naturopath managed to help me and yet they didn't."*

Catherine's point of view was: *"There was no point telling my surgeon that I was taking herbs and homeopathy as he wouldn't have been supportive of it, and I knew that those remedies weren't going to do me any harm."*

Quite a few people were unsure about complementary therapies, but with ongoing health issues related to the cancer, they were interested in different options. Rodney was one of these sceptics but, having been told by his specialist that his neuropathy was unlikely to improve, he was open to trying something new. Before he did so — like most of the other people interviewed — he discussed the possibility with his GP.

---

[1] Tissue salts are tablets made from inorganic salts that are found in the body. Their founder believed that if there was an imbalance of these salts in the body, ill-health would result.[15]

Rodney's Story

"I was diagnosed with Burkitt's lymphoma,[m] *which required aggressive chemotherapy over a five-month period. I was hospitalised for three of those months. The chemotherapy left me with a mild form of neuropathy, and two years after I was first diagnosed, I still had slight numbness in my feet and trouble solving problems quickly. At times I felt as though I was very simple, especially when I was tired. My specialist felt that I was unlikely to improve.*

Two years later I met a fellow patient in hospital who told me he was a faith healer. He offered to treat me a couple of times by laying his hands on me. While I didn't feel that he cured me, I did feel that he helped me. This was interesting because initially I was a real sceptic.

Later I was talking to an acquaintance about my experience with the healer. She said she understood what I was talking about, and then told me she was a reflexologist. This was the first time that I had heard of this form of treatment.

That same night, I received a phone call from a friend who was undergoing treatment for breast cancer. She indicated that some of her fellow patients, also suffering from neuropathy, had received some benefit from reflexology. I looked up reflexology on the Internet and then spoke with my GP, who was supportive of me trying it. I rang the reflexologist for an appointment.

I have now been having treatment with the reflexologist for three years. I have had about 20 sessions over that period. The neuropathy has improved, although not completely. I have also suffered from depression, and the reflexologist's support has complemented other treatments for this condition.

I've found reflexology to be a positive part of my recovery from the effects of the treatment. I found myself to be at complete peace and fully relaxed during the treatment sessions. I wish I had started the treatment earlier, and I feel that as a private patient in a public hospital, I would have appreciated the opportunity to have the reflexology treatment while I was in hospital having the chemotherapy."

Although most people thought about using complementary therapies some time after they learnt they had cancer, it was

[m] Burkitt's lymphoma is a rare type of non-Hodgkin's lymphoma affecting B cells.

actually Lena's naturopath who suspected there was something wrong with her and encouraged her to follow this up with her GP. This reflects the vigilance of Sarah's TCM therapist who strongly urged her not to shun conventional treatment, and suggests that complementary therapists can play an important role in channelling ambivalent or resistant patients into conventional health-care that they might otherwise put off or avoid altogether.

Lena's Story

One day when Lena was having a massage, she told her naturopath that she felt very bloated and had been feeling this way for a while. She had seen her GP, who had recommended some tests but she hadn't got around to having them yet because she was too busy. The naturopath encouraged her to get the tests done. But before she managed to get back to the GP, she was admitted to hospital with excruciating abdominal pain, which she thought was appendicitis.

The doctors discovered Lena actually had a very rare bowel cancer so she had surgery immediately and was then prescribed medication.

The sudden diagnosis and cancer treatment were a huge shock and Lena was incredibly fearful that the cancer would return. She went back to her naturopath to get some nutritional support but, during the consultation, it became clear to the naturopath that Lena needed help on a psychological level as well. It was like she had given up on life and just wanted a miracle cure.

The naturopath's treatment plan involved addressing Lena's emotions through counselling and the use of Bach flower essences[n] for her shock, exhaustion and fear. Lena also started yoga to reduce her stress and anxiety. This approach seemed to be beneficial, as her fear diminished within a few weeks, and she became much more realistic about her situation.

---

[n] Bach flower remedies are essences made from flowers. Their philosophy is that underlying emotional problems contribute to physical disease so, if these are addressed, ailments may clear up.[7]

ART THERAPY

Another mind–body technique for which there are positive psychological outcomes is art therapy. This form of psychotherapy is underpinned by the belief that participating in any creative activity can be therapeutic for people.[6] According to the Australian and New Zealand Art Therapy Association, "art therapy uses creative processes, including art making, drama, and movement to improve and enhance physical, mental and emotional well-being".[16]

An art therapist who was conducting a programme at a hospital specifically for people who had completed cancer treatment informed the course participants about Cancer Council's *Understanding Complementary Therapies* book. A number of people offered feedback about the benefits they obtained from the programme.

Marie's Insight

"Making art to reflect on my life has helped me to gain the self-confidence to put aside the difficult time of cancer treatment and look forward to my future."

Sally's Insight

"Art therapy let me verbalise my inner thoughts. It's often easier to discuss something that you have created, rather than to lay open your life and feel exposed."

Christine's Insight

"What I enjoyed most about art therapy was the relaxation and sharing with others who were on a similar journey."

Ray's Insight

"The most significant change that occurred for me from art therapy was finding a way to express difficult feelings. Sometimes there aren't words to describe what you've been through. Yet, art therapy helped me find a way to share my experience. It was very positive."

Alan's Insight

"Art therapy enabled me to finally understand where I was. It helped bring out my feelings. Using the art materials to reflect on my situation has improved my life immensely."

Sue's Insight

"The course helped me deal with issues surrounding my cancer, the death of my sister with breast cancer, teenage children's crises and poor personal boundaries. I was surprised that art could be used to do this. Under the art therapist's directions I created artworks that allowed me to reveal myself in a non-threatening way in a group. I was able to discuss my created work, then, was given the chance to invite the group to offer comments. It was all about the piece of art and the idea we were focusing on, rather than a confronting revelation about me and my problems.

It amazed me that I did reveal things in my art and that they were obvious to me and to the group members. Now, when I look back over the weekly artworks I can see my feelings changing in small, positive ways. I am less anxious and more accepting of my situation, I am sleeping better and thinking more clearly.

The programme was very useful to me and I could see that it also benefited the other members of the group."

ALTERNATIVE THERAPIES

Although the invitation to contribute to Cancer Council's work focused on complementary therapies, people with experience of using alternative therapies were also welcome to contact Cancer Council. Two men did get in touch with stories about natural cancer cures.

One man was the manager of a herbal medicine supply company. He indicated he had a number of testimonials from customers who had used various herbal blends to treat cancer with great success. These blends included herbs such as red clover (*Trifolium pratense*) and burdock (*Arctium lappa*). The testimonials dated back several years.

The second man talked about his grandfather who had used black salve to treat skin cancers. Black salve contains a blend of herbs with actions that are said to be cleansing and warming. The ingredients may vary from supplier to supplier, with common ingredients being sheep sorrel (*Rumex acetosella)*, red clover (*Trifolium pratense*), bloodroot (*Sanguinaria canadensis*), pau d'arco (*Tabebuia spp)*, graviola (*Annona muricata*), galangal (*Alpinia galanga*) and chapparal (*Larrea mexicana)*, along with pine tar, wintergreen oil and zinc oxide. The substance is available for sale on the Internet but it is not approved by the US Food and Drug Administration or the Therapeutic Goods Administration in Australia. It is termed an 'escharotic', meaning a substance that helps form a scab, with the idea that when the salve is applied on a malignant lesion, a scab forms and then drops off, removing the entire cancer.[17]

As the individuals who had used these herbs were not able to be contacted for their experiences to be verified, and because the testimonials came via a business involved in selling herbal medicine, these stories were not pursued for inclusion in the *Understanding Complementary Therapies* book.

CONCLUSION

The preliminary work for *Understanding Complementary Therapies* revealed informative and rich stories about people's reported experiences of using complementary therapies. They showed that a wide range of people think about trying such therapies and that the types of therapies used are varied. Although the initial motivations for trying complementary therapies may have differed, ultimately all of the people sharing their stories had overwhelmingly positive experiences.

Many people experienced significant physical improvements, ranging from the relief of symptoms during chemotherapy, radiotherapy or hormone treatment through to assistance after cancer treatment with ongoing side-effects such as neuropathy or skin complaints. The emotional, psychological and spiritual benefits were also obvious for those who used mind–body approaches such as meditation, qi gong or art therapy. It can also be assumed that, for those people who were focusing on treating physical complaints, the relief of those side-effects must also have helped their emotional states.

An aim in producing *Understanding Complementary Therapies* was to encourage consumers to talk to their mainstream health practitioners about using complementary therapies. It was clear from the stories that the majority in this group of people were already informed enough to have opened up dialogue with their doctors. Those who did not talk to their doctors had made conscious decisions not to.

The responses from the doctors about their patients using complementary therapies were also varied — from disapproval or disinterest through to encouragement and acceptance. It is promising that some specialists were open to their patients trying different therapies and were interested enough to make some safety recommendations (such as using clean needles for acupuncture or not having herbal medicine on chemotherapy days), given there are still many unknowns about how drugs and herbs may interact or how a cancer patient may react to a natural therapy.

Nobody said that they wouldn't use complementary therapies again. In fact, most people continued to use different therapies to help them with their recovery and for other ailments that cropped up after cancer. It is also worth noting that those people with incurable or advanced cancer placed a high value on the ongoing benefits of complementary therapies, perhaps more so than those who went into remission.

There was only one person who had a negative experience of a complementary therapist (a naturopath) who advised against lymph node removal in a mastectomy and taking Tamoxifen. The patient was informed enough to not only decide against this advice but to also change naturopaths! But it serves as a warning that, despite the many complementary therapists who want to work in collaboration with the medical fraternity, there are still practising natural therapists who take a more alternative approach.

It is therefore important that doctors take the time to find out what a patient's views are about complementary and alternative therapies, not only for their safety but also for the health benefits they might gain. By having a non-threatening discussion about a chosen therapy's pros, cons and safety aspects, a person with cancer may be able to add a worthwhile dimension to their multi-disciplinary cancer care that improves their overall well-being.

REFERENCES

1. O'Callaghan V. *Understanding Complementary Therapies — A Guide for People with Cancer, Their Families and Friends*, Cancer Council NSW, Sydney (2008).
2. Girgis A, Adams J, Sibbritt D. The use of complementary and alternative therapies by patients with cancer. *Oncol Res* **15**:281–289 (2005).
3. Eisenberg DA, Davis RB, Ettner SL, *et al.* Trends in alternative medicine use in the United States, 1990–1997: results of a follow up national survey. *JAMA* **280**:1569–1575 (1998).
4. Memorial Sloan-Kettering Cancer Centre. Andrographis (2009). http://www.mskcc.org/mskcc/html/69120.cfm [Accessed 20 September 2010].
5. Memorial Sloan-Kettering Cancer Centre. Glutamine (2008). http://www.mskcc.org/mskcc/html/69240.cfm [Accessed 20 September 2010].
6. Cassileth B. *Integrative Oncology: Complementary Therapies in Cancer Care*, BC Decker Inc., Ontario (2005).
7. American Cancer Society. *Complementary and Alternative Cancer Methods Handbook*, American Cancer Society, Health Content Products, Atlanta (2002).
8. Chevalier D. The role of shiatsu in the treatment of the side effects of chemotherapy. *Shiatsu Society News* Jul–Sep;**62**:16–17 (2007). http://www.shiatsusociety.org/public/newsletter/autumn 2007/chemotherapy.shtml [Accessed 2 July 2010].
9. Memorial Sloan-Kettering Cancer Centre. Reishi mushroom (2008). http://www.mskcc.org/mskcc/html/69353.cfm [Accessed 20 September 2010].
10. Therapeutic Goods Administration. Substances that may be used in listed medicines in Australia, Commonwealth of Australia Department of Health and Ageing (2007). http://www.tga.gov.au/cm/listsubs.pdf [Accessed 20 September 2010].
11. Coyne JC, Pajak TF, Harris J, *et al.* Emotional well-being does not predict survival in head and neck cancer patients — a radiation therapy oncology group study. *Cancer* **110**:2568–2575 (2007).
12. Schofield P, Ball D, Smith JG, *et al.* Optimism and survival in lung carcinoma patients. *Cancer* **100**:1276–1282 (2004).
13. International Association for the Study of Lung Cancer. Lung cancer patients with optimistic attitudes have longer survival, study finds.

2010. http://www.sciencedaily.com/releases/2010/03/100303131656.htm [Accessed 17 September 2010].
14. Jouret J. Psychology — the power of positive thinking. *Lancet Oncol* **11**:230 (2010).
15. Wikipedia. Biochemic cell salts (2010). http://en.wikipedia.org/wiki/Tissue salts [Accessed 22 September 2010].
16. Australian and New Zealand Art Therapy Association. What is art therapy? (2009). www.anzata.org [Accessed 17 September 2010].
17. Barrett S. Don't use corrosive cancer salves (2008). http://www.quackwatch.org/01QuackeryRelatedTopics/Cancer/eschar.html [Accessed 1 July 2010].

20

Evaluating Complementary and Alternative Medicine

Jaklin A. Eliott

ABSTRACT

Popular and scientific interest in complementary and alternative medicine (CAM) appears to increase with every passing year. Despite (or perhaps because of) this, CAM is a highly contested, even controversial, entity, and prompts strong evaluative responses, both positive and negative. In this chapter I examine some of the judgements and debates associated with CAM, CAM users and CAM providers, drawing on published sources including medical and scientific opinion, and research examining media accounts, the perspectives of patients (including users and non-users of CAM), as well as those of medical and CAM practitioners. I begin with a brief examination of the debate regarding the definition of CAM, arguing that this is integral to the different and evolving perceptions and evaluations of CAM. This is followed by an examination of CAM via a very simplistic categorisation of *CAM is good* and *CAM is bad*. Some consideration is also given to the changing position of CAM with regard to the medical profession, particularly as the latter moves to define and promote 'integrative medicine' as incorporating the best of both healthcare systems for the greater good of the populace.

Keywords: Complementary and Alternative Medicine (CAM); Integrative Medicine; Consumers; Practitioners; Review; Evaluation; Judgements; Debate; Integration.

INTRODUCTION

Popular and scientific interest in complementary and alternative medicine (CAM) seems to be increasing with every passing year. As observed by many, survey reports indicate increased use of and increased annual expenditure on CAM within the general populace; CAM has proven a popular media topic in several countries; the number of medical papers discussing or reporting on CAM is on an upward trend; research institutions dedicated to CAM have been an emerging phenomenon; and there appear to be more government and medical institutions specifically allocating funding (in the form of research monies or medical education options) for CAM.[1–12]

Despite, or perhaps because of, this increased interest across a wide cross-section of society, CAM is a highly contested, even controversial, entity. CAM seems to evoke or provoke strong evaluative responses, both positive and negative, with public access to and acceptance of CAM (until recently) in sharp contrast to mainstream medical perceptions. In this chapter I will examine some of the ways in which CAM is characterised, looking at some of the judgements and debates associated with CAM, CAM users and CAM providers. As a qualitative researcher, my work centres on cancer-related topics, and so I acknowledge that this will inform the following discussion. Perhaps fortunately, however, much of the medical and media debate around CAM has been in the context of cancer patients and cancer treatment, and cancer patients are reportedly frequent users of CAM.[1,13,14]

I will begin with a brief examination of the debate regarding definition, as this is integral to the different and evolving perceptions of CAM. Given the aforementioned evaluative component of such perceptions, it seems then logical to undertake an examination of CAM via a very simplistic categorisation of *CAM is good* and *CAM is bad*. Throughout the chapter, I will consider (albeit briefly) how the medical profession has been repositioning itself with regard to CAM, and (it could be argued), in the process, reshaping both itself and CAM as it promotes "integrative medicine" as a necessary merger of the best of both.

DEFINING CAM

Answering the question 'What is CAM?' often takes the form of defining what CAM is not. Thus, for example, CAM is defined as "many different types of therapy ... [that] are not based on scientific findings or theories and not offered in the public healthcare system".[15] CAM is

> a generic name for 'unconventional' methods', distinct from 'conventional methods' that characterise the classical type of academic medicine as taught at academic institutions and Universities and practiced in most clinics and in private doctors offices [sic].[16]

Alternatively, CAM can be thought of as "a group of diverse medical and health care systems, practices, and products that are not generally considered part of conventional medicine".[17] According to such definitions, CAM is not scientific and neither classical nor conventional, neither taught at high-status academic institutions nor practised or endorsed within respected medical systems or settings. Such definitions mark CAM as the 'other' and infer a subordinate status to said conventional or academic medicine.

The World Health Organization (WHO) has observed that CAM "often refers to traditional medicine that is practised in a country but is not part of the country's own traditions", (a singularly unhelpful definition) and is "sometimes used to refer to healthcare that is considered supplementary to allopathic medicine".[18] The WHO acknowledged that this definition "can be misleading" because in, some countries, CAM may have equivalent legal status to allopathic medicine, and may in fact be the major source of primary health-care for many.[18] By this definition, moreover, such health-care practices as ayurvedic medicine or traditional Chinese medicine (TCM) would be considered as CAM in 'Westernised' nations such as Australia, Europe or the US, but not in their country of origin (India and China, respectively).

CAM may thus be seen as a highly ethnocentric term, that in its very naming serves to delineate and subordinate various health-care practices with regard to the *scientific academic medicine* (SAM) that has established itself within 'Western' nations as the dominant profession of modern times.[19] Indeed, the term itself inherently positions CAM in relation to SAM: *complementary* being in addition to, *alternative* being instead of, SAM. This positioning has shaped much of the debate over CAM, regarding both definition and evaluation. Critically, SAM practitioners now recommend the use of those CAMs that have been (scientifically) proven to have positive effects on (measurable) aspects of (various parameters of) patient well-being (e.g.[20–23]). This endorsement, however, applies only when these CAMs make no claim to cure disease, but are used to complement or augment SAM, and specifically to ameliorate disease symptoms or treatment side-effects. As will be further discussed below, SAM remains highly sceptical, even pejorative, about any CAM presented as potentially offering cure, and strongly condemns options or choices to use CAM instead of SAM. Bluntly, (some) complementary is good, (any) alternative is bad.

Not all definitions of CAM, however, centre on distinguishing it from or positioning it in relation to SAM. Some instead assert various uniquely defining features as common to all CAM. As commented upon by many (e.g.[3,13,24]), some suggest that CAM *en masse* espouses concepts of *vitalism*, a metaphysical element that exists beyond the recognised parameters of the physical and biological sciences. CAM advocates typically propose that this life-force essence can be accessed and harnessed by CAM participants to affect illness and health via a mind–body connection. Alternatively, it may be said that CAMs share an emphasis on subjectivity rather than objectivity — holding that the personal experiences and opinions of CAM participants count as 'evidence' of worth, independent of verification of efficacy via scientific testing under carefully controlled conditions. These definitions allude to differences between SAM and CAM, but draw attention to what CAM might offer, rather than what it lacks, perhaps thereby implying some superiority to SAM that fails to recognise a more expansive world-view. CAM is thus implicitly positioned rather more positively than with the exclusionary ('CAM is not…') sorts of definitions.

As a term, however, CAM has been subject to varied criticism. It could be argued that CAM is a meaningless categorical label, because whether a CAM is complementary or alternative depends on how the user uses it (with or instead of SAM), not on the inherent properties of the CAM itself.[25,26] Furthermore, individuals might variably classify different practices or products as CAM or not, for example some patients who use specific foods, relaxation techniques or prayer have considered these to be CAM, whereas others view them specifically not as CAM, but as lifestyle choices.[27] Some SAM writers suggest that, over time, practices or products are either proven to be efficacious (in which case, they are subsumed within SAM) or not (in which case, they ought not to be considered valid 'alternatives' to SAM, specifically with reference to medical, rather than, say, philosophical or spiritual options).[1,15,20]

It is undisputed that CAM "refers to a heterogeneous category, including a wide range of products and practices … encompass[ing] multiple and not always concordant meanings of the body and illness/health", potentially prompting conclusions that "it is of questionable validity to treat all CAM as if equivalent".[24] Precisely because CAM practices and products can be, and have been, differentiated, so they can be differentially evaluated according to various criteria, with potential for disagreement about merit. Accordingly, some have argued that the term CAM unhelpfully combines elements thought sufficiently different to warrant distinction, conveying the impression that generalised conclusions apply to all practices and products within.[1,16,28]

Recognition of differences in merit may underpin an emerging strategy within SAM, namely of demarcation between the components of CAM. The need for such demarcation and difference in evaluation of merit between CAM components is clearly established through claims such as "it is important to separate the objectively helpful complementary entities from the often dangerous and nearly always expensive alternative and unproven remedies and procedures!" [punctuation in original].[16] Nonetheless, although CAM serves as an umbrella term for this vast array of "hugely diverse and paradigmatically disparate"[13] therapeutic practices and products, there is potential to extrapolate judgement from the specific to the general, justifying perceptions that "all less conventional therapies are tarred with the same brush of being alternative" (Brownes Cancer Support Centre[29]) — that is, all CAM are bad.

CAM IS GOOD

Given the reported prevalence rates of CAM use within the general populace, it would seem self-evident that CAM is good or, at least, good for something. The question, however, of 'what is CAM good for?' comes complete with associated debates regarding issues of legitimacy, and the nature of (what counts as) evidence.[13,30,31] At the very least, CAMs are perceived to extend the range of health-care options available to all, to offer choice — and, by so doing, to engage individuals (often cast as consumers in this context) in their own health-care. Given strong culturally-mandated preferences for consumer choice, juxtaposed with beliefs that individuals should manage or take responsibility for their health and that this will have positive outcomes for them,[32,33] CAM emerges as a positive option.

Studies examining patients' reasons for CAM use consistently cite a desire to gain control, whether this be over disease or the meaning of the disease, or to redress a lack of control felt within their encounters with SAM.[32,34–36] This latter is a component of what might be called the 'push' factor.[37] This proposes that patients are pushed towards CAM as a consequence of dissatisfaction with SAM, or SAM professionals. The 'push' factor is implicit in some media accounts of CAM use that depict SAM as reductionist, as focusing "on the disease, not the person", and SAM professionals as failing to care about or for patients' emotional status.[12] Some CAM users and practitioners have characterised SAM similarly, as disempowering, fragmented and impersonal in its approach to patient care.[38] Finally, descriptions of CAM by CAM users such as "it's totally different to the way doctors work ..., they [CAM practitioners] focus on *your* life and your individual stuff and not just the disease and statistics"[13] [emphasis in original] make a clear contrast with SAM to position CAM favourably. To grossly oversimplify and stereotype, it could be said that CAM aims to care for the person, where SAM aims to cure the disease.

There are some dangers, however, for CAM in such judgements. If patients seek CAM because of a perceived lack in SAM, then the obvious solution is to 'fix' SAM, aiming to maximise patient opportunity for involvement in their treatment, improve the interpersonal skills of SAM practitioners, and perhaps promote a 'bio-psycho-social-spiritual' concept of disease and health as normative within SAM — all of which can be discerned within current developments of SAM.

Nonetheless, currently, and in contrast with what is still characterised as an impersonal reductionist SAM, CAM is often judged positively as more holistic and more personalised. As discussed by many (e.g.[13,32,38,39]), within the CAM paradigm, disease and health are considered to be influenced by the life as and where lived, and as comprised of the psychological, social, emotional, spiritual and physical. Disease is further understood to reflect a less-than-optimal functioning or imbalance in one or more of these domains and as located within, affecting and affected by the body as a whole. Therefore, treatment is appropriately focused on the individual as a whole, aiming to restore balance and allow the body to heal. CAM practitioners typically consider environmental, dietary and/or interpersonal factors in the past and the present, requiring that individuals change whatever negative aspects in their lives are deemed to contribute to ill-health. As a consequence, it seems likely that CAM treatment involves relatively large changes in lifestyle,[39,40] with at least some decisions to use CAM characterised by SAM as "... a decision to join a community of shared values and beliefs, akin to a choice of lifestyle, or perhaps even similar to undertaking a religious commitment".[15]

It has been argued, indeed, that people are drawn towards CAM because of its congruence with their personal philosophical beliefs or lifestyle preferences[34,38,41] — a 'pull' factor'.[34] Some have suggested that CAM embodies and reflects various social movements, including individualism, consumerism, and the current ethos of self-responsibility for health; alternatively, that CAM popularity might be attributed to changing social practices (e.g. increased migration and Internet use), changes that increase exposure to medical practices other than that dominant within a culture, or even an increased emphasis on good nutrition and balanced lifestyles.[3,32,38] Compared with SAM, CAM — in attending to the whole interconnected balanced person — may be judged positively to be more congruent with both the current zeitgeist, and contemporary understandings of health and disease, as exemplified in the WHO's definition of health as "a state of complete physical, mental and social well-being and not merely the absence of disease or infirmity".[42]

For many, CAM is also judged to have beneficial consequences on health and well-being, though how and in what domains this is realised is sometimes contentious. Perhaps least contentiously, CAM is perceived to have merit when SAM cannot or fails to provide a (promised) cure. Use of CAM reportedly increases during chronic illness or when dying[43,44] and, currently, some SAM practitioners actively recommend CAM use in the context of cancer and palliative care.[20,45–48] Such positive portrayals of CAM, however, may be a dual-edged sword. There is a danger of an implicit (and sometimes explicit) attitude of 'well it can't do any harm' that works subtly to denigrate or dismiss the value of CAM.[13] Moreover (as previously indicated), official SAM endorsement of any specific CAM in any context rests on evidence of positive outcomes in scientifically-controlled tests. CAM such as hypnosis, meditation, relaxation, acupuncture, transcutaneous electrical nerve stimulation, massage, exercise, and some dietary regimens have, so to speak, passed the tests, and become relatively acceptable in mainstream medical practice.[20,48–50] The vast majority of CAMs, however, have not. Despite this, patients and the public evidently continue to use and approve of many scientifically-unsubstantiated CAMs, often with the justification that they make you "feel better" even if they don't "make you better".[24] As noted earlier, some have suggested that a defining feature of CAM is that the perceptions of those using CAM are deemed at least as salient as any evidence obtained through science. Indeed, anecdotal evidence and personal testimony of various benefits of CAM are a dominant feature of positive media accounts,[12] and of promotional materials presented by CAM advocates (e.g. *www.gawler.org/testimonials/* and *www.naturesalternatives.com/silver/testimonials.html*). They also feature in reasons provided by SAM doctors for why they incorporate particular CAM into their clinical practice; namely, that, even if these CAM aren't scientifically legitimated, they've personally witnessed their clinical efficacy.[13,51] CAM is good, because personal experience tells us so. To challenge, deny or dismiss this perception of CAM therefore is to accuse those holding it of lying or of foolishness — accusations unlikely to promote positive interpersonal relationships, whether between persons or institutions.

CAM is sometimes deemed to counter or to offer an effective antidote against the perils of modern life. It is proposed that, through a combination of things such as poor diet, increased stress, increased use of artificial substances, and neglect of the spiritual or the natural, modern living effectively undermines or depletes the immune system, leaving us prone to disease.[52,53] Therefore, judicious uptake of CAM can redress such modern ills, drawing upon the healing power of nature,[3] and, sometimes, ancient or at least old wisdoms and traditions (e.g. TCM, ayurveda, naturopathy). Some research indicates that, in those already struck down by illness such as cancer, a common reason for undertaking CAM appears to be a desire to strengthen the immune system and permit a natural process of healing.[54,55] 'Natural' appears to be a common descriptor of CAM, as patient, public and media accounts often depict CAM as inherently natural, and therefore CAM practices or products as safe, good and unlikely to cause harm (e.g.[12,53,55]). Again, in such accounts, this positive evaluation of CAM is sometimes strengthened through contrast with the invasive, toxic and debilitating treatments offered by SAM.

Finally, CAM can be a source of hope in the face of serious illness. One of the most commonly cited reasons for CAM use in patients with cancer is to find hope.[36] Given the perception that hope is vital to patient well-being,[56,57] CAM use is thus further open to positive evaluation. For some patients, hope may be centred on the experience of care and support, or the increased perception of control provided through CAM.[58] In such instances, patients, CAM practitioners and SAM practitioners will find common ground that CAM provides positive outcomes. Such accord disappears, however, in the not-uncommon cases where patients turn to CAM in the hope that it will cure their disease.[43,55,59,60] Although this can be depicted as a rational choice to pursue all and any options that might successfully treat disease,[60] it is often troublesome to SAM, specifically as SAM considers achieving cure as a consequence of using CAM to be unlikely,[22,23] to put it mildly. Concerns arise that CAM is providing unrealistic or false hope — and, as having or providing false hope is rarely positively perceived,[5] CAM is evaluated as bad. I now turn to a consideration of this and other ways in which CAM is negatively evaluated.

CAM IS BAD

The perception that CAM use is prompted by false hope is a regular feature of negative judgements about CAM users and providers. Disapproval is most pronounced, however, where it is perceived that CAM use is motivated exclusively by the search for cure of life-threatening disease. For example, Australian media accounts of using CAM to treat cancer have described CAM practitioners (specifically offering alternative rather than complementary therapies) as exploitative

> 'peddlers of false hope' ... who take 'advantage of vulnerable cancer battlers' ... [who are] typically depicted as innocent victims that, through no fault of their own due to their desperate situation, ... [are] exploited by 'rogues peddling bogus cancer cures'.[12]

Harsh words indeed and, given that the media both reflects and shapes public attitudes, they indicate the extent to which CAM can elicit strong negative evaluation within the general public.

Judgements about CAM can appear particularly damning when CAM use results in either delays in seeking, or complete refusal to access treatment provided by SAM (e.g.[16]). This may be because, unlike CAM, SAM can cite statistical evidence to support the claim that it provides curative treatment.[13,16] Patients who eschew SAM are therefore readily interpreted as decreasing their chances of survival, as "risking their lives".[12] Some medical professionals have thus identified CAM providers as fraudulently exploiting those with "incurable or fatal disease who ... suspend their normal commonsense judgement because of the desperate situation in which they find themselves",[21] and CAM users as "prepared to do what no rational person would do because ... [of] their irrational situation, ... facing something that's going to kill them".[61] Similarly, CAM providers have been described by Australian suburbanites as exploiting those who are desperately ill,[53] and cancer patients who specifically identified themselves as non-users of CAM characterised those who did use CAM as "that gullible that they'll do anything" or as prepared to "grasp at anything".[24] In the eye of the beholder, the distinction between a person's 'rational choice' to try any measures to treat disease, and a 'desperate grasping at anything' may be difficult to sustain, particularly at the end of life. Thus, the positive perception of CAM as empowering patients in their search for health can easily be reframed as exploiting them — and a hope offered as fundamentally just a hoax.[62]

Many of the aforementioned negative accounts include a concern regarding the financial cost of CAM, particularly as the vast majority must be paid for by the patient.[14,16,20] Concern or disapproval regarding costs is implied through the use of terms above such as 'fraudulent' 'peddlers' 'exploiting' the vulnerable; in medical observations that CAM is a highly organised commercial enterprise raising "considerable profits";[21] and in media descriptions of CAM as a "multi-million-dollar industry", and naming of the large sums paid by some CAM users to no avail.[12] Disapproval is made more explicit in medical claims that CAM practitioners are "greedy ghouls ... in it for the money",[63] and assertions by non-users of CAM that using CAM is a "waste of money" and that users are simply "shelling out money"[24] — with 'for nothing' implied.

Similar concerns can be found regarding the cost of CAM in terms of time. Some CAMs require significant effort and time commitments, and medical professionals worry that this might be excessive,[22] whereas some patients dismiss CAM as a waste of time, particularly when patients might have little time left.[24] Judgements about monies and time spent, however, often rely on judgements about the aims and outcomes of CAM use; if the aims are achieved, costs become less relevant.[24] One might also challenge the basis of such negative views of CAM with observations that SAM is rarely subject to the same evaluative judgements. Particularly at the end of life, many costly SAM practices and products fail to achieve the desired outcome, yet are not usually condemned as a waste of time or money.

One of the most common reasons why CAM is identified as bad is because of its potential for harm. Harm might be indirect, realised via the above factors (raising false hope, wasting time or money), but both the media and SAM cite instances of actual physical harm, ranging from toxicity and negative interactions with SAM prescriptions through to malnutrition, physical injury, and even death.[12,22,47] The extent of scientific evidence of actual harm caused by specific CAMs, however, is relatively small compared with the vast array of CAMs on offer, and this is due in part to the paucity of research examining the effects of CAM.[14] Some reasons given for this lack include reluctance of SAM clinicians to undertake, or of ethical committees to endorse, CAM research; difficulties in gaining research funding; and multiple problems with designing appropriate and feasible projects, that are, moreover, acceptable to both CAM and SAM proponents.[14] Somewhat ironically, this lack of evidence can further engender and justify doubt about the value of CAM, as manifest, for example, in media claims that "their benefits and harms are not known" and "many ... [are] of questionable efficacy".[12] Furthermore, given the priority placed upon scientific evidence (at least in theory), SAM practitioners can and do justify considerable scepticism about CAM[13] with assertions that CAMs are "considered unproven or of questionable efficacy and toxicity"[16] alongside cautionary arguments that "until adequately tested, *no* treatment can be considered safe or effective"[22] [italics in original] working to undermine confidence in the-mostly-untested CAM.

Many, however, have asserted that scientific tests (fundamental to the scientific research process) cannot adequately assess CAM. Drawing on the holistic cornerstone of CAM, it can be argued that, if CAM efficacy is the product of "a complex mix [of factors] ... with no single element that can be isolated and attributed to the remedy alone", then scientific practices of testing will interfere with or fundamentally change CAM,[64] rendering testing meaningless. Some CAM practitioners have consequently resisted the process of scientific research claiming that it

> doesn't mesh well with the integrative healing philosophy of whole person care. As clinicians, we evaluate patients as whole people, the sum of all parts, whereas outcomes research seems to want to break everything into individual parts.[65]

Such assertions invoke ideas of holism and personalised care to position CAM resistance to testing positively, as part of the greater 'healing' and 'holistic' philosophy underpinning CAM, and as consequential on the altruistic motives of caring practitioners. Some SAM practitioners, however, have described both those resisting and resistance to scientific testing more negatively, asserting that CAM proponents

> often reject scientifically based testing or proclaim their own, sometimes obscure principles of attesting benefits … . [They] do not accept — or even actively fight — mainstream academic medicine and often tend to distract patients from curative treatments … . [They] use their own specific nomenclature, rules of clinical assessment, interpretation of results, and statistical evaluation and public exclusively in their own publication media outside the general scientific community.[16]

Here, CAM and CAM practitioners are positioned as extremist 'others' and as unreasonable, insular, isolated and dangerous; qualities singularly ill-suited for or desirable in providers of health-care, and ones that work to justify SAM concern for patients' well-being. In addition, this description functions to cast considerable doubt upon the status of CAM, and specifically to render any 'results' and 'statistical evaluation' (i.e. research) provided by CAM and, by extrapolation, CAM as an enterprise, as both unacceptable and untrustworthy.

Moreover, even when scientific testing of specific CAM can and has occurred to a standard considered acceptable by the SAM community, concern is not necessarily eradicated. The safety and efficacy of individual CAM products, practices or practitioners can (almost) always be called into question. To illustrate how this is achieved: following on from observations regarding the effectiveness of St. John's wort and evidence that other CAM botanicals (e.g. ginseng and echinacea) appear marginally beneficial or at least not harmful (a description that appears to damn with faint praise), a closing argument is presented that "scientific evaluations of CAM products have shown that standardisation is so poor that preparations might not contain ingredients noted on the product label".[21] Doubt is sometimes linked to the fact that CAMs, with very few exceptions, stand outside processes of judicial regulation. Claims that "inadequate quality control of manufacturing and packaging in this unregulated industry and absence of requirements for and governmental regulation of safety and efficacy",[20] and warnings to patients that "labelling regulations do not ensure that what is on the bottle corresponds to what is on the label"[50] strongly convey the impression that CAM is fundamentally untrustworthy, allowing arguments to centre on an always-present potential for harm. This sometimes, but not always, takes the form of a contrast with the stringently-regulated SAM, as the media report that CAM, "the multi-million-dollar industry [is] not subject to the same level of scrutiny" as SAM, such that one "should be very cautious of stepping outside the conventional medical system, which has many inbuilt safeguards".[12]

Of course, one solution is to make CAM more like SAM — more regulated, codified, standardised, and subject to independent 'objective' review. Some have argued that this process is already occurring,[2] and it may both reflect and help to establish an increased legitimacy of and acceptance of CAM, particularly by SAM. Along with the strategy of reshaping SAM to incorporate valued CAM features (e.g. holistic personalised care), this may have contributed to the emergence of attempts within SAM to meld SAM and CAM or, more specifically, to incorporate approved CAM practices and products into SAM as the mainstream medical paradigm, thus creating a new category of 'integrative medicine'.[14] Some SAM affiliates champion the integration of mainstream SAM with "safe, efficient, and effective" CAM as "an ideal situation [where] individual patients, as well as the whole community would be the beneficiaries of integrated, holistic care".[2] Nonetheless, any proposed integration is very much upon terms dictated by SAM, with integrated CAM being confined to (as discussed above) those with scientifically-proven efficacy and safety. This caveat necessarily limits acceptable CAM to those amenable to such testing. In opinion and recommendation, as well as in practice, SAM acts as the gatekeeper, limiting which and how much CAM can be integrated into mainstream medical care.[13] Some caution therefore that integration of CAM and SAM may

> actually mean subjugation, disintegration, or marginalisation ... and may fundamentally alter CAM … . If part of the attraction of CAM is its uniqueness, or its non-biomedical conception of health and disease, then integration might result in the loss of this alternative, or … [the] expansion of conventional medical, as it absorbs evidence-based CAM and the reshaping, shrinking and marginalisation of the CAM modalities that remain.[47]

Similar sentiments (both positive and negative) about the possibilities of integration are voiced by CAM users and providers.[13,38]

CONCLUSION: CAM IS …

In perusing the (expanding) field of research into, claims regarding, or commentary upon CAM, I am struck by the plethora of contradictory judgements that abound, only a few of which I have delved into here. Depending on where you look, or who you believe, CAM is seen: to empower or exploit; to be natural, yet highly commercialised; to be grounded in experience, yet ineffable; to heal or harm; to offer cure or care; as a new social phenomenon and an ancient tradition; as effective and efficacious, or useless if not harmful; as a hope or a hoax; as a rational health-care option or a desperate and ill-informed choice; as good, as bad, and so on. Given that many of these judgements are emotionally or ideologically loaded, it seems likely that CAM will continue to evoke or provoke strong evaluative responses and heated debate. It seems equally likely that, despite, or perhaps in part because of this, CAM will remain a moveable feast that resists categorisation and definition, but will continue to constitute a significant feature of modern individualised health-care.

REFERENCES

1. Cassileth BR, Deng G. Complementary and alternative therapies for cancer. *Oncologist* **9**:80–89 (2004).
2. Cohen MM. CAM practitioners and 'regular' doctors: is integration possible? *Med J Aust* **180**:645–646 (2004).
3. Coulter ID, Willis EM. The rise and rise of complementary and alternative medicine: a sociological perspective. *Med J Aust* **180**:587–589 (2004).
4. Gaster B, *et al*. What should students learn about complementary and alternative medicine. *Acad Med* **82**:934–938 (2007).
5. Goldbeck-Wood S, *et al*. Complementary medicine is booming worldwide. *Br Med J* **313**:131–133 (1996).
6. Harris P, Rees R. The prevalence of complementary and alternative medicine use among the general population: a systematic review of the literature. *Complement Ther Med* **8**:88–96 (2000).

7. MacLennan AH, Wilson DH, Taylor AW. The escalating cost and prevalence of alternative medicine. *Prev Med* **35**:166–173 (2002).
8. Milazzo S, Ernst E. Newspaper coverage of complementary and alternative therapies for cancer — UK 2002–2004. *Support Care Cancer* **14**:885–889 (2006).
9. Raschetti R, *et al.* Complementary and alternative medicine in the scientific literature. *J Altern Complement Med* **11**:209–212 (2005).
10. Richardson M. Biopharmacologic and herbal therapies for cancer: research update from NCCAM. *J Nutr* **131**(suppl 11):3037S–3040S (2001).
11. Weeks L, Verhoef M, Scott C. Presenting the alternative: cancer and complementary and alternative medicine in the Canadian print media. *Support Care Cancer* **15**:931–938 (2007).
12. Mercurio R, Eliott JE. Trick or treat? Australian newspaper portrayal of complementary and alternative medicine for the treatment of cancer. *Support Care Cancer* **19**:67–80 (2011).
13. Broom A, Tovey P. *Therapeutic Pluralism: Exploring the Experiences of Cancer Patients and Professionals*, Routledge, London (2008).
14. Robotin MC, Penman AG. Integrating complementary therapies into mainstream cancer care: which way forward? *Med J Aust* **185**:377–379 (2006).
15. Hansen K. The proper role of evidence in complementary/alternative medicine. *J Med Philos* **35**:7–18 (2010).
16. Diel V. The bridge between patient and doctor: the shift from CAM to integrative medicine. *Hematol Am Soc Hematol Educ Program* **2009**:320–325 (2009).
17. National Center for Complementary and Alternative Medicine (NCCAM). *Get the Facts: What is Complementary and Alternative Medicine?* NCCAM, National Institute of Health, Bethesda, MD (2007). http://nccam.nih.gov/health/whatiscam/#sup2 [Accessed 5 March 2008].
18. World Health Organization (WHO). *Legal Status of Traditional Medicine and Complementary/Alternative Medicine: A Worldwide Review,* WHO Department of Essential Medicines and Pharmaceutical Policies, Health Systems and Services Cluster, Geneva (2001). http://apps.who.int/medicinedocs/en/d/Jh2943e/ [Accessed 20 April 2010].
19. Freidson E. *Profession of Medicine: A Study of the Sociology of Applied Knowledge,* The University of Chicago Press, Chicago, IL (1988).

20. Deng G, Cassileth BR, Yeung KS. Complementary therapies for cancer-related symptoms. *J Support Oncol* **2**:419–429 (2004).
21. Dwyer JM. Good medicine and bad medicine: science to promote the convergence of 'alternative' and orthodox medicine. *Med J Aust* **180**:647–648 (2004).
22. Ernst E. Complementary cancer treatments: hope or hazard? *Clin Oncol* **7**:259–263 (1995).
23. Society for Integrative Oncology. Integrative oncology practice guidelines. *J Soc Integr Oncol* **5**:65–84 (2007).
24. Eliott JA, Kealey CP, Olver IN. (Using) complementary and alternative medicine: the perceptions of palliative patients with cancer. *J Pall Med* **11**:58–67 (2008).
25. Cassileth BR, Chapman CC. Alternative and complementary cancer therapies. *Cancer* **77**:1026–1034 (1996).
26. Tataryn DJ. Paradigms of health and disease: a framework for classifying and understanding complementary and alternative medicine. *J Altern Complement Med* **86**:877–892 (2002).
27. Balneaves LG, Kristjanson LJ, Tataryn D. Beyond convention: describing complementary therapy use by women living with breast cancer. *Patient Educ Couns* **38**:143–153 (1999).
28. Caspi O, *et al.* On the definition of complementary, alternative, and integrative medicine: societal mega-stereotypes vs. the patients' perspectives. *Altern Ther Health Med* **9**(6):58–62 (2003).
29. Parliament of Australia Senate Community Affairs References Committee. *The Cancer Journey: Informing Choice. Report on the Inquiry into Services and Treatment Options for Persons with Cancer*, Commonwealth of Australia, Senate Printing Unit, Parliament House, Canberra (2005). http://www.aph.gov.au/Senate/committee/clac_ctte/cancer/report/index. htm [Accessed 22 April 2010].
30. Caspi O, Koithan M, Criddle MW. Alternative medicine or "Alternative" patients: a qualitative study of patient-oriented decision-making processes with respect to complementary and alternative medicine. *Med Decis Making* **24**:64–79 (2004).
31. Verhoef M, *et al.* Assessing the role of evidence in patients' evaluation of complementary therapies: a quality study. *Integr Cancer Ther* **6**:345–353 (2007).
32. McClean S. 'The illness is part of the person': discourses of blame, individual responsibility and individuation at a centre for spiritual healing in the North of England. *Sociol Health Illn* **27**:628–648 (2005).

33. Schneider CE. *The Practice of Autonomy: Patients, Doctors, and Medical Decisions*, Oxford University Press, New York (1988).
34. Astin JA. Why patients use alternative medicine: results of a national study. *JAMA* **279**:1548–1553 (1998).
35. Richardson MA, *et al.* Complementary/alternative medicine use in a comprehensive cancer center and the implications for oncology. *J Clin Oncol* **18**:2505–2514 (2000).
36. Verhoef M, *et al.* Reasons for and characteristics associated with complementary and alternative medicine use among adult cancer patients: a systematic review. *Integr Cancer Ther* **4**:274–286 (2005).
37. Furnham A, Smith C. Choosing alternative medicine: a comparison of the beliefs of patients visiting a general practitioner and homeopath. *Soc Sci Med* **26**:685–689 (1988).
38. Barrett B, *et al.* Themes of holism, empowerment, access, and legitimacy define complementary, alternative, and integrative medicine in relation to conventional biomedicine. *J Altern Complement Med* **9**:937–947 (2003).
39. Salkeld EJ. Holistic physician's clinical discourse on risk: an ethnographic study. *Med Anthropol* **24**:325–347 (2005).
40. Broom A, Tovey P. Exploring the termporal dimension in cancer patients' experiences of nonbiomedical therapeutics. *Qual Health Res* **18**:1650–1661 (2008).
41. Taylor MD, *et al.* Complementary and alternative medicines versus prescription drugs: perceptions of emergency department patients. *Emerg Med J* **23**:266–268 (2006).
42. World Health Organization (WHO). *WHO Definition of Health*, Preamble to the Constitution of the World Health Organization as adopted by the International Health Conference, New York, 19–22 June 1946; signed on 22 July 1946 by the representatives of 61 States (Official Records of the World Health Organization, no. 2, p. 100) and entered into force on 7 April 1948. http://www.who.int/about/definition/en/print.html [Accessed 24 April 2010].
43. Correa-Velez I, *et al.* Use of complementary and alternative medicine and quality of life: changes at the end of life. *Palliat Med* **17**:695–703 (2003).
44. Miller MF, *et al.* Dietary supplement use in individuals living with cancer and other chronic conditions: a population-based study. *J Am Diet Assoc* **108**:483–494 (2008).

45. Ernst E, Filshie J, Hardy J. Evidence-based complementary medicine for palliative cancer care: does it make sense? *Palliat Med* **17**:704–707 (2003).
46. Kellehear A. Complementary medicine: is it more acceptable in palliative care practice? *Med J Aust* **179** (suppl 6):S46–S58 (2003).
47. Kerridge IH, McPhee JR. Ethical and legal issues at the interface of complementary and conventional medicine. *Med J Aust* **181**:164–166 (2004).
48. Mansky PJ, Wallerstedt DB. Complementary medicine in palliative care and cancer symptom management. *Cancer J* **12**:425–431 (2006).
49. Vitetta L, Sali A. Complementary medicine in palliative care. *Aust Fam Physician* **35**:783 (2006).
50. Weiger WA, *et al.* Advising patients who seek complementary and alternative medical therapies for cancer. *Ann Intern Med* **137**:889–903 (2002).
51. Eastwood HL. Complementary therapies: the appeal to general practitioners. *Med J Aust* **173**:95–98 (2000).
52. Baer HA. The drive for legitimation in Australian naturopathy: successes and dilemmas. *Soc Sci Med* **63**:1771–1783 (2006).
53. Conner LH. Relief, risk and renewal: mixed therapy regimens in an Australian suburb. *Soc Sci Med* **59**:1695–1705 (2004).
54. Boon H, *et al.* Breast cancer survivors' perceptions of complementary/alternative medicine (CAM): making the decision to use or not to use. *Qual Health Res* **9**:639–653 (1999).
55. Correa-Velez I, Clavarino A, Eastwood H. Surviving, relieving, repairing, and boosting up: reasons for using complementary/alternative medicine among patients with advanced cancer: a thematic analysis. *J Palliat Med* **8**:953–961 (2005).
56. Eliott JA, Olver IN. Hope, life, and death: a qualitative analysis of dying cancer patients' talk about hope. *Death Stud* **3**:609–638 (2009).
57. Eliott JA, Olver IN. The discursive properties of 'hope': a qualitative analysis of cancer patients' speech. *Qual Health Res* **12**:173–193 (2002).
58. Truant T, Bottorff JL. Decision making related to complementary therapies: a process of regaining control. *Patient Educ Couns* **38**:131–142 (1999).
59. Boon H. Men with prostate cancer: making decisions about complementary/alternative medicine. *Med Decis Making* **23**:471–479 (2003).
60. Yates PM, *et al.* Patients with terminal cancer who use alternative therapies: their beliefs and practices. *Sociol Health Illn* **15**:199–216 (1993).

61. Broom A, Adams J. Oncology clinicians' accounts of discussing complementary and alternative medicine with their patients. *Health* **13**:317–336 (2009).
62. Young P. Laetrile: hope for cancer patients, or just a hoax? *Natl Obs* **May 16**:1+ (1997).
63. Kennedy BJ. Use of questionable methods and physician education. *J Cancer Educ* **8**:129–131 (1993).
64. Walach H. Reinventing the wheel will not make it rounder: controlled trials of homeopathy reconsidered. *J Altern Complement Med* **9**:7–13 (2003).
65. Verhoef MJ, *et al*. Identifying the barriers to conducting outcomes research in integrative health care clinic settings — a qualitative study. *BMC Health Serv Res* **10**:14 (14 Jan 2010). http://www.biomedcentral.com/1472-6963/10/14 [Accessed 24 April 2010].

21

Complementary and Alternative Medicine: The Perspective of a Cancer Patient

Loretta Marron

ABSTRACT

Now growing at a rate of over 5% per annum, the $3 billion 'alternative health therapies' business is now positioned in the top ten growth industries in Australia. With poor regulation of both therapeutic goods and the unregistered therapists who promote them, cancer patients may well be putting their health at risk when they place their faith in many so-called 'natural' or 'traditional' treatments. With a focus on what complementary therapists refer to as 'energy medicine' and 'nutritional medicine', this chapter explores the risks and benefits of some of the more popular alternative health-care choices. While investigating their histories, it outlines what influences cancer patients to try these unproven therapies, and the conflict and contrast in information relating to the claims made for them and the conclusions of evidence-based research. Although there are a number of complementary therapies that are of benefit to some patients, both during and after their cancer treatments, 'natural' does not always equal 'safe', may be expensive and may even compromise their health. More patients now want a greater say in their choices of treatment, and selecting complementary therapies that may help is another of the many challenges faced in trying to make informed choices, as we navigate along our individual roads on our journeys to recovery.

Keywords: Acupressure; Aloe Vera; Aromatherapy; Australian Competition and Consumer Commission; Bio-energy Field Mapping; Bio-feedback; Bio-impedance; Black Cohosh; Blood; Blood Type; Breuss Cancer Cure; CAM; Chakras; Chelation; Complementary Medicines; Department of Fair Trading; Diagnostics; Doctors; eBooks; Electrical Resistance; Energy Medicine; Gerson Diet; Ginger; Hair; Herbal Remedies; Holistic; Homeopaths; Homeopathy; Hydrotherapy; Hypnosis; Kinesiology; Massage; Medical Devices; Medicines; Meridian; Music; Natural; Natural Therapists; Naturopaths; Nutritional Medicines; National Prescribing Service; Painting; Pharmacists; Pilates; Pills; Public Summary; Qi; Quack; Reflexology; Regulation; Reiki; Relaxation; Scams; Sigma; Skeptics; Supplements; Tai Chi; TGA; Traditional; Urine; VEGA; Vital Force; Vitamins; Yoga.

INTRODUCTION

Alternative therapists are spreading unchecked and unchallenged into the heart of our communities. Trumpeting the benefits of tradition, these unregulated and uninsured health practitioners are setting up makeshift clinics everywhere from homes in quiet backstreets to glamorous high-street locations. Although some offer proven therapies, others provide questionable holistic treatments, and claim they can cure nearly every real and imaginary health condition with an inexhaustible and continually mutating toolbox of scientifically implausible treatments and remedies.

Many patients may just want support to help them on their cancer journey, but a growing number of them, feeling confused, frightened and abandoned after long treatments, are walking out of oncology wards heading for these practitioners, encouraged by references in booklets from well-meaning support groups and friends. Of real concern to me is that books and websites or even information provided by Cancer Councils may provide patients with the impetus to try these treatments.

Others, frightened by the severity of surgery, chemotherapy and radiotherapy, or influenced by unsubstantiated conspiracy theories[1] against modern medicine, or sadly, because they have run out of conventional treatment options, are turning to heavily promoted unproven energy and nutrition-based 'natural' cancer cures.

So what works and what doesn't? What helps and what harms? Who do we trust and what do we ask? We need to know before we make any health-related decisions, so I propose here to summarise relevant information on some of the complementary and alternative medicines (CAMs) in common use by cancer patients.

ALTERNATIVE MEDICINES

'Energy Medicines'

What is 'Energy Medicine'?

'Energy medicine' is increasing in popularity with a growing number of cancer patients. Based on the concept that you are sick as a result of the depletion of your body's 'vital force' or qi,[2] (caused by illness-induced meridian blockages), CAM practitioners claim that you can be cured by manipulating your body's 'energy fields'.

According to Professor Edzard Ernst and Professor Michael Baum, in *The American Journal of Medicine*, energy-based alternative therapies "are based on obsolete or metaphysical concepts of human biology and physiology that have to be described as absurd with proponents who will not subject their interventions to scientific scrutiny or if they do, are not found wanting, suggest that the mere fact of critical evaluation is sufficient to chase the healing process away".[3]

These therapies include reiki, reflexology and homeopathy. Even though some of them are offered in high-profile cancer wellness centres, the concept of these therapies would "advocate re-writing the laws of physics"[4] but they also have no known basis in human physiology.

Reiki[5] is a spiritual practice developed in 1922 by Mikao Usui, who claimed to have the ability of healing without energy depletion. A form of palm healing, it is a therapy whereby practitioners believe they are moving 'healing energy' (a form of qi) through their palms to cure their patients. There is no scientific evidence for the existence of healing energy, life force, vital force, qi or meridians[6] in the body, or any mechanism for its manipulation, and a systematic review of randomised clinical trials conducted in 2008 did not support the efficacy of reiki or its recommendation for use in the treatment of any condition.

Reflexology[7] (a type of zone therapy) is based on the principle that there are reflexes in feet that correspond to every part, gland and organ of the body and that applying pressure to specific parts of patient's feet can improve their health through the manipulation of their qi. Reflexology is based on an absurd theory with no proven efficacy and has not been demonstrated to influence the course of any illness. Reflexology, at best, provides the same benefits as an ordinary extended foot massage.

Homeopathy[8] is a very lucrative belief system "based on an absurd concept that denies progress in physics and chemistry". It was expounded by German physician Samuel Hahnemann in 1796, who treated his patients with preparations diluted to a point where no molecules of the base remedy were left "in the bottle of substance which the patient is given".

Arnica Montana, for example, is a yellow flower that, when you rubbed on your body, turns the skin slightly purple. To homeopaths this is evidence that a dilution of Arnica Montana flowers cures bruising. The homeopathic philosophy states that 'like cures like', which means that their preparations are based on substances that cause certain symptoms in healthy individuals (the purple colour seen on normal skin) and which are then diluted and used as the treatment for patients exhibiting similar symptoms (the bruise). Dilutions of 'Berlin wall' (stops you feeling oppressed) are used for the treatment of schizophrenia and Spanish spider therapy for attention deficit/hyperactivity disorders in children.[9]

Once a base remedy is identified, the homeopathic preparations go through a process of serial dilution which Hahnemann believed increased the remedy's vital force, thereby improving the effect of the treatment.

Dilution often continues until none of the original substance remains, the theory being that the water continues to contain the memory of the original substance. Not only is there no evidence for the existence of memory in water but homeopathy is implausible "because of the extreme dilutions of the allegedly active substances" and because of the claims that "the more dilute it is, the more potent it is" to a point "way beyond where there is going to be any molecules at all".[10]

Naturopaths, homeopaths and many other CAM practitioners claim that variations in the patient's qi can identify any underlying medical conditions they may have. Although the scientifically implausible techniques of kinesiology[11] and homeopathy may be used to identify these variations (which are supposedly caused by allergies), acupressure, homeopathic or herbal remedies are recommended to clear them, which some practitioners claim also cures cancer.[12]

What are Electronic 'Qi' Mapping Devices?

In the 21st century an increasing number of CAM practitioners are incorporating high-tech equipment into their practices for diagnosis and treatments. Using hand-held probes (which they position on specific acupuncture points) or hand scanners to input information into a computer, small electrical currents are passed through the body, which measure electrical resistance. The associated software interprets these measurements and outputs a medical assessment that is displayed on a computer monitor for the patient to see. This usually includes a list of health problems including organ disorders, vitamin/mineral deficiencies, allergies, food sensitivities, psychological stress, fungi/parasites, viral/bacterial infections, pesticide/insecticide contamination and heavy metal intoxication.

The manufacturers of some of these devices state that they produce results superior to even the most sophisticated and expensive laboratory and imaging tests. Computer software may also be used which they claim will modify these 'qi' fields by sending them back to re-establish the energy balance. According to the manufacturers of these devices, the computer-generated remedies are then tested and imprinted with safe frequencies to match the patient's meridian flow. This may result in a list of natural remedies that patients need to buy, which they claim will restore their health.

With the modern-day computerisation of medical records, patients readily believe what they see on a computer screen and these devices produce a convincing professional-looking and graphic description of the state of the patient's health, accompanied by a recommended list of homeopathic and other supplemental remedies. With consultations at $150 per hour and follow-up appointments necessary, this has become easy money for these practitioners. With machines and homeopathic vials (used as part of the diagnostic testing) costing them around $30,000, even with only 10 patients per week, within a year the machines are paid off.

VEGA-Type Device Testing — What's the Evidence?

One popular device in Australia is the VEGA machine, but there are many other brands such as MORO, BICOM-2000, Orion, E4Q Listen System, Avatar, NES, The Beamer Generator, FHD Biometer, Core System Radionics and QXCI/SCIO. In 1991, a *Medical Journal of Australia* position paper on a report from The Australian College of Allergy on VEGA testing,[13] found that there were no controlled trials to support the usefulness of these types of machines and that using them could "lead to inappropriate treatment and expense to the patient and community". Other medical professionals have stated that these machines "diagnose nonexistent health problems, select inappropriate treatment, and defraud insurance companies. The practitioners who use them are either delusional, dishonest, or both. These devices should be confiscated and the practitioners who use them should be prosecuted".[14]

Devices like VEGA, which use resistance measurements for diagnostic or treatment purposes, can no longer be marketed in the US[15] and it's even illegal[16] to import them there, as the US Food and Drug Administration (FDA) found that they had no scientific basis for the claims they make.

However, these words of warning continue to fall on deaf ears here in Australia and so it remains a free-for-all.

The Therapeutic Goods Administration (TGA) was set up to safeguard public health safety in Australia by regulating goods including medical devices. However, more concerned about safety than efficacy, they are still approving bio-impedance,[17] bio-feedback[18] and bio-energy field mapping[19] devices that make similar disproven diagnostic claims. Listed for 'bio-electronic regulation diagnosis', some of the sponsors claim their machines offer a full range of information about the location and causes of ill-health and that this quickly allows the practitioner to get to the root causes of illness and that these practitioners will often find factors that even the most sophisticated and expensive laboratory and imaging tests cannot detect.

The TGA has a risk classification system that is characterised on the risk to the patient, the user and the environment. It is meant to protect consumers from therapies that may lead to misdiagnosis, which could see individuals not seeking appropriate medical treatment. The Therapeutic Goods Act 1989 only requires that, at the time of an application for a listing, sponsors certify that they hold information or have evidence to support any claim the applicant makes about their goods. However, once approval is given by the TGA, there is no transparent mechanism available for consumers to use to get these goods delisted.

Despite worldwide research that they provide no health benefits, there are hundreds of these diagnostic machines used in some pharmacies, in most naturopathic clinics and in wellness centres across Australia, where their owners can legitimately claim that their machines have Government approval for this purpose.

While the VEGA has now been cancelled by the TGA, it continues to be extensively used by practitioners some of whom are located in pharmacies, because its Aust L number maintains "currency", so despite the cancellation, for them it remains business as usual.

'Nutritional Medicine'

What is 'Nutritional Medicine'?

'Nutritional medicine' continues to be heavily promoted by those CAM practitioners who actively target cancer patients.

Recommending a diet, similar to the one that was developed by Dr Max Gerson (who claimed that diseases including cancer could be cured by eliminating toxins), these CAM practitioners attract patients whose immune systems may already be severely compromised from chemotherapy or from the cancer itself. The diet consists of copious amounts of organic vegetable and fruit juice, supplemented by raw liver juice, daily mega-dose vitamin injections, natural remedies and regular coffee enemas.

Despite an independent review by the National Cancer Institute, which concluded that the research available "did not prove the regimen had benefit,"[20] and considerable research that shows that large doses of some vitamins can increase the risk of some cancers, this dietary regimen continues to be heavily promoted. Other diets that may be recommended are those described as eating according to blood type, high pH therapies or the other highly restrictive metabolic diets such as the Livingston–Wheeler therapy, and these diets may be accompanied by long periods of meditation or may require patients to continually repeat positive affirmations.

What Diagnostic Tests do CAM Practitioners Use?

Many CAM practitioners also offer hair, blood and urine analysis; however, Although these tests have a role in environmental and forensic toxicology, the diagnoses made by CAM practitioners based on these tests are neither standardised nor reproducible and consequently remain controversial. Even so, they may also be used to convince patients that they need their imaginary toxins removed by intravenous chelation and to increase the sale of additional supplements.

Many nutritional therapies offered as cures for cancer result in extreme diets accompanied by unnecessary expenses on vitamins, supplements and homeopathic and herbal remedies that offer no proven health benefits, at a time when patients may have compromised immune systems and limited funds.

THE GROWTH IN CANCER SCAMS AND SCAMMERS

Books and eBooks on CAM

It's not just CAM practitioners who encourage cancer patients to undertake extreme diets. Books and eBooks promoting cancer-curing diets, once released on the Internet, soon become best-sellers.

'The Breuss Cancer Cure',[21] is based on the theory that restricting your diet to just drinking the juice of fruits, vegetables and herbs will starve the cancer cells to death and this will cure your cancer. Worldwide, this book has now sold nearly 1 million copies.

Even though the author, Dr Hulda Clarke, recently died of cancer, worldwide over 4 million copies of her book '*The Cure for All Cancer*'[22] have now been sold. Clarke claimed that cancer was caused by a parasitic infection, and could be cured in just a few days, by using an electromagnetic field-generating machine that she invented and that continues to be marketed by her website, by supposedly killing the parasite that caused the cancer.

The Role of the Internet

The explosion in Internet usage is also providing new ways to target vulnerable and desperate cancer patients and dragging along with it many of the new and old cancer scams such as avemar, cesium, essiac/sheep sorrel, gravioli, human growth hormone, hydrazine sulphate, laetrile, maritime pine bark extract, maroon bush tea, noni juice, paw paw, protocol, shark cartilage, ukraine, wheat grass and zeolite. Some CAM practitioners and support groups are registering as charities to promote their remedies. Sometimes they are run by influential practitioners, who push the boundaries into legitimising these unproven, highly profitable therapies.

In Australia, medical ecology centres, small businesses and individuals are also setting up cancer clinics and wellness centres. Sometimes charging up to $100,000[23] for treatments, they offer a variety of products and services that may also include high pH therapy, devices called parasite/energy zappers, Rife machines, Zen Chi massages, magnetic pulsers, coffee enemas, ozone therapy, diets described as eating according to blood type, live blood analysis and thermal imaging.

The Federal Court has upheld complaints against some of these practitioners and the Australian Competition and Consumer Commission (ACCC)[24] and the Department of Fair Trading continue to investigate them but, sadly, too late for many of their patients.

In their search for a natural cure, cancer patients want desperately to believe in any type of treatment they find on websites or in testimonials that they are led to believe may work for them and so they willingly listen to anyone who gives them hope.

Deregistered Doctors and CAM

Offering useless treatments to terminally ill patients has long been, and continues to be, a big money-spinner for some CAM practitioners and now some doctors have joined their ranks.

Unlike CAM practitioners, doctors are required to be registered. Although some doctors promoting alternative cancer cures are deregistering themselves or have lost their registrations, others are using the loopholes in registration guidelines to avoid scrutiny. Doctors who promote expensive and unproven cancer treatments may do the initial consultation with their patients before introducing them to their team of CAM practitioners. Cancer patients are often so traumatised by their condition, the severity of their surgery and chemotherapy and so desperate for a cure that, when they see a doctor or someone dressed like one, they assume that what they offer is backed by evidence-based medicine.

Some of these doctors have faced disciplinary action from medical boards, but that takes a long time and requires the patient harmed to lodge a complaint, and it is extremely unlikely that cancer patients will take them on.

Not only are alternative cancer cures ineffective, they may cause harm to patients. When the benefits claimed are not realised, family conflict may arise when little time may be left for the patient. Of great concern is that improperly or undiagnosed conditions can lead to considerable health risks, by delaying or compromising proven treatments. Some patients also travel long distances to spend months away from their families at great personal expense, after which they are told that their "long term prospects are very very good",[25] only to die a few months later.

THE GROWTH IN CAM PRODUCTS

The Role of the TGA and CAM

High-profile media and sports personalities relentlessly bombard the airways, promoting the benefits of vitamins, supplements and herbal remedies reinforcing the myth that natural remedies are both safe and have contributed to good health for hundreds of years so they don't need to be tested.

Consumers can pay up to $1000 per kilo for products that display a TGA approval (AUST L number),[26] pills containing garden weeds for therapeutic benefits based on unsubstantiated third-world traditions. Even when science is referred to, it may involve research on two rats and a guinea pig, could be written in another language and does not have to be peer-reviewed.

Because the TGA is "forced to cover costs of its own regulation",[27] I am concerned that too much of its funding comes from the industry that it is regulating and that this can create the perception of a potential conflict of interest. As the regulator of all therapeutic goods, when it comes to CAM products, the TGA does not subject them to the scrutiny of conventional drugs and lists them in a different way, which I find has an ambiguous and misunderstood definition of evidence that appears to let sponsors put traditional evidence over science.

"The claim used must reflect the truth"[28] is a phrase from their guidelines but which I believe is not being applied. There are now over 16,000 medicines listed and many of them fail when tested. I am concerned that the TGA gets millions of dollars from annual fees from the exponential growth in the numbers of these products. It's now become an over $3 billion industry.

Only one in five newly listed complementary medicines are checked through a random audit and with 'assists in well-being' as an acceptable indication, and a growing number of consumers eager to try anything that they are told will maintain or improve their health, new products continue to be developed by creative sponsors. For most people, at least these products are safe, for others, there is always the fine print on the labels.[29]

My concern is that sponsors will undoubtedly keep targeting vulnerable and gullible consumers, to sell them unproven goods that claim to treat real and imaginary conditions and yet appear to have TGA approval based on scientific evidence.

Pharmacies and CAM

High-profile product sponsors speak at conferences where they tell pharmacists to capitalise on consumer sentiment by expanding shelf space for 'alternative' therapies to boost their profits. Pharmacists have positioned themselves as the frontline agents of primary care at a time when health reform is widely expected to shoot primary care to new prominence but, when it comes to CAM, I believe they are too readily influenced by health-care services companies who set them up and whose reward schemes[30] are very generous.

It is my contention that some universities, who I believe have questionable standards, set up health courses based on scientific nonsense to send out poorly trained graduates in ever-increasing numbers. A growing number of distance education businesses, offering training on a wide range of pseudo-scientifically-based natural therapies, are advertised on a regular basis in every major newspaper. Armed with a certificate, their graduates may work in pharmacies to enable them to get around guidelines of evidence-based pharmacy practice[31] that require their staff to be trained in the products they promote. Pharmacists have a long history of capitalising on consumer trust and optimism, and with the increase in consumer demand for CAM, this may be challenged.

With direct access to patients, CAM practitioners are sometimes encouraged to diagnose imaginary conditions in gullible people who believe that what they buy in pharmacies works. When they see a diagnosis on a computer screen they may buy the mostly useless and always expensive remedies recommended. Improving 'well-being' or boosting one's immune system to prevent disease can only be done by swallowing bottles of pills; or so it seems.

Sponsors troll antique books in forgotten libraries searching for traditional cures from common plants to keep up the increasing demand for new products. Launched with expensive advertising campaigns, supported with emotive testimonials, these products soon convert into considerable profits; after all, "it works for me" is a very convincing argument.

An ever-changing tsunami of brightly coloured bottles, packets and pads, brandishing impossible and implausible health claims, are stacked tight and tempting in strategic locations in pharmacies where they proudly flash newly acquired computer-generated Government approval numbers. Supermarkets are also packing their shelves because they want their share of these profits.

FIGHTING FOR GOOD INFORMATION

'Expert Committee on Complementary Medicine'

Nearly two-thirds of Australians are now taking complementary medicines. In 2003, an Expert Committee on Complementary

Medicines[32] identified the need for accurate, reliable and independent information about complementary medicines to help consumers and health professionals make informed choices.

In 2008, the independent and non-profit National Prescribing Service funded a study[33] to get out good information on CAM to both health professionals and consumers, but no date has been set for its delivery or even if such a database will ever be made available to consumers.

The Complementary Health Care Council resists regulation changes claiming that this would deny consumers their "rights to self manage their health in an entirely appropriate way".[34] However, this enables the continued growth of unproven and disproven products by unethical sponsors.

Recommending the inclusion of supporting scientific evidence is viewed by this self-interested industry as "unbalanced and verging on fanaticism"[35] or as conspiracy theories about consumer groups and 'big pharma agents' plotting together against the complementary medicine industry.

Improving regulation would have a positive impact on the industry, bringing legitimacy and consumer confidence but, with more products failing to provide the benefits claimed when tested, it may not be good for the 'bottom line'.

Some traditional remedies may hold the key to major illness cures, but these products remain lost in a quagmire of lies, deceit and false claims. It's more profitable to let consumers wallow in ignorance.

Can you Trust All Doctors who Recommend CAM?

Although offering useless treatments to terminally ill patients has long been, and continues to be, a big money-spinner for a growing number of CAM practitioners, now it's some of our doctors who are on the make. Seeing easy money slipping by, they are plugging the financial leak and they too are turning their backs on science.

Doctors selling books are endorsing websites that are thinly disguised fronts for the promotion of CAM. Claims that ingredient-free, energy-based remedies can not only cure cancer, but prevent swine flu, whooping cough and malaria are attractive to parents and young adults, confused about the safety of modern medicine.

Some doctors are collaborating with CAM practitioners, joining them in Holistic Medical Centres — a type of 'one stop shop' for all your medical needs; which in my opinion gives them access to a share of the profits from products that they are not allowed to sell.

They may also deregister themselves so they can slip under the radar of their registration boards to pursue lucrative careers as CAM practitioners, riding on the coat-tail of the evidence-based medical profession, attracting desperately ill people into believing that they may be cured.

CAM IN THE FUTURE

The Growth in CAM Therapies

Private health insurance fund managers, seeking to boost their dwindling membership, are offering substantial rebates on CAM therapies to attract younger, healthier members. It's now fashionable to have your own CAM practitioner who you see weekly and who you can talk to on a first-name basis.

A recent study by IBISWorld[36] has identified CAM therapies as the No. 7 growth industry for 2010, "projecting the sector will experience growth of 5.1% in 2010 to total $3.36 billion" they also predict an increase in employment of CAM therapists by 4.2%.

The Future of Evidence-Based CAM

Cancer patients who use CAM tend to be younger, of higher social class and female and their satisfaction with it includes finding "psychological benefits, including hope and optimism".[37]

Natural remedies such as aloe vera gel are recommended for radiotherapy burns, ginger helps with nausea and the outcomes of research into other therapies such as hypnosis, relaxation, massage, yoga, pilates, aromatherapy, painting, music, Tai Chi and hydrotherapy are encouraging.

The overall rise in CAM worldwide has also led to an increase in funding for research into the efficacy of these products and therapies. Some of them are now clinically proven to help patients through and after their treatment, but many are now known to offer little more than hope without proof at often substantial costs in both time and money and sometimes at great risk.

MAKING INFORMED CAM CHOICES

Before including CAM, cancer centres need to have a robust credentialling process for both individuals and for their disciplines and only those interventions for which a good evidence base exists should be offered or recommended. Any organisation or individual who provides advice to cancer patients should be clear about the level of efficacy of individual CAMs and this information should be readily available to patients, their families and their health practitioners, to assist with their decision-making. Although in some cases these data may not yet be available, it also opens another line of reasoning as to whether using traditional medicines of uncertain efficacy but no evidence of harm over centuries has any justification in today's world.

Whether it works or it doesn't, whether it may help or harm, whether you want your chakras balanced or you'd just like a good massage, when it comes to CAM, it should be all about bringing forward evidence-based research to cancer patients so they can make informed choices.

ACKNOWLEDGEMENTS

I wish to acknowledge the contribution of Dr Peter Arnold to the preparation of this chapter.

REFERENCES

1. Higgins M. Is there really a conspiracy to suppress cancer cures? *Cancer Treatment Watch.* http://www.cancertreatmentwatch.org/q/conspiracy.shtml [Accessed 26 May 2010].
2. Reiki. *Wikipedia.* http://en.wikipedia.org/wiki/Reiki [Accessed 26 May 2010].
3. Baum M, Ernst E. Should we maintain an open mind about homeopathy? *AMJMED Blog*. http://amjmed.blogspot.com/2009/11/should-we-maintain-open-mind-about.html [Accessed 26 May 2010].

4. Baum M, Dawkins R. Prof. Michael Baum Interview (2/6) — Richard Dawkins [Video]. http://www.youtube.com/watch?v=zNloBfx3E-w [Accessed 26 May 2010].
5. Reiki. *Wikipedia.* http://en.wikipedia.org/wiki/Reiki [Accessed 26 May 2010].
6. Ernst E. The ancient Chinese theories are not correct. *Opposing Views.* http://www.opposingviews.com/arguments/the-ancient-chinese-theories-are-not-correct [Accessed 26 May 2010].
7. Reflexology. *Wikipedia.* http://en.wikipedia.org/wiki/Reflexology [Accessed 26 May 2010].
8. Homeopathy. *Wikipedia.* http://en.wikipedia.org/wiki/Homeopathy [Accessed 26 May 2010].
9. Ullman D. The homeopathic treatment of attention deficit disorder and attention deficit/hyperactivity disorder (ADD/ADHD). *The Free Library by Farlex.* http://www.thefreelibrary.com/The+homeopathic+treatment+of+attention+deficit+disorder+and+attention...-a0213722865 [Accessed 26 May 2010].
10. Baum M, Dawkins R. Prof. Michael Baum Interview (2/6) — Richard Dawkins [Video]. http://www.youtube.com/watch?v=zNloBfx3E-w [Accessed 26 May 2010].
11. Kinesiology. *Wikipedia.* http://en.wikipedia.org/wiki/Kinesiology [Accessed 26 May 2010].
12. Therapy Cons. Homeopathy investigated [video]. http://www.blip.tv/file/2747331 [Accessed 26 May 2010].
13. Katelaris CH, Weiner JM, Heddle RJ, *et al.* Vega testing in the diagnosis of allergic conditions. *eMJA.* http://www.mja.com.au/public/guides/vega/vega.html.**155**:113–114 (1991) [Accessed 26 May 2010].
14. Barrett S. Quack "electrodiagnostic" devices. *Quack Watch.* http://www.quackwatch.org/01QuackeryRelatedTopics/electro.html [Accessed 26 May 2010].
15. Vegatest scams. A cure for no diseases, Canadian style. *Canadian Quackery Watch.* http://www.healthwatcher.net/Quackerywatch/Quack-machines/Vegatest/index.html [Accessed 26 May 2010].
16. Barrett S. Regulatory actions related to EAV devices. *Quack Watch.* http://www.quackwatch.org/02ConsumerProtection/eav.html [Accessed 26 May 2010].
17. Life4Ever Pty Ltd — Bio-energy mapping system sensor/device, active. Summary for ARTG Entry: 164353. Public Summary. Department of Health and Ageing Therapeutic Goods Administration.

Australian Government. https://www.ebs.tga.gov.au/servlet/xmlmillr6?dbid=ebs/PublicHTML/pdfStore.nsf&docid=164353&agid=(PrintDetailsPublic)&actionid=1 [Accessed 26 May 2010].

18. Integrated Functional Medicine Pty Limited — Biofeedback system. Summary for ARTG Entry: 164353. Public Summary. Department of Health and Ageing Therapeutic Goods Administration. *Australian Government.* https://www.ebs.tga.gov.au/servlet/xmlmillr6?dbid=ebs/PublicHTML/pdfStore.nsf&docid=148828&agid=(PrintDetailsPublic)&actionid=1 [Accessed 26 May 2010].
19. Inner Glow Health Products Pty Ltd — Bio-energy field mapping device. Summary for ARTG Entry: 117193. Public Summary. Department of Health and Ageing Therapeutic Goods Administration. *Australian Government.* https://www.ebs.tga.gov.au/servlet/xmlmillr6?dbid=ebs/PublicHTML/pdfStore.nsf&docid=117193&agid=(PrintDetailsPublic)&actionid=1 [Accessed 26 May 2010].
20. Questions and answers about the Gerson therapy. Gerson Therapy (PDQ®). *National Cancer Institute.* http://www.cancer.gov/cancertopics/pdq/cam/gerson/Patient/page2 [Accessed 26 May 2010].
21. The Breuss Cancer Cure. *Alternative Health Supplies (Australia).* http://www.alternativehealth.com.au/Books/breuss.htm [Accessed 26 May 2010].
22. Clark HR. The cure for all cancers: including over 100 case histories of persons cured. *Amazon.com.* http://www.amazon.com/Cure-All-Cancers-Including-Histories/dp/1890035009 [Accessed 26 May 2010].
23. Treatment: Warning on 'quack' remedies for cancer. cancer in the news April 2009. *Cancer Voices SA.* http://www.cancervoicessa.org/_docs/Cancer%20in%20the%20News%20April%2009.pdf.
24. ACCC obtains court injunctions over the RANA system cancer treatment. Media Centre. *ACCC.* http://www.accc.gov.au/content/index.phtml/itemId/771894 [Accessed 26 May 2010]. ACCC acts quickly to temporarily restrain alleged misleading cancer treatment claims. Media Centre. *ACCC.* http://www.accc.gov.au/content/index.phtml/itemId/917765 [Accessed 26 May 2010].
25. Letter from Barry Gomersall. Help from Men of League. Magazine October–November 2006. *Men of League.* http://webcache.googleusercontent.com/search?q=cache:6zRsZRV0CTIJ:www.menofleague.com/Joomla/index2.php%3Foption%3Dcom_docman%26task%3Ddoc_view%26gid%3D11%26Itemid%3D67+%22men+of+

league%22+gomersall+magazine+october+november+2006&cd=1&hl=en&ct=clnk&gl=au [Accessed 26 May 2010].
26. McEwen J. What does TGA approval of medicines mean? *Australian Prescriber.* http://www.australianprescriber.com/magazine/27/6/156/8/ [Accessed 26 May 2010].
27. Korczak V. Comments. Is regulation on complementary medicine marketing a joke? Croakey. *Crikey.* http://www.crikey.com.au/Blogs/Croakey/Is-regulation-of-complementary-medicine-marketing-a-joke.html [Accessed 26 May 2010].
28. Guidelines for levels and kinds of evidence to support indications and claims for non-registerable medicines, including complementary medicines, and other listable medicines. Department of Health and Ageing Therapeutic Goods Administration. *Australian Government.* http://www.tga.gov.au/docs/pdf/tgaccevi.pdf [Accessed 26 May 2010].
29. Black cohosh, New label requirement. Department of Health and Ageing Therapeutic Goods Administration. *Australian Government.* http://www.tga.gov.au/cm/0705blkcohosh.htm#newlabel [Accessed 26 May 2010].
30. Sigma rewards. *Sigma.* http://www.sigmaco.com.au/rewards.cfm [Accessed 26 May 2010].
31. McInerney G. Commentary. Skeptics, pharmacists and the evidence Base. *Information to Pharmacies.* http://archive.i2p.com.au/?page=site/article&id=1274 [Accessed 26 May 2010].
32. Expert Committee on Complementary Medicines in the Health System. Department of Health and Ageing. *Therapeutic Goods Administration.* http://www.tga.gov.au/docs/html/cmreport.htm [Accessed 26 May 2010].
33. Highest quality complementary resources identified. Media Release. *NPS.* http://www.nps.org.au/news_and_media/media_releases/repository/Highest_quality_complementary_medicines_resources_identified [Accessed 26 May 2010].
34. Complementary Medicine Regulation Protects Consumers. Media Release. *CHC.* http://www.chc.org.au/view/document.shtml?v13023-jqrvdff [Accessed 26 May 2010].
35. Harvey K. Is regulation of complementary medicines marketing a joke? Croakey. *Crikey.* http://www.crikey.com.au/Blogs/Croakey/Is-regulation-of-complementary-medicine-marketing-a-joke.html [Accessed 26 May 2010].

36. Bryant R. Which industries will sink & soar in 2010? *Smart Company.* http://www.smartcompany.com.au/index.php?option=com_content&task=view&id=36510&Itemid=282 [Accessed 26 May 2010].
37. Clinical Practice Guidelines for the Management of Melanoma in Australia and New Zealand. *Cancer Council Australia.* http://www.cancer.org.au/File/HealthProfessionals/ClinicalPracticeGuidelines-ManagementofMelanoma.pdf [Accessed 26 May 2010].

22

Complementary and Alternative Medicine Use by Adult Cancer Patients: An Overview

Carlo Pirri

ABSTRACT

Complementary and alternative medicine (CAM) continues to evoke fierce debate and divergent views within the medical community, yet complementary medicine is used by 14–65% of Australian adults diagnosed with cancer (with estimates as high as 80–91% in the US and Europe), and alternative medicine by 8–14%. Cancer patients who use CAM are typically female, younger, better educated and of higher socio-economic status. Whereas surgery, chemotherapy and radiotherapy have proven increasingly successful but still have limited curative potential, these conventional approaches are generally more invasive, aggressive and associated with greater toxicity than CAMs, which tend to take a slower, gentler approach by attempting to bolster constructive forces (e.g. the immune system) rather than battling the destructive forces of growing cancer cells. They focus on symptom control and patients are generally encouraged to be active participants in the management of their illness. This patient-centred approach, which is more easily accessible, contributes to the appeal of CAM. Many CAMs, however, have drawn steadfast opposition from cancer physicians, primarily because they remain unproven in clinical trials and pose potential safety risks and financial or psychological harm to their patients. Research indicates that 33–77% of patients do not disclose CAM use to their physicians, often because of a perceived negative response. The perception that CAMs are more "natural" and, by association, safer than conventional treatments is problematic. Indeed, they may pose direct safety risks because of their potential adverse effects or interactions with conventional oncology treatments. Alternative therapies promoted as "cures" in place of conventional treatments have the potential to cause patients harm. It is therefore imperative that those involved in the medical care of cancer patients are equipped with the skills and knowledge to help patients appropriately evaluate complementary and alternative therapies, and be aware of interactions with conventional anticancer therapies, in order to increase the likelihood that patients avoid harm and, where possible, receive benefit should they choose to use CAM.

Keywords: Complementary and Alternative Medicines; Interactions; Natural.

INTRODUCTION

Complementary and alternative medicine (CAM) continues to evoke fierce debate and divergent views within the medical community. It remains an attractive and commonly used treatment option for many cancer patients, regardless of whether their clinicians like it or believe in it. Consequently, it divides health professionals providing conventional cancer care and CAM practitioners offering unconventional care.

BACKGROUND

Definitions

The US National Institutes of Health's National Center for Complementary and Alternative Medicine defines CAM as 'a group of diverse medical and health care systems, practices and products that are not presently considered part of conventional medicine'.[1] Complementary and alternative therapies must be distinguished, however. "Complementary therapies" are *adjuncts* to conventional medical treatment increasingly perceived as an important part of supportive care;[2,3] they are often used for symptom management and to enhance quality of life (QoL) and overall patient care.[4] "Alternative therapies", in contrast, are clinically unproven and are used *instead* of conventional treatments.[2] This is particularly damaging for cancer patients, as delay or outright refusal of conventional treatment often compromises their likelihood of cure or remission.[5] More recently, the term "integrative oncology" has emerged and involves a standard of care for cancer patients that utilises safe, evidence-based complementary therapies *in conjunction* with conventional anticancer treatments via a multi-disciplinary approach designed to evaluate and treat the whole person rather than the disease *per se*.[6]

Prevalence and Cost of CAM Use

In 2004, an estimated 52.2% of the Australian population used CAM, which was at least equivalent to prescription drug use[7,8] and cost AUD$1.8 billion (approximately four times the public contribution to the Pharmaceutical Benefits Scheme).[7] More recent surveys in 2005/06, however, revealed a significant increase in prevalence to an estimated 67%[9] and out-of-pocket spending of AUD$4.13 billion, with as many visits being made to CAM practitioners as medical practitioners (approximately 68 million each).[10]

CAM use is quite prominent in oncology, with the prevalence often being higher in cancer patients than in the general and other chronic disease populations.[11–15] In adult cancer patients, a systematic review of 21 studies worldwide reported an average prevalence of CAM use of 31.4% (range: 7–64%),[16] whereas a more recent European survey of 13 countries found an average prevalence of 35.9% (range: 14.8–73.1%).[17] Other studies report an even higher prevalence, depending on the CAM definitions used and cancer populations studied. For instance, the 2002 Datamonitor Survey encompassing the US and Europe revealed an 80% prevalence amongst adult cancer patients,[18] whereas 91% of US patients reported CAM use (including prayer and exercise) during treatment in another study.[19] In Australia, CAM use by cancer patients has varied widely from 14.5%[20] to 65%.[21] More specifically, 22–52% of medical oncology,[21–24] 40% of palliative[25] and 46% of paediatric oncology patients[26] report CAM use.

CAM USE BY CANCER PATIENTS

Profile of CAM Users

Studies have consistently shown that cancer patients who use CAM are typically female, younger, better educated and of higher socio-economic status than those who do not.[2,17,24,27–29] This mimics the basic trend observed in the general population.[30] CAM use is also associated with being married,[31] medical comorbidity,[24] advanced cancer,[31–33] longer disease/treatment,[24,28] greater symptoms,[31,87] psycho-social distress and poor QoL,[24,27,33] and engaging in self-help groups and other active coping strategies.[32–35]

Attraction of Cancer Patients to CAMs and the Motivation to Use Them

The underlying philosophy of most CAMs primarily focuses on health and improving well-being (e.g. Cohen *et al.*)[36] rather than on the disease itself. Conventional treatments are generally invasive and aggressive, whereas CAMs tend to take a slower, gentler approach, by attempting to bolster constructive forces (e.g. the immune system), rather than battling the destructive forces of growing cancer cells. Patients are generally encouraged to be active participants in the management of their illness, as opposed to being passive spectators in the case of taking prescribed medical treatment. These ingredients culminate in a highly empowering holistic treatment approach that is tailored to patients and preserves a sense of hope, which makes CAM, like the patient-centred approach *per se*, very attractive.

There are many reasons why cancer patients use CAM. Common reasons include cancer cure or prolongation of life;[22,23,25,26,37–42] relief from cancer symptoms and conventional treatment side-effects;[29,40,43,44] to assist conventional treatments;[23,38] boosting immunological function or energy;[24,29,40,43] enhancing physical, emotional and spiritual well-being;[17,24,45,46] and maintaining a sense of control or hope.[22–25,29,32,37,38,45] Other motivations for patients to use CAM include perceptions that CAMs are natural/non-toxic, beneficial and, at worst, will do no harm; strong encouragement from family, friends, other cancer patients/survivors and the media;[29,34,41,47–50] congruence with cultural values and beliefs;[46] poor prognosis resulting in limited conventional treatment options;[51] strengthening the body to cope with conventional treatments in surgery, chemotherapy and radiotherapy; improving QoL; to prevent recurrence following conventional treatment;[52,53] high accessibility of CAMs (e.g. due to non-prescription or self-referral);[54] greater individual attention from CAM practitioners; dissatisfaction with some aspects of conventional medical care;[54] and a poor doctor–patient relationship.[54]

PATIENT–CLINICIAN COMMUNICATION AND DECISION-MAKING

Concerns and Attitudes of Cancer Physicians Relating to CAM Use

Conventional treatments do not always relieve cancer symptoms adequately, nor do prescribed medications provide total coverage against their side-effects. Some CAMs (e.g. acupuncture, relaxation, massage) have received medical endorsement for use as complementary therapies alongside conventional treatments, due to their proven efficacy in relieving disease symptoms/treatment side-effects or enhancing QoL/psychosocial functioning, as well as the minimal health risks they pose to patients.[6,55,56] Other CAMs (e.g. herbs, nutritional supplements, antioxidants), however, have drawn steadfast opposition from oncologists, primarily because they remain unproven in clinical trials (particularly as curative alternative therapies replacing conventional treatments); possess greater health risks due to adverse interactions with prescribed cancer treatments or medications (e.g. CAM–drug interactions, surgical complications such as bleeding); and as they may delay or reduce the efficacy of conventional treatments such as chemotherapy and radiotherapy and, subsequently, compromise the likelihood of cure/remission and shorten survival time.[57] Additionally, concerns are held that CAMs may inflict financial or psychological harm (e.g. by creating false hope in medically hopeless situations); precipitate the abandonment of conventional treatment; lead patients to confuse a physician's willingness to discuss and support their decision to use CAMs with actual medical support for them; and result in litigation against physicians in instances of failure if they (appear to) advocate CAM use.[58]

Disclosure of CAM Use by Patients and Barriers to Open Communication Between Cancer Physicians and Their Patients about CAM

Despite the empirical benefits of some CAMs and greater endorsement of their use as complementary therapies, support is far from universal[17] with many oncologists exhibiting dismissive attitudes and negative views towards them.[59] Indeed, although one study revealed that cancer patients expected their physicians to be supportive, caring, accepting and non-judgemental about CAM use and to inspire a sense of hope in them,[60] several studies have demonstrated that the reality is frequently different.

Oncologists consistently underestimate their patients' use of CAM.[61,62] Discussions about CAM are also uncommon and most likely to be initiated by patients, rather than physicians.[63–65] Research has shown that 33–77% of patients do not disclose CAM use to their physicians,[66] with one Australian study reporting that 40% of cancer patients did not inform their oncologist.[22] Another study has revealed that only 54% of cancer patients disclosed CAM use to their doctor, whereas medical treatments were discussed with their CAM practitioner in 94% of instances.[67] Patients do not tell their doctors for several reasons, including anticipation of a negative response to their CAM use (e.g. fears that physicians will discontinue their health-care, will not support their CAM use, or try to dissuade them from using CAM);[66–69] the belief that it is unimportant for physicians to know due to perceptions that CAM is entirely natural and safe and irrelevant to the course of conventional treatment;[67] perceived inability or unwillingness of physicians to provide useful information about CAM due to inadequate training or bias against CAM use;[67] physicians simply not asking about CAM use or appearing disinterested (35% of patient attempts to initiate CAM discussions were ignored by oncologists in one Australian study);[66–69] physicians' emphasis on scientific evidence;[69] and patients' uncertainty about the benefits of CAM.[68]

Although cancer patients typically do not inform their physicians about their CAM use, patients and their doctors report that it usually enhances their relationship when it is being discussed and patients exhibit greater satisfaction and treatment compliance.[63,70] Nevertheless, few oncologists feel comfortable discussing CAM with their patients, with one survey of 291 oncology health professionals revealing that only 34% thought they could effectively communicate with patients using CAM and 42% believing that they lacked the skills to help patients maintain hope.[70] In another survey, cancer physicians and nurses were significantly less likely to instigate CAM discussions with patients than social workers.[64]

Many CAM studies have examined patient perspectives, but few have investigated the barriers to effective communication from oncologists' viewpoints. Major obstacles to physicians initiating such discussions with patients include the lack of proven efficacy for many individual CAMs in clinical trials,[71–74] limited time for patient consultations[68,70] and a lack of knowledge of specific CAMs (including benefits and adverse effects) preventing them from sufficiently addressing patient questions or concerns.[68,71] Indeed, an Australian study of 161 oncologists reported self-identified gaps in their knowledge of CAMs used by some patients, and highlighted the need for including education about them in medical training in order to provide adequate advice to patients.[75] Other barriers to effective physician–patient communication about CAM also include limited physician resources for patient referral (e.g. information about qualified CAM practitioners, knowledge of CAM practitioner specialties),[76] and distrust of CAM practitioners to educate them about non-biomedical therapies.[71]

Making the Decision to Use CAM Alongside Conventional Anticancer Treatment and the Information Sources and Types of Evidence Used by Patients to Make Such Decisions

Cancer patients may make the decision to use CAM upon diagnosis, during conventional treatment, in response to disease progression or recurrence, or during remission/survivorship. In contrast to information needs and decision-making for conventional treatments, relatively little is understood about how information is utilised and evaluated by cancer patients in their decisions about whether to use CAM and which therapies to undertake. The decision to use CAM is a highly personal and individual one (as patients differ in their

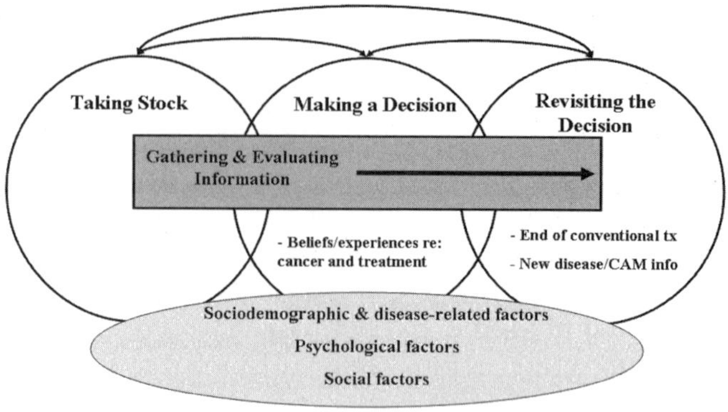

Fig. 1. Factors involved in the decision-making process utilised by cancer patients to use CAM. Used with publisher's permission from "Patient decision-making about complementary and alternative medicine in cancer management: context and process" by Balneaves LG *et al. Curr Oncol* **15**(suppl 2):s94–s100 (2008).[104]

perceptions of the benefits and risks of available treatment options), and is complex and dynamic in nature.

CAM decisions are influenced throughout the cancer experience by a number of demographic, disease-related psychological and social factors, many of which have been discussed above. Several decision-making models describing the complex interaction between these factors and the cognitive processes underpinning decision-making have evolved from CAM research that has predominantly involved breast and prostate cancer patients. A recent qualitative review of such studies has identified four main stages within the CAM decision-making process of cancer patients: (1) taking stock of treatment options, (2) gathering and evaluating CAM information, (3) making a decision, and (4) revisiting the decision (Fig. 1).

Making the Decision to Forego Conventional Anticancer Treatment in Favour of Alternative Therapies and Physician Responses to Patients Making Such Decisions

A study of CAM use amongst breast cancer patients[41] revealed that few patients distinguish explicitly between conventional treatments and CAMs, and perceive their treatment options as a menu from which to choose a unique treatment protocol or package. Although most cancer patients utilising CAM employ them alongside conventional treatments as *complementary therapies*,[20,23,77] others decline all conventional treatments and substitute them with *alternative therapies*. Clinicians often view such choices made by patients as irrational and non-compliant in nature, especially when the proposed conventional treatment is curative.[78,79] They find such decisions difficult to accept and particularly troubling, given the reduced likelihood of cure and shorter survival time that delay/complete refusal of conventional treatment often confers to patients and the potentially greater health risks, poorer QoL and expense associated with unproven alternative therapies.[5,75,79–83] Clinicians, however, consider CAM to be more likely to help patients treated palliatively than curatively,[75] and thus have less difficulty accepting the patient's decision to decline conventional treatment in favour of alternative therapies in palliative contexts.[78]

How many cancer patients decline conventional treatment is largely unknown, but some researchers and clinicians (particularly in Australia) appear comfortable in dismissing the figure as being very low (1–2%) in the absence of any real supportive evidence. The few studies that have attempted to gauge this, however, suggest that the number is likely to be substantial enough to demand much greater attention and concern than is currently being shown, with prevalence estimates ranging from 8–14%.[84,85]

Given the escalating popularity of CAM, it is quite likely that the prevalence of cancer patients who refuse conventional treatment will increase. Understanding how patients come to such decisions, however, will allow clinicians to offer them the best possible care and guidance that will probably prevent them from discontinuing with conventional cancer care altogether. Fortunately, a number of studies have examined why cancer patients decline conventional treatment and adopt alternative therapies instead. A qualitative review of these studies identified prior negative experiences with conventional medicine, the death of close family or friends to cancer while receiving conventional treatment, pre-existing alternative therapy use, and a strong belief system invested in the holistic approach as the most important predisposing factors.[82] Factors influencing decisions to refuse treatment following diagnosis include poor doctor–patient communication, psychosocial distress resulting from diagnosis (e.g. fear, anger), perceived severity of conventional treatment side-effects, a strong desire for control in decision-making, great belief in holistic approaches and the mind–body–spirit connection, and beliefs about conventional medicine (e.g. incompatibility with QoL, treatment of symptoms rather than the underlying disease or whole person, reduced capacity for cure) and the causes of cancer (e.g. lifestyle factors such as diet caused their cancer).[78,82,86]

Few studies have investigated physicians' responses to cancer patients making decisions to forego conventional treatment. One study of oncologists and general practitioners, however, found that physicians naturally adopt a goal-orientated medical viewpoint for decision-making, whereas patients rely predominantly on personal values and experiences to make decisions.[78] Consequently, a patient's decision to decline conventional treatment appears irrational to doctors, especially when the proposed treatment is curative. Besides the distinctions between curable/non-curable disease and rational/irrational treatment decisions, physicians differentiate between patients who assume passive and active roles in decision-making.[79] Although most patients are fairly passive decision-makers and follow the medical advice of their doctors, patients who adopt active stances are perceived as being different and may be inclined to forego conventional treatment and seek alternative therapies.

Unsurprisingly, patients who reject conventional treatment in favour of alternative therapies are viewed by some doctors as difficult, irrational, non-compliant, desperate, and in need of more time to reach a sensible decision. In these circumstances, physicians often experience much inner conflict in accepting the patient's decision and about the role they should play, with interviews of medical and radiation oncologists in one study revealing common themes of uncertainty (e.g. what approach to take in this situation with patients, about their ability to effectively communicate with patients), failure (e.g. to understand the patient or resolve their difference of opinion), helplessness and concern (i.e. about the patient's well-being and the implications of his/her treatment decision).[79] The authors concluded that the tendency of physicians to categorise patient decisions as rational or irrational may contribute to their feelings of uncertainty and concern, and that this may interfere with their ability to respond with appropriate sensitivity and understanding to patients who decline conventional treatment in favour of alternative therapies.[79]

In the search to make informed treatment decisions, family, friends and CAM practitioners were identified in two qualitative studies as the most valuable sources of support by cancer patients who declined conventional treatment.[82,87] Cancer physicians were also cited, but more support was forthcoming from general practitioners within the conventional health realm. Patients who perceived that their oncologist was trying to coerce them into accepting conventional treatment (i.e. by pressuring them, equating alternative therapies to a "death sentence" or making disparaging remarks about CAM) were more likely to cease conventional cancer care altogether. Conversely, patients highly valued oncologists who could openly communicate and were open-minded enough to support them and provide ongoing follow-up care, despite disagreeing with their decision to decline conventional treatment.

The decision to decline conventional treatment is not necessarily born from distrust of the health system or the preceding medical care provided by cancer physicians, but may reflect the personal characteristics of individual cancer patients. What clinicians must remember is that treatment decisions are not limited to a single point in time, nor are they absolute. Patients who substitute conventional treatments with alternative therapies want to keep their options open,[82] and evidence suggests that some patients ultimately decide to utilise some form of conventional treatment.[87] The need for effective, supportive, open-minded/non-judgemental and respectful communication is the most common and important theme identified across the studies in this area.[86,88] Understanding what categories of patients are likely to use alternative therapies as surrogates for conventional treatment and what their motivations are is likely to help improve the communication between cancer physicians and their patients, and enhance the overall quality of cancer care offered by oncologists providing conventional treatment.

EFFICACY AND SAFETY OF CAM

Collectively, there is a lack of scientific evidence for the efficacy of CAMs in oncology.[16,89–91] A useful distinction, however, is that between *cancer cure* and *cancer care*.[92] Some CAMs (e.g. mind–body techniques, massage and touch therapies) have proven effective in relieving disease symptoms/treatment side-effects or enhancing QoL/psychosocial functioning and, thus, are important in caring for cancer patients and alleviating the physical and emotional burden experienced during cancer and its treatment.[4,6,55,56,93,94] To date, however, no CAM has proven effective in reliably curing or suppressing any form of cancer.[6] Nevertheless, with the growing popularity of CAM, patients have become increasingly aware that commonly used chemotherapy drugs and other medications used in Western medicine were originally derived from natural sources[95] and hence they are investigating natural products in their search to make informed treatment decisions.

In one population survey, 75% of people agreed that combining conventional medical treatment and CAMs was preferable to using either alone.[96] Although use of CAMs may be problematic, they are often perceived by patients as being more "natural" and, by association, safer than conventional treatments. CAMs can directly harm patients via toxic or allergic reactions resulting from their use alone, interactions with chemotherapy agents and prescribed medications, or contaminants in their manufacturing or from the environment (e.g. heavy metals, pesticides, bacteria, fungi).[57,97] Some herbs, nutritional supplements and other botanical agents, for instance, have toxic and potentially life-threatening effects (e.g. kava, comfrey and black cohosh may cause hepatotoxicity, laetrile/amygdalin causes cyanide toxicity and dermatitis and high-dose beta-carotene increases lung cancer incidence and cancer mortality in smokers).[97–99] Other botanical preparations can interact with chemotherapy and prescription drugs (e.g. St. John's wort interferes with drug metabolism via the cytochrome P450 pathway and may result in serotonin syndrome or lethargy when taken with antidepressants, as well as reducing the efficacy of chemotherapy drugs, particularly irinotecan and imatinib; botanical agents with oestrogenic properties including red clover, soy and dong quai/female ginseng may interfere with the treatment of hormone-sensitive conditions such as breast cancer and endometriosis)[57,98] or cause complications during surgery (e.g. garlic, ginkgo biloba and ginseng may increase bleeding; ephedrine alkaloids such as ephedra/ma huang may cause cardiovascular events including hypertension, tachycardia, heart attack and stroke) and radiotherapy (e.g. limited evidence suggests that high-dose supplementation of antioxidants such as vitamin E and beta-carotene during radiotherapy may protect tumour cells along with healthy cells, thus shortening survival of cancer patients).[57,100]

CAMs may also cause indirect harm to patients. Resultant delays in conventional treatment potentially compromise treatment outcomes, QoL and survival.[80,81] Clinical trial outcomes, particularly those involving advanced disease patients with poor prognosis, may also be compromised when positive or negative effects of CAM are misattributed to the new conventional treatment being investigated.[101,102] Financial or emotional burden (e.g. prolonged denial), or the simple squandering of precious, limited time that some patients have left also constitute indirect harm.

Finally, patients may be harmed as a result of the unsafe practices of CAM practitioners with inadequate training and competence, often owing to the absence of self-regulatory bodies and unsatisfactory government legislation protecting health consumers. Furthermore, harm may be exacerbated by regulatory absence or deficiencies in monitoring of the biological potency of herbal crops (causing wide variation in therapeutic efficacy) or the use of incorrect plant species; product standardisation in terms of purity and dosage (resulting in possible substitution/adulteration and incorrect dosing or preparation); and product labelling or advertising.[103]

ACKNOWLEDGEMENTS

I would like to thank Professor Ian Olver (editor), Professor Peter Drummond and Mr Paul Katris for their comments on early drafts of this chapter. Finally, I would like to thank my loved ones for the patience they showed during the writing of this chapter.

REFERENCES

1. National Center for Complementary and Alternative Medicine (NCCAM). CAM basics: what is CAM? http://nccam.nih.gov/health/whatiscam/D347.pdf [Accessed 28 July 2009].

2. Cassileth BR. Complementary and alternative cancer medicine. *J Clin Oncol* **17**:44–52 (1999).
3. Cancer Council New South Wales (NSW). *Understanding Complementary Therapies: A Guide for People with Cancer, Their Families and Friends*, 2nd edn, Cancer Council NSW, Woolloomooloo (2009).
4. Deng G, Cassileth BR, Yeung KS. Complementary therapies for cancer-related symptoms. *J Support Oncol* **2**:419–426 (2004).
5. Cassileth BR, Deng G. Complementary and alternative therapies for cancer. *Oncologist* **9**:80–89 (2004).
6. Deng GE, Frenkel M, Cohen L, *et al*. Evidence-based clinical practice guidelines for integrative oncology: complementary therapies and botanicals. *J Soc Integr Oncol* **7**(3):85–120 (2009).
7. MacLennan AH, Myers SP, Taylor AW. The continuing use of complementary and alternative medicine in South Australia: costs and beliefs in 2004. *Med J Aust* **184**:27–31 (2006).
8. Australian Bureau of Statistics. *Australian Social Trends 1998*, Australian Bureau of Statistics, Canberra (1998).
9. National Prescribing Service. NPS National consumer survey no. 5. http://www.nps.org.au/__data/assets/pdf_file/0009/26874/cons_survey_5_exec.pdf [Accessed 22 January 2010].
10. Xue CC, Zhang AL, Lin V, *et al*. Complementary and alternative medicine use in Australia: a national population-based survey. *J Altern Complement Med* **13**(6):643–650 (2007).
11. Saydah SH, Eberhardt MS. Use of complementary and alternative medicine among adults with chronic diseases: United States 2002. *J Altern Complement Med* **12**(8):805–812 (2006).
12. Mao JJ, Farrar JT, Xie SX, *et al*. Use of complementary and alternative medicine and prayer among a national sample of cancer survivors compared to other populations without cancer. *Complement Ther Med* **5**(1):21–29 (2007).
13. Habermann TM, Thompson CA, LaPlant BR, *et al*. Complementary and alternative medicine use among long-term lymphoma survivors: a pilot study. *Am J Hematol* **84**(12):795–798 (2009).
14. Thomas KJ, Nicholl JP, Coleman P. Use and expenditure on complementary medicine in England: a population based survey. *Complement Ther Med* **9**(1):2–11 (2001).
15. Hyodo I, Amano N, Eguchi K, *et al*. Nationwide survey on complementary and alternative medicine in cancer patients in Japan. *J Clin Oncol* **23**(12):2645–2654 (2005).

16. Ernst E, Cassileth BR. The prevalence of complementary/alternative medicine in cancer. *Cancer* **83**:777–782 (1998).
17. Molassiotis A, Fernadez-Ortega P, Pud D, *et al*. Use of complementary and alternative medicine in cancer patients: a European survey. *Ann Oncol* **16**(4):655–663 (2005).
18. Datamonitor. Complementary and alternative medicines in cancer therapy. Publication BFHC0462, http://www.datamonitor.com/all/reports/product_summary.asp?pid=BFHC0462 [Accessed 13 June 2006].
19. Yates JS, Mustian KM, Morrow GR, *et al*. Prevalence of complementary and alternative medicine use in cancer patients during treatment. *Support Care Cancer* **13**(10):806–811 (2005).
20. Sibbritt D, Adams J, Easthope G, *et al*. Complementary and alternative medicine (CAM) use among elderly Australian women who have cancer. *Support Care Cancer* **11**(8):548–550 (2003).
21. Oh B, Butow P, Mullan B, *et al*. Patient-doctor communication: use of complementary and alternative medicine by adult patients with cancer. *J Soc Integr Oncol* **8**(2):56–64 (2010).
22. Begbie SD, Kerestes ZL, Bell DR. Patterns of alternative medicine use by cancer patients. *Med J Aust* **165**(10):545–548 (1996).
23. Miller M, Boyer MJ, Butow PN, *et al*. The use of unproven methods of treatment by cancer patients: frequency, expectations and cost. *Support Care Cancer* **6**:337–347 (1998).
24. Pirri C, Katris P, Trotter J, *et al*. Use of complementary and alternative therapies by Australian cancer patients. *Asia-Pac J Clin Oncol* **4**(3):161–169 (2008).
25. Yates PM, Beadle G, Clavarino A, *et al*. Patients with terminal cancer who use alternative therapies: their beliefs and practices. *Sociol Health Illn* **15**(2):199–216 (1993).
26. Sawyer MG, Gannoni AF, Toogood IR, *et al*. The use of alternative therapies by children with cancer. *Med J Aust* **160**:320–322 (1994).
27. Burstein HJ, Gelber S, Guadagnoli E, *et al*. Use of alternative medicine by women with early-stage breast cancer. *N Engl J Med* **340**:1733–1739 (1999).
28. Girgis A, Adams J, Sibbritt D. The use of complementary and alternative therapies by patients with cancer. *Oncol Res* **15**:281–289 (2005).
29. Verhoef MJ, Balneaves LG, Boon HS, *et al*. Reasons for and characteristics associated with complementary and alternative medicine

use among adult cancer patients: a systematic review. *Integr Cancer Ther* **4**(4):274–286 (2005).
30. MacLennan AH, Wilson DH, Taylor AW. The escalating cost and prevalence of alternative medicine. *Prev Med* **35**(2):166–173 (2002).
31. Fouladbakhsh JM, Stommel M, Given BA, *et al*. Predictors of use of complementary and alternative therapies among patients with cancer. *Oncol Nurs Forum* **32**(6):1115–1122 (2005).
32. Söllner W, Maislinger S, DeVries A, *et al*. Use of complementary and alternative medicine by cancer patients is not associated with perceived distress or poor compliance with standard treatment but with active coping behavior: a survey. *Cancer* **89**(4):873–880 (2000).
33. Paltiel O, Avitzour M, Peretz T, *et al*. Determinants of the use of complementary therapies by patients with cancer. *J Clin Oncol* **19**(9):2439–2448 (2001).
34. Boon H, Westlake K, Stewart M, *et al*. Use of complementary/alternative medicine by men diagnosed with prostate cancer: prevalence and characteristics. *Urology* **62**(5):849–853 (2003).
35. Nagel G, Hoyer H, Katenkamp D. Use of complementary and alternative medicine by patients with breast cancer: observations from a health-care survey. *Support Care Cancer* **12**(11):789–796 (2004).
36. Cohen L, Cohen MH, Kirkwood C, *et al*. Discussing complementary therapies in an oncology setting. *J Soc Integr Oncol* **5**(1):18–24 (2007).
37. Richardson MA, Sanders T, Palmer JL, *et al*. Complementary/alternative medicine use in a comprehensive cancer center and the implications for oncology. *J Clin Oncol* **18**(13):2505–2514 (2000).
38. Boon H, Stewart M, Kennard MA, *et al*. Use of complementary/alternative medicine by breast cancer survivors in Ontario: prevalence and perceptions. *J Clin Oncol* **18**(13):2515–2521 (2000).
39. Correa-Velez I, Clavarino A, Barnett AG, *et al*. Use of complementary and alternative medicine and quality of life: changes at the end of life. *Palliat Med* **17**(8):695–703 (2003).
40. Correa-Velez I, Clavarino A, Eastwood H. Surviving, relieving, repairing, and boosting up: reasons for using complementary/alternative medicine among patients with advanced cancer: a thematic analysis. *Palliat Med* **8**(5):953–961 (2005).
41. Boon H, Brown JB, Gavin A, *et al*. Breast cancer survivors' perceptions of complementary/alternative medicine (CAM): making the decision to use or not to use. *Qual Health Res* **9**(5):639–653 (1999).

42. Sparber A, Bauer L, Curt G, *et al*. Use of complementary medicine by adult patients participating in cancer clinical trials. *Oncol Nurs Forum* **27**(4):623–630 (2000).
43. Shen J, Andersen R, Albert PS, *et al*. Use of complementary/alternative therapies by women with advanced-stage breast cancer. *BMC Complement Altern Med* **2**:8 (2002).
44. Harris P, Finlay IG, Cook A, *et al*. Complementary and alternative medicine use by patients with cancer in Wales: a cross sectional survey. *Complement Ther Med* **11**(4):249–253 (2003).
45. Scott JA, Kearney N, Hummerston S, *et al*. Use of complementary and alternative medicine in patients with cancer: a UK survey. *Eur J Oncol Nurs* **9**(2):131–137 (2005).
46. Singh H, Maskarinec G, Shumay DM. Understanding the motivation for conventional and complementary/alternative medicine use among men with prostate cancer. *Integr Cancer Ther* **4**(2):187–194 (2005).
47. Ohlén J, Balneaves LG, Bottorff JL, *et al*. The influence of significant others in complementary and alternative medicine decisions by cancer patients. *Soc Sci Med* **63**(6):1625–1636 (2006).
48. Evans M, Shaw A, Thompson EA, *et al*. Decisions to use complementary and alternative medicine (CAM) by male cancer patients: information-seeking roles and types of evidence used. *BMC Complement Altern Med* **7**:25 (2007).
49. Bonevski B, Wilson A, Henry DA. An analysis of news media coverage of complementary and alternative medicine. *PLoS One* **3**(6): e2406 (2008).
50. Mercurio R, Eliott JA. Trick or treat? Australian newspaper portrayal of complementary and alternative medicine for the treatment of cancer. *Support Care Cancer* **19**(1):67–80 (2011).
51. Broom A, Tovey P. Therapeutic pluralism? Evidence, power and legitimacy in UK cancer services. *Sociol Health Illn* **29**(4):551–569 (2007).
52. Eng J, Ramsum D, Verhoef M, *et al*. A population-based survey of complementary and alternative medicine use in men recently diagnosed with prostate cancer. *Integr Cancer Ther* **2**(3):212–216 (2003).
53. Hann D, Baker F, Denniston M, *et al*. Long-term breast cancer survivors' use of complementary therapies: perceived impact on recovery and prevention of recurrence. *Integr Cancer Ther* **4**(1):14–20 (2005).

54. Ernst E. The role of complementary and alternative medicine in cancer. *Lancet Oncol* **1**:176–180 (2000).
55. Deng G, Cassileth BR. Integrative oncology: complementary therapies for pain, anxiety, and mood disturbance. *CA Cancer J Clin* **55**(2):109–116 (2005).
56. Devine EC, Westlake SK. The effects of psychoeducational care provided to adults with cancer: meta-analysis of 116 studies. *Oncol Nurs Forum* **22**(9):1369–1381 (1995).
57. Seely D, Oneschuk D. Interactions of natural health products with biomedical cancer treatments. *Curr Oncol* **15**(suppl 2):s109.es81–10.es86 (2008).
58. O'Beirne M, Verhoef M, Paluck E, *et al*. Complementary therapy use by cancer patients. Physicians' perceptions, attitudes, and ideas. *Can Fam Physician* **50**: 882–888 (2004).
59. Lee RT, Hlubocky FJ, Hu JJ, *et al*. An international pilot study of oncology physicians' opinions and practices on complementary and alternative medicine (CAM). *Integr Cancer Ther* **7**(2):70–75 (2008).
60. Verhoef MJ, Hilsden RJ, O'Beirne M. Complementary therapies and cancer care: an overview. *Patient Educ Couns* **38**(2):93–100 (1999).
61. Kao GD, Devine P. Use of complementary health practices by prostate carcinoma patients undergoing radiation therapy. *Cancer* **88**(3):615–619 (2000).
62. Joyce E, Gallagher J, Tenhover J, *et al*. *Complementary Therapies: Knowledge, Attitudes and Use Among Providers*. Poster presented at the Association of Oncology Social Workers Annual Conference, Washington DC (2004).
63. Roberts CS, Baker F, Hann D, *et al*. Patient–physician communication regarding use of complementary therapies during cancer treatment. *Psychosocial Oncol* **23**(4):35–60 (2005).
64. Hann DM, Baker F, Denniston MM. Oncology professionals' communication with cancer patients about complementary therapy: a survey. *Complement Ther Med* **11**(3):184–190 (2003).
65. Schofield PE, Juraskova I, Butow PN. How oncologists discuss complementary therapy use with their patients: an audio-tape audit. *Support Care Cancer* **11**(6):348–355 (2003).
66. Robinson A, McGrail MR. Disclosure of CAM use to medical practitioners: a review of qualitative and quantitative studies. *Complement Ther Med* **12**(2–3):90–98 (2004).

67. Adler S, Fosket J. Disclosing complementary and alternative medicine use in the medical encounter. *J Family Pract* **48**(6):453–458 (1999).
68. Richardson MA, Mâsse LC, Nanny K, *et al*. Discrepant views of oncologists and cancer patients on complementary/alternative medicine. *Support Care Cancer* **12**(11):797–804 (2004).
69. Tasaki K, Maskarinec G, Shumay DM, *et al*. Communication between physicians and cancer patients about complementary and alternative medicine: exploring patients' perspectives. *Psycho-Oncology* **11**(3):212–220 (2002).
70. Roberts C, Benjamin H, Chen L, *et al*. Assessing communication between oncology professionals and their patients. *J Cancer Educ* **20**(2):113–118 (2005).
71. Broom A, Adams J. Oncology clinicians' accounts of discussing complementary and alternative medicine with their patients. *Health (London)* **13**(3):317–336 (2009).
72. Hyodo I, Eguchi K, Nishina T, *et al*. Perceptions and attitudes of clinical oncologists on complementary and alternative medicine: a nationwide survey in Japan. *Cancer* **97**(11):2861–2868 (2003).
73. Weiger WA, Smith M, Boon H, *et al*. Advising patients who seek complementary and alternative medical therapies for cancer. *Ann Intern Med* **137**(11):889–903 (2002).
74. Lerner IJ, Kennedy BJ. The prevalence of questionable methods of cancer treatment in the United States. *CA Cancer J Clin* **42**(3):181–191 (1992).
75. Newell S, Sanson-Fisher RW. Australian oncologists' self-reported knowledge and attitudes about non-traditional therapies used by cancer patients. *Med J Aust* **172**(3):110–113 (2000).
76. Bourgeault IL. Physicians' attitudes toward patients' use of alternative cancer therapies. *CMAJ* **155**(12):1679–1685 (1996).
77. van der Weg F, Streuli RA. Use of alternative medicine by patients with cancer in a rural area of Switzerland. *Swiss Med Wkly* **133**(15–16):233–240 (2003).
78. van Kleffens T, van Leeuwen E. Physicians' evaluations of patients' decisions to refuse oncological treatment. *J Med Ethics* **31**(3):131–136 (2005).
79. Madjar I, Kacen L, Ariad S, *et al*. Telling their stories, telling our stories: physicians' experiences with patients who decide to forgo or stop treatment for cancer. *Qual Health Res* **17**(4):428–441 (2007).

80. Bagenal FS, Easton DF, Harris E, *et al.* Survival of patients with breast cancer attending Bristol Cancer Help Centre. *Lancet* **336**(8715): 606–610 (1990).
81. Cassileth BR, Lusk EJ, Guerry D, *et al.* Survival and quality of life among patients receiving unproven as compared with conventional cancer therapy. *N Engl J Med* **324**(17):1180–1185 (1991).
82. Verhoef MJ, Rose MS, White M, *et al.* Declining conventional cancer treatment and using complementary and alternative medicine: a problem or a challenge? *Curr Oncol* **15**(suppl 2):s101–s116 (2008).
83. Ernst E. Intangible risks of complementary and alternative medicine. *J Clin Oncol* **19**(8):2365–2366 (2001).
84. Cassileth BR, Lusk EJ, Strouse TB, *et al.* Contemporary unorthodox treatments in cancer medicine. A study of patients, treatments, and practitioners. *Ann Intern Med* **101**(1):105–112 (1984).
85. Simmons K, Lindsay S. Psychological influences on acceptance of postsurgical treatment in cancer patients. *J Psychosom Res* **51**(1): 355–360 (2001).
86. Shumay DM, Maskarinec G, Kakai H, *et al.* Why some cancer patients choose complementary and alternative medicine instead of conventional treatment. *J Fam Pract* **50**(12):1067 (2001).
87. White MA, Verhoef MJ, Davidson BJ, *et al.* Seeking mind, body and spirit healing: why some men with prostate cancer choose CAM (complementary and alternative medicine) over conventional cancer treatments. *Integr Med Insights* **3**:1–11 (2008).
88. Montbriand MJ. Abandoning biomedicine for alternate therapies: oncology patients' stories. *Cancer Nurs* **21**(1):36–45 (1998).
89. Ernst E. A primer of complementary and alternative medicine commonly used by cancer patients. *Med J Aust* **174**:88–92 (2001).
90. Schraub S. Unproven methods in cancer: a worldwide problem. *Support Care Cancer* **8**:10–15 (2000).
91. Risberg T, Lund E, Wist E, *et al.* Cancer patients use of non-proven therapy: a 5-year follow-up study. *J Clin Oncol* **16**:6–12 (1998).
92. Ernst E. Complementary cancer treatments: hope or hazard? *Clin Oncol (R Coll Radiol)* **7**(4):259–263 (1995).
93. Joske DJ, Rao A, Kristjanson L. Critical review of complementary therapies in haemato-oncology. *Intern Med J* **36**(9):579–586 (2006).
94. Newell SA, Sanson-Fisher RW, Savolainen NJ. Systematic review of psychological therapies for cancer patients: overview and recommendations for future research. *J Natl Cancer Inst* **94**(8):558–584 (2002).

95. Coseri S. Natural products and their analogues as efficient anti-cancer drugs. *Mini Rev Med Chem* **9**(5):560–571 (2009).
96. Eisenberg DM, Kessler RC, Van Rompay MI, *et al*. Perceptions about complementary therapies relative to conventional therapies among adults who use both: results from a national survey. *Ann Intern Med* **135**(5):344–351 (2001).
97. Cassileth B, Yeung KS, Gubili J. Herbs and other botanicals in cancer patient care. *Curr Treat Options Oncol* **9**(2–3):109–116 (2008).
98. Shord SS, Shah K, Lukose A. Drug-botanical interactions: a review of the laboratory, animal, and human data for 8 common botanicals. *Integr Cancer Ther* **8**(3):208–227 (2009).
99. Milazzo S, Ernst E, Lejeune S, *et al*. Laetrile treatment for cancer. *Cochrane Database Syst Rev* **2**:CD005476 (2006).
100. Lawenda BD, Kelly KM, Ladas EJ, *et al*. Should supplemental antioxidant administration be avoided during chemotherapy and radiation therapy? *J Natl Cancer Inst* **100**(11):773–783 (2008).
101. Hlubocky FJ, Ratain MJ, Wen M, *et al*. Complementary and alternative medicine among advanced cancer patients enrolled on phase I trials: a study of prognosis, quality of life, and preferences for decision making. *J Clin Oncol* **25**(5):548–554 (2007).
102. Dy GK, Bekele L, Hanson LJ, *et al*. Complementary and alternative medicine use by patients enrolled onto phase I clinical trials. *J Clin Oncol* **22**(23):4810–4815 (2004).
103. Robotin MC, Penman AG. Integrating complementary therapies into mainstream cancer care: which way forward? *Med J Aust* **185**(7): 377–379 (2006).
104. Balneaves LG, Weeks L, Seely D. Patient decision-making about complementary and alternative medicine in cancer management: context and process. *Curr Oncol* **15**(suppl 2):s94–s100 (2008).

Index